Food Factors in Health Promotion and Disease Prevention

ACS SYMPOSIUM SERIES **851**

Food Factors in Health Promotion and Disease Prevention

Fereidoon Shahidi, Editor
Memorial University of Newfoundland

Chi-Tang Ho, Editor
Rutgers, The State University of New Jersey

Shaw Watanabe, Editor
Tokyo University of Agriculture

Toshihiko Osawa, Editor
Nagoya University

Sponsored by the
ACS Division of Agricultural and
Food Chemistry

American Chemical Society, Washington, DC

Library of Congress Cataloging-in-Publication Data

Food factors in health Promotion and disease prevention / Fereidoon Shahidi, editor, [et al.] ; sponsored by the ACS Division of Agricultural and Food Chemistry.

p. cm.—(ACS symposium series ; 851)

"Part of the 221st National American Chemical Society meeting at San Diego, California, April 2001"—Pref.

Includes bibliographical references and index.

ISBN 0–8412–3807–3

1. Functional foods—Congresses. 2. Phytochemicals—Therapeutic use—Congresses. 3. Nutrition—Congresses.

I. Shahidi, Fereidoon, 1951- II. American Chemical Society. Division of Agricultural and Food Chemistry. III. American Chemical Society. Meeting (221st : 2001 : San Diego, Calif.) IV. Series.

QP144.F85F665 2003
613.2—dc21 2003043738

The paper used in this publication meets the minimum requirements of American National Standard for Information Sciences—Permanence of Paper for Printed Library Materials, ANSI Z39.48–1984.

Distributed by Oxford University Press

PRINTED IN THE UNITED STATES OF AMERICA

Foreword

The ACS Symposium Series was first published in 1974 to provide a mechanism for publishing symposia quickly in book form. The purpose of the series is to publish timely, comprehensive books developed from ACS sponsored symposia based on current scientific research. Occasionally, books are developed from symposia sponsored by other organizations when the topic is of keen interest to the chemistry audience.

Before agreeing to publish a book, the proposed table of contents is reviewed for appropriate and comprehensive coverage and for interest to the audience. Some papers may be excluded to better focus the book; others may be added to provide comprehensiveness. When appropriate, overview or introductory chapters are added. Drafts of chapters are peer-reviewed prior to final acceptance or rejection, and manuscripts are prepared in camera-ready format.

As a rule, only original research papers and original review papers are included in the volumes. Verbatim reproductions of previously published papers are not accepted.

ACS Books Department

Contents

Biomarker and Animal Models

Antioxidants

Fruits and Vegetables

Other Food Factors

Preface

Food factors, also known as bioactive compounds in foods, are considered to be critical for human health. Overwhelming evidence from epidemiological studies indicate that diets rich in fruits and vegetables are associated with lower risk of several degenerative ailments, such as cancer and cardiovascular disease. Moreover, the advances and applications in genomic science as well as molecular and cell biology have helped in the understanding of the relationship between food bioactives and diseases.

The symposium upon which this book is based was developed to bring together the leading scientists from academia and industry to present their state-of-the-art research information about the chemistry, biochemistry, molecular biology and nutrition aspects of food factors. This four day symposium, *Food Factors in Health Promotion and Disease Prevention,* was a part of the 221st National American Chemical Society (ACS) meeting at San Diego, California, April 2001. It was co-sponsored by the ACS Division of Agricultural and Food Chemistry, Inc. and the International Society of Food Factors. The intent of the book is to disseminate recent developments in this rapidly expanding field.

The book includes an introductory overview on food factors and then perspective chapters on bioavailability of catechins and chemistry of structured and nutraceutical lipids. Subsequent sections cover signal transduction, gene modulation, biomarker, and animal model studies as affected by food bioactives. Finally, the chemistry and bioactivity of antioxidative compounds associated fruits, vegetables, and other plants are presented.

We thank all the authors for their contributions and efforts in the preparation of this book. We also extend our sincere gratitude to the many scientists who reviewed the chapters found herein.

Fereidoon Shahidi
Department of Biochemistry
Memorial University of Newfoundland
St. John's, Newfoundland, A1B 3X9
Canada

Chi-Tang Ho
Department of Food Science
Rutgers University
New Brunswick, NJ 08901–8520

Shaw Watanabe
Department of Nutritional Science
Tokyo University of Agriculture
Tokyo 156–8502
Japan

Toshihiko Osawa
Nagoya Graduate School of Bioagricultural Sciences
Nagoya University
Chikusa, Nagoya 4640–8601
Japan

Overview and Perspectives

Chapter 1

Food Factors in Health Promotion and Disease Prevention

Fereidoon Shahidi[1] and Chi-Tang Ho[2]

[1]Department of Biochemistry, Memorial University of Newfoundland, St. John's, Newfoundland A1B 3X9, Canada
[2]Department of Food Science, Rutgers, The State University of New Jersey, New Brunswick, NJ 08903–8520

Food factors represent a myriad of different classes of compounds present mainly in plant foods and exert a positive effect in disease prevention and health promotion. The chemicals of interest are present as a mixture and their mechanism of action may be varied and dependent on the presence of other compounds in the "soup" or "cocktail" of extracts under investigation. The compounds involved many function cooperatively and synergistically in exerting their effects on health and disease.

The importance of food factors in health promotion and disease prevention has been an issue of interest since antiquity as evidenced by the Chinese concept of Ying and Yang and the famous saying of Hypocrates "Let food be thy medicine and medicinal be thy food". However, many of the beneficial food factors, at some point, were regarded as "antinutrients" because of their demonstrated effect in lowering nutritive value of food by "protein precipitation" or by toxic effects and growth depression when consumed in relatively large quantities. More recently, the concept of "nutraceuticals", "functional foods", "phytochemicals" and "bioactives" has brought about a better understanding of the health promoting activity of many of the minor components of foods as well as certain plant products in the entirety. Thus, effects of food bioactives on gene regulation, signal transduction and modulation of different mechanistic pathways have been studied in relation to their preventive affect on a number of chronic diseases such as cancer, coronary heart disease, diabetes, immune and others. Although the mechanisms of action of bioactives are varied, often antioxidant activity of food components is an issue of interest in supplementing body's ability to neutralize excess free radicals in the elderly and in those suffering from certain diseases and ailments. The food factors of importance to health may be classified into several groups, but not limited to those listed below:

- terpenoids and saponins
- enzyme inhibitors
- glucosinolates and their breakdown products
- essential fatty acids, including long-chain omega-3 fatty acids
- phenolics and polyphenolics
- carotenoids
- lignans and related compounds

While each plant material may be dominated by the presence of one group of phytochemicals, often several classes of bioactives are present in a certain plant. These compounds/classes of compounds provide a "cocktail" or "soup" that may function in a "cooperative" and "synergistic" manner to exert the beneficial health effects related to the particular material under consideration.

Terpenoids and Saponins

The terpenoids are a class of secondary plant metabolites that are lipophilic in nature and represent the largest and most diverse class of plant compounds (*1,2*). The common biosynthetic pathway in their production involves combination of isopentenyl pyrophosphate (IPP) and dimethylallyl pyrophosphate to yield geranyl pyrophosphate which affords monoterpenes (C10) followed by further combination with more IPP molecules to afford sesquiterpenes (C15), triterpenes (C30) and tetraterpenes (C40). Terpenoids act as allelopathic chemicals and hence have insecticidal activity as well as attraction of insects as pollinators. Some important plant hormones such as abscisic acid and gibberelli acid also belong to the sesquiterpene and diterpene group of compounds, respectively (*2*). Some important plant terpenoids in food components are myrecene from bay leaves, geraniol from roses and citronella, and menthol from peppermint, linalool from coriander, pinene and limonene from conifers as well as the widely spread saponins (*1,3*).

Saponins are made of a triterpene or a steroid attached to a sugar moiety and may be distributed in a wide variety of plants. Many types of saponins have been isolated from soybean seeds and these may be divided into two groups; group A and DDMP (2,3-dihydro-2,5-dihydroxy-6-methyl-4H-pyran-4-one) saponins. Group A saponins are present only in the soybean hypocotyl, while DDMP saponins are widely distributed in leguminous seeds and are present in both hypocotyl and coltedon. From pharmacological or health point of view, saponins have been reported to exhibit various effects such as hypolipidemic, antioxidative and HIV infection inhibitory properties. The hypocholesteralenic effect of saponins is quite strong, especially when fed in the presence of cholesterol.

Enzyme Inhibitors

There are numerous proteins in higher plants that inhibit enzymes found in plants, animals including humans and microorganisms. These may serve endogenous physiological functions in plant or serve a protective role. There are different classes of enzyme inhibitors amongst which protease inhibitor and amylase inhibitors might be most important. Bowman-Birk inhibitors are best known for their health effects, especially against anglogenesis. They are also known to inhibit or prevent the development of chemically-induced cancer of the liver, lung, colon, oral and oesophagus. Lectins from many plant seed extracts are capable of agglutination of erythrocytes and exhibit a wide variety of biological effects. These include possible preferential agglutination of tumor cells, inhibition of tumor growth, inhibition of fungal growth and insecticidal action, among others (*4*). The unique property of lectins in binding specific sugar residues located on the surface of cells resulting in agglutination is responsible for these effects (*5*).

Glucosinolates and their Breakdown Products

Glucosinolsates are found universally in the family of Brassicaceae in some other angiosperm families (*6*). Glucosinolates are found in plants along with the enzyme myrosinase which catalyzes their degradation once the plant material is macerated. Although glucosinolates as such are non-toxic, some of their breakdown products may have toxic effects. The biological activity of glucosinolates in most cases is dependent on their hydrolysis and production of certain degradation products. The role of glucosinolates in plants is for defense purposes. The breakdown products of glucosinolates may disturb the fluidity of biomembranes and bind to some enzymes, receptors or other macromolecules such as DNA (*7*). Some major glucosinolates and their respective breakdown products include glucobrassicin giving rise to indole-3-carbinol, gluconasturtin producing phenethyl isothiocyanate, and glucoraphanin affording sulforaphane, among others. Several isothiocyanates have also been shown to inhibit or block tumors induced by chemical carcinogens and 1-isothiocyanate-4-(methylsulfinyl) butane or sulforaphane, isolated from broccoli is a potent inhibitor of mammary tumors. Indolyl glucosinolates and their breakdown products, such as indole-3-carbinol play a major role in cancer prevention.

Essential Fatty Acids

The essential fatty acids are those that are not produced by the body and need to be acquired from dietary sources. Thus, while saturated and monounsaturated fatty acids may be prepared in the body, polyunsaturated fatty acids containing two or more double bonds have to be obtained from food and possibly supplements. The main polyunsaturated fatty acid groups are parented by linoleic acid (18:2 n-6) and linolenic acid (18:3 n-3). Each of these fatty acids could undergo a series of chain elongation and desaturation to produce other important fatty acids which are important in the body. In particular, production of arachidonic acid (20:4 n-6) from linoleic acid and that of eicosapentaenoic acid (EPA, 20:5 n-3) and docosahexaenoic acid (DHA, 20:6 n-3) from linolenic acid is important. Other conditionally essential fatty acids are GLA (gamma-linolenic acid) and CLA (conjugated linoleic acid), among others. The C20 polyunsaturated fatty acids are precursors to eicosanoids and play multifunctional roles in the human body. The importance of long-chain omega-3 fatty acids from marine and algal sources in health and disease has been well explained in the literature (*8,9*).

Phenolics and Polyphenolics

Phenolic and polyphenolic compounds are found in relatively large quantities and in a variety of chemical forms in plant foods and serve as secondary metabolites that protect plant tissues against injuries, insect and animal attack. They also serve as UV filters, signaling agents and free radical scavengers. These belong to the phenylpropanoid (C_6-C_3) family and are derivatives of cinnamic acid; these are produced from phenylalanine and to a lesser extent in some plants from tyrosine. Benzoic acid derivatives may subsequently be formed from C_6-C_3 compounds via the loss of a two-carbon moiety. Condensation of C_6-C_3 compounds with malonyl co-enzyme leads to the formation of chalcones which cyclize under acidic conditions to flavonoids and isoflavonoids, among others. Tocopherols and tocotrienols are another group of phenolics found in plants (*10*).

Phenolic acids, phenylpropanoids and flavonoids may occur in the free form, but are often glycosylated with different sugars, especially glucose. While the presence of sugar moieties in such compounds is responsible for their specific characteristics, they do not have any significant effect on the biological activity of compounds involved, once ingested. Phenolic acids may also be present in the esterified as well as bound forms.

Phenolic compounds have a myriad of health benefits related to cancer prevention, effects on cardiovascular disease by inhibition of cholesterol oxidation and other mechanisms and the process of aging, among others (*11,12*).

Carotenoids

Carotenoids are among the most widely distributed class of compounds in nature, particularly among organisms that are exposed to light. They possess a C_{40}-backbone and may be acyclic or have a cyclic end-group. In food, dietary carotenoids have been mostly studied for their protective effect against a variety of degenerative diseases, such as cancer (*13*), cardiovascular disease (*14*), and age-related macular degeneration (*15*). The mechanisms of cancer chemopreventive action of carotenoids are varied and include upregulation of the gene expression and gap junction proteins. The anti-inflammatory properties, anti-tumor promoting property and induction of the phase 2 detoxification enzymes are among mechanisms by which carotenoids function. Thus formulation of mixtures, as nutraceuticals, which could closely resemble those present in the healthy individuals who consume a diet rich in fruits and vegetables might prove beneficial.

Lignans and Related Compounds

Lignans are present in higher plants including cereals, legumes, oilseeds, fruits and vegetables. Lignans are a group of diphenolic compounds formed by the union of two cinnamic acid residues and comprised of a dibenzylbutane backbone (*13*).

The lignan, secoisolariciresorsinol diglycoside (SDG) is found in a relatively large amount in flaxseed (*16*). Flax lignans act as natural anticancer agents. Thus the total number of aberrant crypts and reductions in early risk markers for mammary tumors and tumors size were demonstrated in rats fed a high-fat diet supplemented with flaxseed.

Other Food Factors

There are many other food factors that are of interest with different biological activities and potential beneficial health effects. These include biopeptides, carbohydrates, cyanogenic glycosides, tetrahydro-ε-carboline derivatives as well as sulfur-containing compounds from garlic, among others. In addition, pre- and probiotics are of interest in view of their effects on health and disease prevention.

References

1. Brielmann, H.L., Jr. In *Natural Products from Plants.* P.B. Kaufman, L.J. Cseke, S. Warber, J.A. Duke and H.L. Brielmann, Eds. CRC Press: Boca Raton, FL. **1999**, pp. 1-36.
2. Harborne, J.B. In *Chemicals from Plants: Perspectives on Plant Secondary Metabolites.* N.J. Walton and D.E. Brown, Eds. Imperial College Press: London, UK. **1999**, pp. 45-59.
3. Gershenzon, J.; Kreis, W. In *Biochemistry of Plant Secondary Metabolism.* Annual Plant Reviews, Volume 2. M. Wink, Ed. Sheffield Academic Press: Sheffield, UK. **1999**, 222-299.
4. Liener, I.E. In *Herbivors: Their Interaction with Secondary Metabolites. Volume 1. The Chemical Participants.* G.A. Rosenthal and M.R. Berenbaum, Eds. Academic Press: San Diego, CA. **1991**, pp. 327-353.
5. Harborne, J.B. In *Secondary Plant Products: Antinutritional and Beneficial Actions in Animal Feeding.* J.C. Caygill and I. Mueller-Harvey, Eds. Nottingham University Press: Nottingham, UK. **1999**, pp. 7-16.
6. Shahidi, F.; Daun, J.K.; DeClercq, D.R. In *Antinutrients and Phytochemicals in Food.* ACS Symposium Series 662. F. Shahidi,

Ed. American Chemical Society: Washington, D.C. **1997**, pp. 31-43.

7. Selmar, D. In *Biochemistry of Plant Secondary Metabolism, Annual Plant Reviews, Volume 2,* M. Wink, Ed. Sheffield Academic Press: Sheffield, UK. **1999**, pp. 79-150.
8. Shahidi, F.; Finley, J.W. *Omega-3 Fatty Acids: Chemistry, Nutrition and Health Effects.* ACS Symposium Series 788. American Chemical Society: Washington D.C.
9. Shahidi, F.; Kim, S-K. In *Bioactive Compounds in Foods: Effects of Processing and Storage.* ACS Symposium Series 816. T-C. Lee and C-T. Ho, Eds. American Chemical Society: Washington, D.C. **2002**, pp. 1-13.
10. Shahidi, F. Nahrung **2000**, *40*, 158-163.

11. Shahidi, F. *Natural Antioxidants: Chemistry, Health Effects and Applications.* AOCS Press: Champaign, IL, **1997**, pp. 1-414.
12. Shahidi, F.; Ho, C-T. *Phytochemicals and Phytopharmaceuticals.* AOCS Press: Champaign, IL. **2000**, pp. 1-431.
13. Ziegler, R.G. *Am. J. Clin. Nutr.* **1991**, 53 (Supp.), 251S-259S.
14. Morris, D.L.; Kritchevsky, S.B.; Davis, L.E. *J. Am. Med. Assoc.* **1994**, 272, 1439-1441.
15. Bernstein, P.S.; Khachik, F.; Carvalho, L.S.; Muir, G.J.; Zhao, D.Y.; Katz, N.B. *Exp. Eye Res.* **2001**, 72, 215-223.
16. Rickard, S.E.; Thompson, L.V. In *Antinutrients and Phytochemicals in Food.* ACS Symposium Series 662. Shahidi, F., Ed. American Chemical Society: Washington, D.C. **1997**, pp. 273-293.

Chapter 2

Bioavailability and Biological Activity of Tea Polyphenols

Hong Lu, Xiaofeng Meng, Mao-Jung Lee, Chuan Li, Pius Maliakal, and Chung S. Yang

Laboratory for Cancer Research, College of Pharmacy, Rutgers, The State University of New Jersey, Piscataway, NJ 08854–8020

Tea polyphenols have biological activities including modulation of key signal transduction pathways. The possible significance of these activities in inhibition of carcinogenesis *in vivo* depends on the bioavailabilities of the polyphenols. After oral administration of tea to rats, about 14% of (-)-epigallocatechin (EGC), 31% of (-)-epicatechin (EC), and <1% of (-)-epicatechin-3-gallate (EGCG) appeared in the blood. In mice, the bioavailability of EGCG was higher. After administration of 3 g of decaffeinated green tea to humans, the C_{max} for EGCG, EGC, and EC were 0.57, 1.60, and 0.6 μM, respectively. Tea catechins undergo extensive methylation and glucuronidation. These reactions, the efflux pumps, and other transportors may play key roles in determining the bioavailability of tea catechins. These metabolites and ring fission metabolites of catechins have been identified by LC-MS with significant quantities in blood and urine. The biological activities of these catechin metabolites need to be investigated.

Introduction

The consumption of tea *(Camellia sinensis)* has a long history and is believed to have beneficial health effects. In recent years, progress has been made concerning the biological effects of green and black tea. Consumption of green tea has been suggested to prevent cancer (*1*), heart disease (*2*), and Parkinson's disease *(3,4)*; however, convincing data are lacking.

Whereas cancer preventive effect of drinking tea has been demonstrated with different models (e.g. skin, lung, esophagus, stomach, liver, pancreas, colon, bladder, prostate, and mammary glands), the epidemiologic data on the association between drinking tea and cancer risk is inconsistent (*5-13*). Such inconsistency could be due to the high doses of tea used in animal studies. There is a general lack of understanding of the relationship between tissue levels of tea constituents and inhibition of carcinogenesis. A careful study on the biotransformation and bioavailability of major active constituents of tea is warranted for extrapolating animal data to human and for rational design of future human studies.

The major characteristic constituents of green tea are catechins including (-)-epicatechin-3-gallate (EGCG), (-)-epigallocatechin (EGC), epicatechin-3-gallate (ECG), and (-)-epicatechin (EC), which account for up to 30% of the dry weight of the water extractable material in brewed tea. In black tea, a large portion of the catechins is converted to theaflavins and thearubigens through oxidation and polymerization.

We herein report recent studies on the biological activities and bioavailability of tea polyphenols.

Results and Discussion

Biological Activities

The inhibitory activity of tea constituents against tumorigenesis has been demonstrated in many studies with animal models (*1*). Nevertheless, the molecular mechanisms of such inhibition are not clearly understood. Many investigators have used cell lines to elucidate the biological activities that may be related to the inhibition of carcinogenesis and shown that EGCG, the major catechin in tea, has the following activities (reviewed in (*1*)):

1) Inhibition of MAP-kinase related signal transduction pathways as well as transcription factor (such as AP-1) activities; 2) preventing the degradation of IκB and thus the activation of NFκB; 3) modulating cell cycle regulation by

affecting the levels or activities of cdk2/4,Rb, p16^{INK4a}, p21^{WARF1}, and p53; 4) interfering the ligands binding to receptors in system such as EGF, PDGF, FGF, and protein kinase C; 5) inhibiting cell proliferation and enhancing apoptosis; and 6) inhibiting angiogenesis and tumor cell invasion. Nevertheless, the relevance of some of these activities to the inhibition of tumorigenesis *in vivo* is uncertain, because of the rather high concentrations of EGCG (usually >20 μM) used in comparison to the plasma and tissue levels of EGCG observed in humans and animals (usually <1 μM) after tea ingestion. A clear understanding of the bioavailability, biotransformation, and biological activities of tea constituents is vital for elucidating the mechanisms of inhibition of carcinogenesis by tea.

Recent studies in our laboratory demonstrated some of the aforementioned activities in a lung tumorigenesis model in A/J mice (*unpublished*). In this study, A/J mice were injected a dose of 4-methylnitrosamino-1-(3-pyridyl)-1-butanone (NNK) (i.v., 100 mg/kg) and were given green tea (0.6% green tea solid) as the sole source of drinking fluid. After 16 weeks, the mean number of lung tumors formed per mouse was decreased by 40% in the tea-treated group. The number of microvessels (as determined by immunohistochemistry with Factor VIII-related antibody) formed per tumor was significantly lower in the tea-treated group. The VEGF staining score was also lower in the tea-treated group. Enhanced apoptosis due to tea treatment was observed in the tea-treated group based on morphological analysis and TUNEL assay. The immunochemical staining for phosphorylated c-jun in the lung tumors was less intense in the tea-treated group than the control, suggesting the inhibition of the phosphorylation of c-jun by the tea treatment. These preliminary results are interesting and further investigation is warranted.

Pharmacokinetics of Tea Polyphenols

After *i.v.* administration of decaffeinated green tea to rats, the $t_{1/2}$ of EGC and EC (the total concentrations of the conjugated and non-conjugated forms) were 40-45 min, and that of EGCG was about 5 times longer (*14*). EGC and EC were excreted from the urine, but EGCG was excreted through the bile to the intestine. With oral administration, about 14% EGC, 31% of EC, and <1% EGCG appeared in the blood. In the mouse, the bioavailability of EGCG was much higher, but it was still lower than EGC. Prolonged oral administration of green tea to rats and mice changed the profile of plasma and urinary levels of catechins, possibly due to enzyme induction (*15*). After administration of 3 g of decaffeinated green tea solids (in water) to humans, the C_{max} for EGCG, EGC, and EC (reached between 1.4-2.4 h) were 0.57, 1.60, and 0.6 μM, respectively. The corresponding $t_{1/2}$ values were 5.0, 2.8, and 3.4 h (*16*). Additional studies indicated that the plasma EGCG is mostly in the non-conjugated form, whereas EGC and EC are mostly in the conjugated (mostly glucuronide) forms (*17*).

Biotransformation of Tea Catechins

Because of the polyphenolic structure, tea catechins do not undergo appreciable Phase I metabolism by enzymes such as cytochromes P450 in animals. Tea catechins, however, undergo Phase II metabolism extensively. After ingestion of tea, over 50 metabolites (mostly in methylated, glucuronidated, and sulfated forms) could be detected by LC-MS (*18*). The catechol-*O*-methyltransferase (COMT)-catalyzed methylation and UDP-glucuronosyltransferase (UGT)-catalyzed glucuronidation have been extensively characterized in mice and rats. Our data show that, for EGC, the major methylation sites are the 4′- and 3′-positions of the B ring, and the major glucuronidation sites are the 7-position of the A ring and 3′-position of the B-ring (Figure 1).

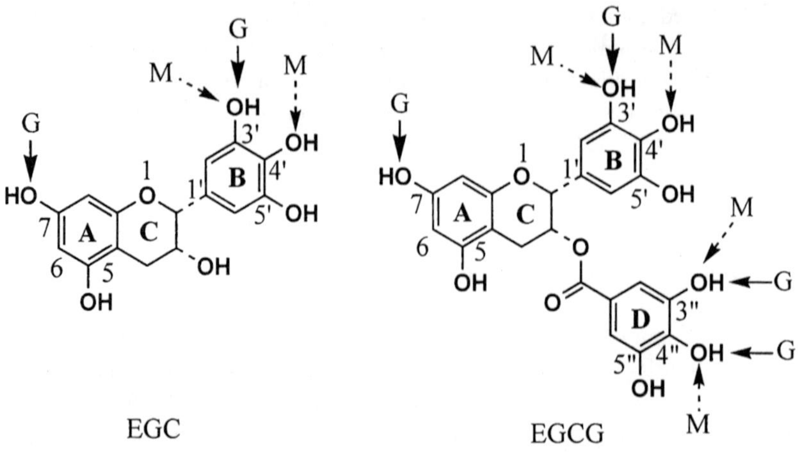

Figure 1. Glucuronidation (G) and methylation (M) of catechins.

The EGC glucuronidation has very similar kinetics in regard to 3′- and 7-position. Glucuronidation of the 3'-position would inhibit the methylation at the 3′- and 4′-positions, whereas glucuronidation at the A-ring does not affect the methylation at the B-ring. As judged by the V_{max} and catalytic efficiency (V_{max}/K_m), the mouse liver microsomes are more efficient than the rat liver microsomes in catalyzing the glucuronidation of EGC both at the 7- and 3′-positions. The rat liver appears to be more active than the mouse liver in the methylation of EGC.

For EGCG, in addition to the above described A- and B-rings, the 3″- and 4″-positions of the D-ring are sites for methylation and glucuronidation (Figure 1). The mouse liver and intestine have higher activities, than the rat counter part, in catalyzing the glucuronidation of EGCG. Of particular interest is the rather high activity in the mouse intestine vs. the very low level of activity in the rat intestine. This may be related to the higher bioavailability of EGCG in the mice than rats. For the methylation of EGCG, the rats have higher activities than the mice. In both species, the methyltransferase activity (V_{max}) toward EGC is 20-30 times higher than toward EGCG in the liver. However, EGCG is a much stronger inhibitor of COMT.

Stability and biological activity of catechin conjugates

We compared the chemical and enzymatic stability of the two EGC glucuronides. 3′-*O*-EGC-glucuronide is much more stable than EGC and 7-*O*-EGC-glcuronide at pH 7.4, further confirming the concept that B-ring is critical for the stability of catechins. 3′-*O*-EGC-glucuronide is a much better substrate than 7-*O*-EGC-glcuronide for beta-glucuronidase in mouse liver homogenates. The two EGC glucuronides are found to retain significant antioxidative activity based on their 1,1-diphenyl-2-picrylhydrazyl radical scavenging activities. 7-*O*-EGC-glucuronide has comparable activity to EGC, in regard to the inhibition of spontaneous release of arachidonic acid and metabolites from HT29 human colon cancer cell line.

4′-*O*-methyl-EGC and 4′,4″-dimethyl-EGCG, the major *in vivo* methylation products of EGC and EGCG, are much more stable than their parent compounds at pH 7.4. They retained comparable activity to their parent compounds in the inhibition of spontaneous release of arachidonic acid and metabolites from HT29 cell line. Since 4′-*O*-methyl-EGC was detected in the urine and plasma in amounts several fold higher than EGC, further study on the biological activities of methylated EGC and other catechins is warranted.

Biotransformation of catechins in the intestine

Tea catechins are also degraded in the intestine by microflora. Several microbial metabolites, including 4-hydroxybenzoic acid, 3,4-dihydroxybenzoic acid, 3-methoxy-4-hydroxy-hippuric acid, and 3-methoxy-4-hydroxybenzoic acid, were observed in human urine samples (*19*). 5-(3′,4′-Dihydroxyphenyl)-γ-valerolactone and 5-(3′,4′,5′-trihydroxyphenyl)-γ-valerolactone were identified in the human urine as the ring fission products of EGC and EC, respectively (*20*). Both metabolites (mainly in the conjugated form) were detected in the urine and plasma in amounts several fold higher than their respective precursors in some individuals. Judging from the di(tri)-hydroxyphenyl and valerolactone structures, these metabolites may possess interesting biological activities.

Concluding Remarks

The antioxidative properties and biological activities of tea polyphenols have been studied extensively *in vitro*. Their biological activities after oral ingestion of tea, however, are determined by the bioavailability and biotransformation. The blood, tissue, and urine levels of tea catechins and their metabolites are beginning to be understood. The demonstration of biological activities of catechin glucuronides and methylated catechins broadens our vision and increases the chance of green tea as effective chemopreventive agent. The extensive interactions of catechins with UGT and COMT could have significant effect on the metabolism of endogenous compounds (Dopa, catechol estrogen, catecholamines, DNA, etc.) and xenobiotics (drugs and carcinogens). The theaflavins from black tea have also been shown to inhibit lung tumorigenesis, even though significant amounts of theaflavins have not been detected in the blood. It is possible that degradation products of theaflavins (and perhaps thearubigens), formed by intestinal microflora, are absorbed and display biological activities. Further studies on the biological activities of these compounds will enhance our understanding on the health effects of tea consumption.

References

1. Yang, C. S.; Maliakal, P.; Meng, X. *Annu. Rev. Pharmacol. Toxicol.* **2002,** *42*, 25-54.
2. Vinson, J. A. *Biofactors* **2000,** *13*, 127-32.
3. Levites, Y.; Weinreb, O.; Maor, G.; Youdim, M. B.; Mandel, S. *J. Neurochem.* **2001,** *78*, 1073-82.
4. Chan, D. K.; Woo, J.; Ho, S. C.; Pang, C. P.; Law, L. K.; Ng, P. W.; Hung, W. T.; Kwok, T.; Hui, E.; Orr, K.; Leung, M. F.; Kay, R. *J. Neurol. Neurosurg. Psychiatry.* **1998,** *65*, 781-4.
5. Inoue, M.; Tajima, K.; Mizutani, M.; Iwata, H.; Iwase, T.; Miura, S.; Hirose, K.; Hamajima, N.; Tominaga, S. *Cancer Lett.* **2001,** *167*, 175-82.

6. Setiawan, V. W.; Zhang, Z. F.; Yu, G. P.; Lu, Q. Y.; Li, Y. L.; Lu, M. L.; Wang, M. R.; Guo, C. H.; Yu, S. Z.; Kurtz, R. C.; Hsieh, C. C. *Int. J. Cancer* **2001,** *92*, 600-4.
7. Nakachi, K.; Matsuyama, S.; Miyake, S.; Suganuma, M.; Imai, K. *Biofactors* **2000,** *13*, 49-54.
8. Imai, K.; Suga, K.; Nakachi, K. *Prev. Med.* **1997,** *26*, 769-75.
9. Ellison, L. F. *Eur. J. Cancer Prev.* **2000,** *9*, 125-30.
10. Bianchi, G. D.; Cerhan, J. R.; Parker, A. S.; Putnam, S. D.; See, W. A.; Lynch, C. F.; Cantor, K. P. *Am. J. Epidemiol.* **2000,** *151*, 377-83.
11. Rosenblatt, K. A.; Thomas, D. B.; Jimenez, L. M.; Fish, B.; McTiernan, A.; Stalsberg, H.; Stemhagen, A.; Thompson, W. D.; Curnen, M. G.; Satariano, W.; Austin, D. F.; Greenberg, R. S.; Key, C.; Kolonel, L. N.; West, D. W. *Cancer Causes Control* **1999,** *10*, 107-13.
12. Hollman, P. C.; Feskens, E. J.; Katan, M. B. *Proc. Soc. Exp. Biol. Med.* **1999,** *220*, 198-202.
13. Hartman, T. J.; Tangrea, J. A.; Pietinen, P.; Malila, N.; Virtanen, M.; Taylor, P. R.; Albanes, D. *Nutr. Cancer* **1998,** *31*, 41-8.
14. Chen, L.; Lee, M. J.; Li, H.; Yang, C. S. *Drug Metab. Dispos.* **1997,** *25*, 1045-50.
15. Kim, S.; Lee, M. J.; Hong, J.; Li, C.; Smith, T. J.; Yang, G. Y.; Seril, D. N.; Yang, C. S. *Nutr. Cancer* **2000,** *37*, 41-8.
16. Yang, C. S.; Chen, L.; Lee, M. J.; Balentine, D.; Kuo, M. C.; Schantz, S. P. *Cancer Epidemiol. Biomarkers Prev.* **1998,** *7*, 351-4.
17. Chow, H. H.; Cai, Y.; Alberts, D. S.; Hakim, I.; Dorr, R.; Shahi, F.; Crowell, J. A.; Yang, C. S.; Hara, Y. *Cancer Epidemiol. Biomarkers Prev.* **2001,** *10*, 53-8.
18. Li, C.; Meng, X.; Winnik, B.; Lee, M. J.; Lu, H.; Sheng, S.; Buckley, B.; Yang, C. S. *Chem. Res. Toxicol.* **2001,** *14*, 702-7.
19. Pietta, P. G.; Simonetti, P.; Gardana, C.; Brusamolino, A.; Morazzoni, P.; Bombardelli, E. *Biofactors* **1998,** *8*, 111-8.
20. Li, C.; Lee, M. J.; Sheng, S.; Meng, X.; Prabhu, S.; Winnik, B.; Huang, B.; Chung, J. Y.; Yan, S.; Ho, C. T.; Yang, C. S. *Chem. Res. Toxicol.* **2000,** *13*, 177-84.

Chapter 3

Structured Lipids Enriched with Omega-3 and Omega-6 Highly Unsaturated Fatty Acids

S. P. J. Namal Senanayake[1,2] and Fereidoon Shahidi[1]

[1]Department of Biochemistry, Memorial University of Newfoundland, St. John's, Newfoundland A1B 3X9, Canada
[2]Current address: Martek Biosciences Corporation, 555 Rolling Hills Lane, Winchester, KY 40391

Structured lipids are triacylglycerols (TAG) that have been modified to change the fatty acid compositions and stereospecific distribution of fatty acids from their native state. These tailor-made lipids may contain mixtures of short-, medium- and long chain fatty acids on the same glycerol molecule, and these can be saturated or unsaturated. They can be designed for nutritional and pharmaceutical purposes targeting specific diseases and pathological conditions. Structured lipids containing n-6 and n-3 polyunsaturated fatty acids (PUFA) were produced with both immobilized and non-immobilized lipases as biocatalysts. Among PUFA, eicosapentaenoic (EPA; 20:5n-3), docosahexaenoic(DHA; 22:6n-3) and γ-linolenic (GLA; 18:3n-6) acids have attracted much attention in recent years due to their beneficial health effects. Structured lipids containing these fatty acids may be desirable in certain health, nutritional and pharmaceutical applications.

Structured lipids are defined as triacylglycerols (TAG) containing mixtures of short- and/or medium- and long-chain fatty acyl residues attached to the glycerol backbone for specific functionality and produced *via* chemical or enzymatic reactions (*1*). The first structured lipids were produced, *via* chemical means, by mixing medium-chain triacylglycerols and long-chain triacylglycerols, allowing hydrolysis to free fatty acids, followed by random transesterification of the fatty acids into mixed triacylglycerol molecules. This results in the production of triacylglycerols containing combinations of short-, medium- and long-chain fatty acid moieties on the single glycerol backbone. These have unique physical, chemical and physiological properties, which differ from simple physical mixtures of the starting lipids. It is now possible to synthesize structured lipids *via* lipase- catalyzed reactions.

As acyl donors for structured lipid production, both n-3 and n-6 polyunsaturated fatty acids (PUFA) may impart desirable benefits. For example, it is known that n-3 PUFA, mainly eicosapentaenoic (EPA; 20:5n-3) and docosahexaenoic (DHA; 22:6n-3) acids, exhibit various physiological functions. The potential health benefits of n-3 fatty acids include reduced risk of cardiovascular disease, hypertension, inflammatory and autoimmune disorders (*2*). EPA is an antagonist of the arachidonic acid cascade and competes with arachidonic acid to produce eicosanoids. It is believed that presence of DHA in both the brain and retina is important for proper nervous system and visual acuity in humans, respectively (*3,4*). The maintenance of adequate levels of DHA may be required for optimum neurological functions throughout the life span. It has been noted that there is a correlation between DHA deficiency and the incidence of Alzheimer's disease. A study of more than thousand elderly individuals indicated that a low DHA level is a significant risk factor in the onset of dementia (*5*). Studies have shown that an early dietary supplementation of DHA is a major determinant of improved performance on the mental development index (MDI) of term infants (*6*). Therefore, n-3 PUFA such as EPA and DHA should be included in the diet, perhaps in the form of structured lipids. Among n-6 PUFA, γ-linolenic acid (18:3n-6; GLA) is an intermediate metabolite in the conversion of linoleic acid (LA; 18:2n-6) to arachidonic acid (AA; 20:4n-6). GLA has the physiological functions of modulating immune and inflammatory response (*7*). GLA has also been used in the treatment of atopic eczema, rheumatoid arthritis, dermatitis, hypertension, diabetic neuropathy, cirrhosis of the liver, and premenstrual syndrome (*8,9*).

Nutritional benefits of structured lipids

Nutritional value and application of structured lipids containing medium-chain fatty acids at the *sn*-1 and *sn*-3 positions and unsaturated fatty acids at the *sn*-2 position have been of much interest. These structured TAG can be easily hydrolyzed by pancreatic lipase. Pancreatic lipase acts mainly on the *sn*-1 and *sn*-3 positions of the TAG molecules to release 2-monoacylglycerols (2-MAG) and free medium-chain fatty acids. These free fatty acids are readily absorbed in the intestine and are transported into the liver to be consumed as a source of energy while the remaining 2-MAG become the source of essential fatty acids.

A study involving two types of structured lipids (randomized *vs.* specific product) revealed that the fatty acids located in the *sn*-2 position of TAG are preferentially absorbed (*10*). The randomized structured lipid used contained EPA, DHA and capric acid randomly distributed in the molecule. The specific structured lipid had EPA and DHA at the *sn*-2 position and capric acid at the *sn*-1 and *sn*-3 positions of TAG. The concentrations of EPA and DHA in lymphatics were higher in the specific structured lipid than in the randomized structured lipid. Rapid hydrolysis and absorption of structured lipids containing medium-chain fatty acids at the *sn*-1 and *sn*-3 positions and long-chain fatty acids at the *sn*-2 position have also been reported (*11*).

Lipase-catalyzed reactions

Lipase-catalyzed modification of TAG may be performed with several benefits over chemically assisted reactions to produced structured lipids. Through enzyme-catalyzed reactions, it is possible to incorporate a desired acyl group onto a specific position of the TAG (*12,13*), whereas chemically assisted reactions do not possess this regiospecificity due to the random nature of the reaction. In lipase-mediated reactions, lipases catalyze either the removal or exchange of fatty acyl groups on the glycerol backbone. Different lipases, however, show a preference for both the position of the fatty acyl group on the triacylglycerol and the nature of the fatty acid. This lipase specificity provides a means of classifying them.

Based on the substrates involved in the lipase-catalyzed reactions, they can be classified into different categories: esterification, hydrolysis, acidolysis, alcoholysis and interesterification (*1*). Direct esterification reaction may be employed for the preparation of structured lipids by reacting free fatty acids with glycerol. However, this process is not commonly used in structured lipid production. The major problem is that the water molecules are formed as a result of the esterification reaction. The water molecules so produced need to be removed in order to prevent the hydrolysis of the product. Hydrolysis is the natural reaction for lipases, producing free fatty acids and glycerol. If a *sn*-1,3-regiospecifc lipase is employed, free fatty acids and 2-monoacylglycerols will be produced. However, a non-specific lipase will catalyze complete hydrolysis of triacylglycerols to free fatty acids and glycerol. Acidolysis is the exchange reaction between an ester and free fatty acids, and the lipase will catalyze the transfer of the alcohol moiety of the ester to the new fatty acid until an equilibrium corresponding to the ratio of ester to fatty acid is obtained. Alcoholysis refers to the reaction of an alcohol with triacylglycerols and produces a new ester with another alcohol moiety. Glycerolysis is an important reaction that is used for the production of mono- and diacylglycerols. During this reaction, a triacylglycerol is reacted with excess glycerol and mono- and diacylglycerols are produced. Interesterification reaction is generally performed by mixing two types of esters and the lipase catalyzes redistribution of fatty acid moieties.

Synthesis of structured lipids *via* acidolysis

For bench-scale synthesis of borage or evening primrose oil-based structured lipids, 297-300 mg oil were mixed with 115 mg EPA and/or 120 mg DHA. The mole ratio was 1:1 for oil to EPA or DHA. The reactions were conducted in 3 mL of hexane or in the absence of any organic solvent. Lipases from *Candida antarctica* (Novozym-435) or *Pseudomonas sp.* (PS-30) were added to the reaction mixture and incubated in an orbital shaker at 37°C for 24 h at 250 rpm.

Structured lipids containing n-6 and n-3 PUFA

Borage, evening primrose, blackcurrant and fungal oils serve as major sources of γ-linolenic acid (18:3n-6; GLA). Among these, borage and evening primrose oils are used most frequently in nutritional and clinical studies. The contents of GLA present in borage and evening primrose oils are 23.5 and 9.1%, respectively (Table I). Borage and evening primrose oils containing GLA are used as ingredients of food materials, health foods, infant formula and cosmetics (*14*). There is evidence for therapeutic benefits of GLA-rich oils in the treatment of atopic eczema, dermatitis, hypertension and premenstrual syndrome (*8*). On the other hand, n-3 PUFA have potential for prevention of cardiovascular disease, arthritis, hypertension, immune and renal disorders, diabetes and cancer (*4*). Structured lipids containing both GLA and n-3 PUFA may be of interest because of their desired health benefits. Structured lipids containing GLA, EPA and/or DHA in the same glycerol backbone using borage and evening primrose oils were successfully produced as the main substrates (*12*,*13*).

Table I. Fatty acid compositions (mole %) of test oils

Major fatty acids	*Borage oil*	*Evening primrose oil*
C16:0	9.6	6.2
C18:0	3.5	1.8
C18:1	15.5	8.7
C18:2n-6	37.8	72.6
C18:3n-6	23.5	9.1
C20:1	4.2	0.3
C22:1	2.3	0.1
C24:1	1.5	ND

ND: not detected

Borage and evening primrose oils were transesterified with DHA at 1:1 mole ratio in hexane catalyzed by an immobilized Novozym-435 from *Candida antarctica* (Table II). The incorporation of DHA into borage and evening primrose oils was 27.4 and 25.2%, respectively. The amounts of GLA retained in the modified oils were 17.0 and 7.6%, respectively.

Table II. Enzymatically transesterified borage (BO) and evening primrose oils (EPO) with DHA to produce structured lipids

Reaction	*Major fatty acids*	*Modified BO*	*Modified EPO*
Novozym-435 lipase, 150 units	C16:0	6.9	4.7
Mole ratio of reactants, 1:1	C18:0	2.6	0.7
Temperature, 37°C	C18:1	11.3	4.2
Incubation time, 24 h	C18:2n-6	27.0	54.3
	C18:3n-6	17.0	7.6
	C22:6n-3	27.4	25.2
	n-3/n-6 ratio	0.6	0.4

The fatty acid compositions of borage and evening primrose oils were also modified by incorporation of EPA using lipase PS-30 from *Pseudomonas sp.* as the biocatalyst (Table III). After acidolysis reaction, modified borage oil contained 26.8% EPA and 15.2% GLA. Meanwhile, modified evening primrose oil had EPA and GLA contents of 25.2 and 7.6%, respectively.

Table III. Enzymatically transesterified borage (BO) and evening primrose oils (EPO) with EPA to produce structured lipids

Reaction	*Major fatty acids*	*Modified BO*	*Modified EPO*
Lipase PS-30, 150 units	C16:0	6.4	4.0
Mole ratio of reactants, 1:1	C18:0	2.6	1.1
Temperature, 37°C	C18:1	12.0	5.6
Incubation time, 24 h	C18:2n-6	25.3	55.6
	C18:3n-6	15.2	7.6
	C20:5n-3	26.8	25.2
	n-3/n-6 ratio	0.7	0.4

In another study, borage and evening primrose oils were modified using combinations of EPA and DHA to produce structured lipids in an acidolysis reaction catalyzed by lipase PS-30 from *Pseudomonas sp.* (Table IV). Borage-oil based structured lipid contained 23.1 and 8.7% EPA and DHA, respectively, and 18.4% GLA. On the other hand, evening primrose oil-based structured lipid had 23.5% EPA, 9.2% DHA and 7.4% GLA. The modified borage and evening primrose oils thus obtained may have potential health benefits.

Lipase-catalyzed acidolysis has been employed for the incorporation of EPA and capric acid (10:0) into borage oil using two immobilized lipases, SP435 from *Candida antarctica* and IM60 from *Rhizomucor miehei* as biocatalysts (*15*). Higher incorporation of EPA (10.2%) and 10:0 (26.3%) was achieved with IM60 lipase, compared to 8.8 and 15.5%, respectively, with SP435 lipase (*15*). By a two-step process, which involved *Candida rugosa* lipase-catalyzed selective hydrolysis of borage oil and subsequent acidolysis of the resulting products with n-3 fatty acids, 72.8% of n-3 and n-6 fatty acids in borage oil acylglycerols was obtained (*16*). The contents of GLA, EPA and DHA in the structured lipid so prepared were 26.5, 19.8 and 18.1%, respectively. The n-3/n-6 ratio increased from 0 to 1.09, following acidolysis (*16*).

Table IV. Enzyme-catalyzed transesterification of borage (BO) and evening primrose oils (EPO) with n-3 fatty acids to produce structured lipids

Reaction	*Major fatty acids*	*Modified BO*	*Modified EPO*
Lipase PS-30, 150 units	C16:0	4.0	3.5
Mole ratio of oil:EPA:DHA,	C18:0	2.0	1.0
1:0.5:0.5	C18:1	10.7	5.9
Temperature, 37°C	C18:2n-6	26.5	49.4
Incubation time, 24 h	C18:3n-6	18.4	7.4
	C20:5n-3	23.1	23.5
	C22:6n-3	8.7	9.2
	n-3/n-6 ratio	0.7	0.6

Stereospecific analyses

The stereospecific distribution of fatty acids in TAG molecules of DHA, EPA and EPA+DHA-enriched structured lipids synthesized in our laboratory was determined. Tables V and VI report the positional distribution of fatty acids in structured lipids examined. The results of this study showed that DHA was randomly distributed over all three positions (34.6% at *sn*-1, 33.5% at *sn*-2 and 35.9% at *sn*-3) of the TAG molecules of DHA-enriched borage oil (Table V). In DHA-enriched evening primrose oil, however, this fatty acid was mainly occupied by the *sn*-2 position (38.2%), followed by *sn*-3 (33.1%) and *sn*-1 (24.5%) positions (Table VI). It should be noted that these DHA-enriched structured lipids were prepared using Novozym-435 from *Candida antarctica* as the biocatalyst. The positional specificity of Novozym-435 depends on the type of substrates used in various reactions. In some reaction systems, this enzyme behaves as a nonspecific lipase whereas in other systems it exhibits *sn*-1,3 regiospecificity (*17*). Based on the reaction conditions employed in this study, Novozym-435 functions as a nonspecific lipase.

The stereospecific distribution of fatty acids in the native borage and evening primrose oils have previously been reported (*18*). In native borage oil, GLA was distributed asymmetrically and preferentially located at the *sn*-2 and *sn*-3 positions (*18*). In native evening primrose oil, GLA was concentrated in the *sn*-3 position (*18*). Linoleic acid (LA; 18:2n-6) was fairly evenly distributed in all positions of native evening primrose oil, but was preferentially located in the *sn*-1 position of native borage oil (*18*). The results of our study showed that in DHA-enriched borage oil, GLA was mainly located in the *sn*-2 (18.4%) and *sn*-3

(19.2%) positions of TAG (Table V). In DHA-enriched evening primrose oil, however, GLA was mainly located in the *sn*-2 (7.5%) position (Table VI). LA was randomly distributed over all three positions of TAG in both oils.

The positional distribution of fatty acids in TAG of EPA-enriched oils (Tables V and VI) was also determined. In this work, EPA-enriched oils were synthesized using lipase PS-30 from *Pseudomonas sp.* as the biocatalyst. The EPA of EPA-enriched borage oil was randomly distributed in the TAG (33.4% at *sn*-1; 32.5% at *sn*-2; 30.9% at *sn*-3) (Table V). In EPA-enriched evening primrose oil, however, this fatty acid was mainly esterified at the primary positions (39.5% at *sn*-1 and 42.1% at *sn*-3) of TAG (Table VI) and was also present in appreciable amounts (23.2%) at the *sn*-2 position. Therefore, it is assumed that *Pseudomonas sp.* lipase shows no specificity and may incorporate EPA in all three positions of TAG of the oils. In both oils, GLA was esterified preferentially at the *sn*-2 position (18.6 and 7.2% in EPA-enriched borage and evening primrose oils, respectively). In EPA-enriched borage oil, LA in TAG was distributed randomly while in EPA-enriched evening primrose oil it was mainly placed at the *sn*-2 position (Tables V and VI).

In another study, the positional distribution of fatty acids in n-3 fatty acids (EPA and DHA)-enriched oils were determined (Tables V and VI). In this study, preparation of EPA+DHA-enriched structured lipids was catalyzed by lipase PS-30 from *Psuedomonas sp.* In EPA+DHA enriched borage oil, GLA was mainly located at the *sn*-2 position (32.9%) (Table V). However, EPA and DHA were preferentially esterified at the primary positions (*sn*-1 and *sn*-3) of TAG molecules (Table V) and their quantities were EPA, 26.1 and 30.8%; and DHA, 8.3 and 9.8%, respectively. In EPA+DHA enriched evening primrose oil, GLA was located mainly at the *sn*-2 (10.8%) and *sn*-3 (9.0%) positions of TAG (Table VI). EPA was preferentially esterified at the *sn*-1 (31.5%) and *sn*-3 (24.1%) positions while approximately half of the DHA was located in the *sn*-3 position (10.5%) (Table VI). Therefore, lipase PS-30 from *Pseudomonas sp.*, under the reaction conditions employed in this study, has the ability to incorporate n-3 fatty acids (EPA and DHA) preferentially at the *sn*-1 and *sn*-3 positions of the TAG molecules.

Oxidative Stability

Structured lipids containing n-3 fatty acids were highly susceptible to oxidation probably because they lost some of the endogenous antioxidants, such as tocopherols, present in borage and evening primrose oils used for the synthesis (*19*) and also partly due to the increase in their degree of unsaturation. Therefore, it is suggested that appropriate antioxidants of choice be added back to structured lipids as this may improve their oxidative stability and preserve the integrity of nutritionally important n-3 and n-6 fatty acid components present.

Table V. Stereospecific distribution of fatty acids (mole %) in modified and unmodified borage oils

Positional distribution	*C18:2n-6*	*C18:3n-6*	*C20:5n-3*	*C22:6n-3*
Unmodified borage oil[a]				
sn-1	38.5	3.5	ND	ND
sn-2	53.4	32.2	ND	ND
sn-3	34.2	17.4	ND	ND
DHA-enriched				
sn-1	23.9	13.2	ND	34.6
sn-2	22.8	18.4	ND	33.5
sn-3	25.3	19.2	ND	35.9
EPA-enriched				
sn-1	23.6	11.5	33.4	ND
sn-2	21.2	18.6	32.5	ND
sn-3	20.2	13.4	30.9	ND
EPA+DHA-enriched				
sn-1	22.9	4.1	26.1	8.3
sn-2	26.2	32.9	15.2	3.8
sn-3	15.3	15.1	30.8	9.8

[a]Reference (*18*)

ND: not detected

Table VI. Stereospecific distribution of fatty acids (mole %) in modified and unmodified evening primrose oils

Positional distribution	*C18:2n-6*	*C18:3n-6*	*C20:5n-3*	*C22:6n-3*
Unmodified evening primrose oil[a]				
sn-1	70.0	4.9	ND	ND
sn-2	81.5	10.3	ND	ND
sn-3	71.6	10.2	ND	ND
DHA-enriched				
sn-1	45.1	5.5	ND	24.5
sn-2	44.9	7.5	ND	38.2
sn-3	41.5	4.8	ND	33.1
EPA-enriched				
sn-1	39.1	4.4	39.5	ND
sn-2	48.4	7.2	23.2	ND
sn-3	37.5	4.8	42.1	ND
EPA+DHA-enriched				
sn-1	40.1	4.2	31.5	5.8
sn-2	61.0	10.8	17.2	4.8
sn-3	32.6	9.0	24.1	10.5

[a]Reference (*18*)

ND: not detected

References

1. Senanayake, S.P.J.N.; Shahidi, F. In *Seafood in Health and Nutrition. Transformation in Fisheries and Aquaculture: Global Perspectives*; Shahidi, F., Ed.; ScienceTech Publishing Company, St. John's, 2000; pp 29-44.
2. Weber, P.C.; Leaf, A. *World Rev. Nutr. Diet.* **1991**, *66*, 218-232.
3. Linko, Y.-Y.; Hayakawa, K. *Trends Food Sci. Technol.* **1996**, *7*, 59-63.
4. Senanayake, S.P.J.N.; Shahidi, F. *J. Food Lipids* **2000**, *7*, 51-61.
5. Soderberg, M.; Edlund, C.; Kristensen, K. *Lipids* **1991**, *26*, 421-425.
6. Birch, E.E.; Farfield, S.; Hoffman, D.R.; Uauy, R.; Birch, D.G. *Dev. Med. Child. Neurol.* **2000**, *42*, 174-181.

7. Wu., D.; Maydani, S.N. In *γ-Linolenic Acid: Metabolism and Its Roles in Nutrition and Medicine*; Huang, Y.-S.; Mills, D.E., Eds.; AOCS Press: Champaign, IL, 1996; pp 106-117.
8. Bugnariu, S. *Farmacia* **1996**, *44*, 3-4.
9. Senanayake, S.P.J.N.; Shahidi, F. *J. Am. Oil Chem. Soc.* **1999**, *76*, 1009-1015.
10. Christensen, M.S.; Hoy, C.E.; Becker, C.C.; Redgrave, T.G. *Am. J. Clin. Nutr.* **1995**, *61*, 56-61.
11. Jandacek, R.J.; Whiteside, J.A.; Holcombe, B.N.; Volpenhein, R.A.; Taulbee, J.D. *Am. J. Clin. Nutr.* **1987**, *45*, 940.
12. Senanayake, S.P.J.N.; Shahidi, F. *J. Agric. Food Chem.* **1999**, *47*, 3105-3112.
13. Senanayake, S.P.J.N.; Shahidi, F. In *Omega-3 Fatty Acids: Chemistry, Nutrition and Health Effects*; Shahidi, F.; Finley, J.W., Eds.; ACS Symposium Series 788, American Chemical Society, Washington, D.C., 2001; pp 162-173.
14. Crozier, G.L.; Secretin, M.-C. In *γ-Linolenic Acid: Metabolism and Its Roles in Nutrition and Medicine*; Huang, Y.-S.; Mills, D.E., Eds.; AOCS Press: Champaign, IL, 1996; pp 246-251.
15. Akoh, C.C.; Moussata, C.O. *J. Am. Oil Chem. Soc.* **1998**, *75*, 697-701.
16. Ju, Y.; Huang, F.-C.; Fang, C.H. *J. Am. Oil Chem. Soc.* **1998**, *75*, 961-965.
17. Novo Nordisk Biochem North America, Inc., Product Sheet. B 606c-GB, Franklinton, NC, 1999.
18. Redden, P.R.; Lin, X.; Fahey, J.; Horrobin, D.F. *J. Chromatogr. A.* **1995**, *704*, 99-111.
19. Senanayake, S.P.J.N.; Shahidi, F. *J. Food Sci.* **2002** (In Press).

Chapter 4

Effects of Tea Polyphenols on Arachidonic Acid Metabolism in Human Colon

Jungil Hong and Chung S. Yang*

Laboratory for Cancer Research, College of Pharmacy, Rutgers, The State University of New Jersey, Piscataway, NJ 08854–8520

Tea has been suggested to be a possible cancer chemopreventive agent, and tea polyphenols are believed to be responsible for its anti-carcinogenic effect. Since modulation of arachidonic acid metabolism has been demonstrated to be an important target for cancer chemoprevention, the effects of green and black tea polyphenols on human colonic enzymes involved in arachidonic acid metabolism were investigated. At a concentration of 30 μg/mL, (-)-epigallocatechin-3-gallate (EGCG), (-)-epigallocatechin (EGC), and (-)-epicatechin-3-gallate (ECG) from green tea and theaflavins from black tea inhibited lipoxygenase (LOX)-dependent activity by 30 to 75%. Tea polyphenols (30 μg/mL) inhibited cyclooxygenae (COX)-dependent arachidonic acid metabolism in microsomes from normal colon mucosa by 37 to 62%. EGCG and ECG (50 μM) inhibited cytosolic phospholipase A_2 ($cPLA_2$) activity by 15 and 30%, respectively. Theaflavins (50 μM) inhibited $cPLA_2$ activity by 10–45%. The inhibition of arachidonic acid metabolism at multiple levels by tea polyphenols may decrease the risk of human colon cancer.

Introduction

Environmental factors are important in the causation of cancers. Diet is believed to account for about one-third of cancer cases in the United States (*1*). Dietary modification has been suggested as an important way for cancer chemoprevention. Many dietary factors have been studied as possible cancer chemopreventive agents. Among them, tea polyphenols have shown some promise.

Tea (*Camellia sinensis*) is one of the most commonly consumed beverages in the world. Green tea contains polyphenols including (-)-epigallocatechin-3-gallate (EGCG), (-)-epigallocatechin (EGC), epicatechin-3-gallate (ECG) and (-)-epicatechin (EC), which account for up to 30 % of dry weight of the water extractable material in brewed tea. In black tea, through an oxidation and polymerization process, a significant portion of the catechins is converted to theaflavins (TFs) such as TF, TF monogallates (TF3-G, and TF3'-G), TF digallate (TFdi-G), and higher molecular weight polymers which are responsible for the dark brown color of the black tea (*2*).

Among the many biological effects of tea, the anticarcinogenic effect has been extensively investigated. The inhibitory action of tea and tea constituents against chemically-induced carcinogenesis has been demonstrated in many animal models including those for the skin, lung, esophagus, stomach, liver, small intestine, pancreas, colon, bladder, prostate, and mammary glands (*3-7*). Several epidemiological studies also support a protective role of tea against development of colorectal, uterine, and gastric cancers (*3,8,9*). A variety of mechanisms have been suggested for the anticarcinogenic effect of tea polyphenols, including antioxidative activities, inhibition of many enzymes related to the tumor promotion such as ornithine decarboxylase, protein kinase C, cycloxygenase and lipoxygenase, inhibition of activator protein-1, and the inhibition of angiogenesis (*3,10-15*).

Colorectal cancer is one of the most frequent types of cancer in the Western countries, and remains the second leading cause of cancer death in the United States (*16*). The importance of archidonic acid metabolism in colorectal carcinogenesis has been demonstrated by the observation that individuals regularly using nonsteroidal anti-inflammatory drugs (NSAIDs), which are inhibitors of COX, showed significantly low incidence and mortality rates of colorectal cancer (*17*). Arachidonic acid is metabolized by three types of enzymes; COXs, LOXs and cytochromes P450. Arachidonic acid metabolism is frequently elevated in various tumors and its inhibitors effectively suppressed tumorigenesis. Consequently, the modulation of arachidonic acid metabolism has become a potentially important approach for cancer chemoprevention. The overall scheme of arachidonic acid metabolism is shown in Figure 1. In this

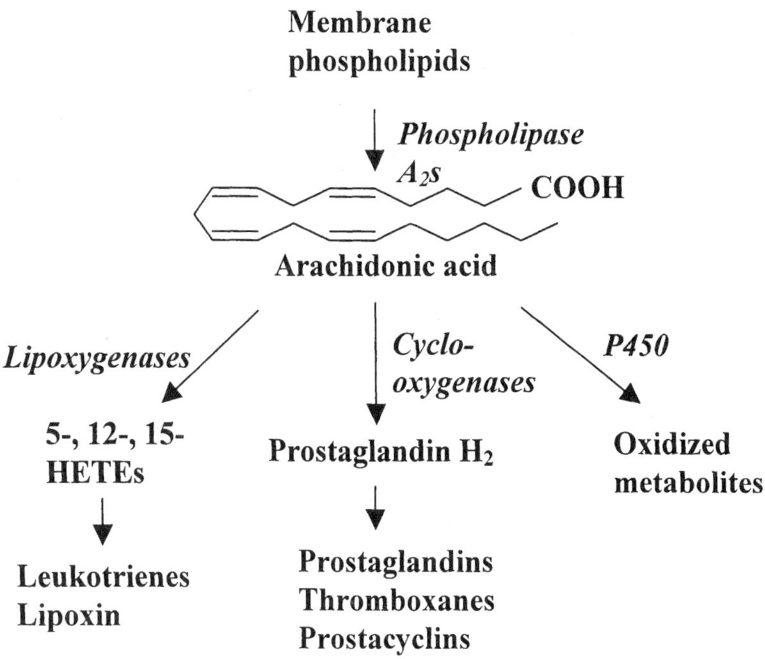

Figure 1. *The overall scheme of arahcidonic acid metabolism.*

study, the effects of tea polyphenols on several important enzymes involved in arachidonic acid metabolism in human colon have been investigated.

Results and Discussion

Tea polyphenols and Lipoxygenase

LOXs catalyze the oxygenation of arachidonic acid to produce hydroxyeicosatetraenoic acids (HETEs). 5-LOX, 12-LOX and 15-LOX have been identified in humans. HETEs and their metabolites are reported to be important regulators in proliferation and apoptosis in cancer cell lines (*18–20*).

The effects of tea polyphenols and nordihydroguiaretic acid (NDGA) on LOX- dependent arachidonic acid metabolism in human colon are shown in

Figure 2. In the current assay system, 15, 12, and 5-HETEs were produced during incubation of human colon cytosol with [^{14}C]-arachidonic acid, which were inhibited almost completely by NDGA, a general LOX inhibitor, implying that the metabolites are LOX-dependent. Tea polyphenols (30 μg/mL) inhibited LOX-dependent arachidonic acid metabolism by 30–74%. ECG showed the most potent inhibitory effects, whereas black tea TFs displayed relatively weaker activity on a weight basis. Tea polyphenols inhibited the formation of 5, 12, and 15-HETEs to about the same extent.

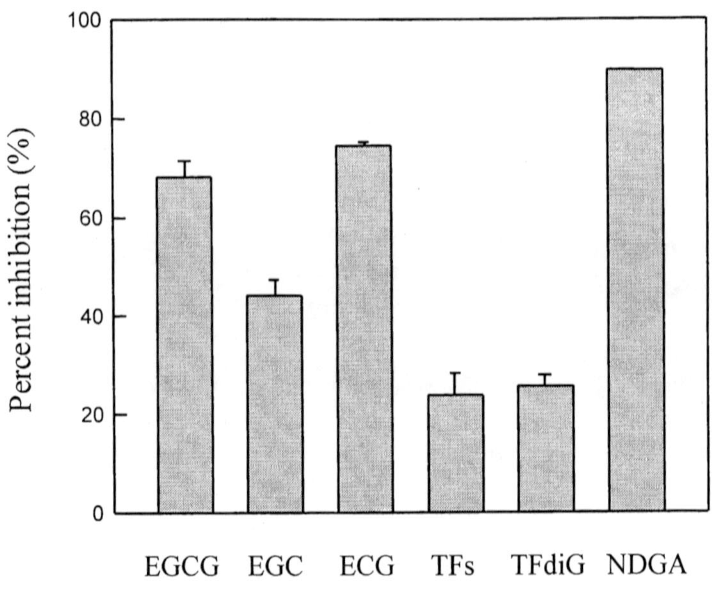

***Figure 2**. The inhibitory effect of tea polyphenols and nordihydorguiaretic acid (NDGA) on LOX-dependen arachidonic acid metabolites in cytosols from human colon. The incubation mixture contained 0.6 mg cytosolic protein, 20 μM (0.22 μCi) arachidonic acid and 2 mM $CaCl_2$ with or without 30 μg/mL tea polyphenols or 20 μM NDGA in 100 mM Tris-HCl buffer, pH 7.4. The reactions (200 μL) were performed at 37°C for 30 min. The reaction products were analyzed by HPLC. Percent inhibition was calculated based on the sum of the total metabolites. The data are the mean ± S.E. from 3 independent experiments. The result of NDGA is the mean of duplicate experiments (Data from reference 13).*

Although there are some conflicting reports regarding the role of 15-LOX in carcinogenesis (*21*), inhibition of LOXs is generally considered to decrease tumor formation (*22*). LOXs are regulated at several different stages such as expression, up-regulation by cellular signal cascades, and activation by 5-LOX activating protein (FLAP). In addition to the catalytic inhibition observed herein, tea polyphenols may interrupt the multiple steps in the regulation of LOXs.

Tea polyphenols and Cycloxygenases

COX metabolizes arachidonic acid to prostaglandin G_2 (PGG_2), which is subsequently reduced to prostaglandin H_2 (PGH_2). PGH_2 is further metabolized to eicosanoids such as prostaglandins, prostacyclin, and thromboxane by prostaglandin synthase, prostacyclin synthase and thromboxane synthase, respectively. Two COX isoforms, COX-1 and COX-2, have been identified. Overexpression of COX-2, an inducible COX isoform, has been observed in various types of cancers, including colorectal cancer (*23–27*). Prostaglandin E_2 (PGE_2), a major metabolite derived from COX- catalyzed arachidonic acid metabolism, was reported to be involved in cell hyperproliferation, mitogenesis, tumor cell invasiveness, and angiogenesis as well as in the inhibition of apoptosis (*28–31*). Many experimental animal studies using NSAIDs also support the idea that inhibition of COX is an important approach for prevention of cancers.

As shown in figure 3, tea polyphenols (30 μg/mL) inhibited COX-dependent arachidonic acid metabolism in microsomes from normal colon mucosa by 37–62 %. Among the metabolites, thromboxane and 12-hydroxyheptadecatrienoic acid were inhibited to a greater extent. ECG also exhibited strongest inhibitory action (on a weight basis), displaying non-competitive inhibition with a K_i value of 16.9±1.3 μM by using ovine COX-1 (*13*). The IC_{50} values (in μM) of each tea polyphenol in COX-dependent arachidonic acid metabolism in normal colon mucosa follow the order of TFdiG (41.8) < ECG (54.9) < EGCG (72.1) < TFs (92.8) < EGC (152.8).

The inhibitory effect of tea polyphenols was generally less pronounced in colon tumor tissues (Figure 3). Black tea polyphenols with TF backbone enhance PGE_2 formation in tumor (not normal) microsomes (*13*). The enhancement appears to be dependent on COX-2, which is frequently overexpressed in tumor tissues. Since all TFs showed the inhibitory effect on isolated ovine COX-2, the increase in PGE_2 might not be the result of direct activation of COX-2 but due to the stimulation of an interaction between COX-2 and other microsomal factors. Black tea has shown relatively weaker anti-carcinogenic effects compared to green tea or no effects (*32*). The enhancing effect on the formation of PGE_2, one

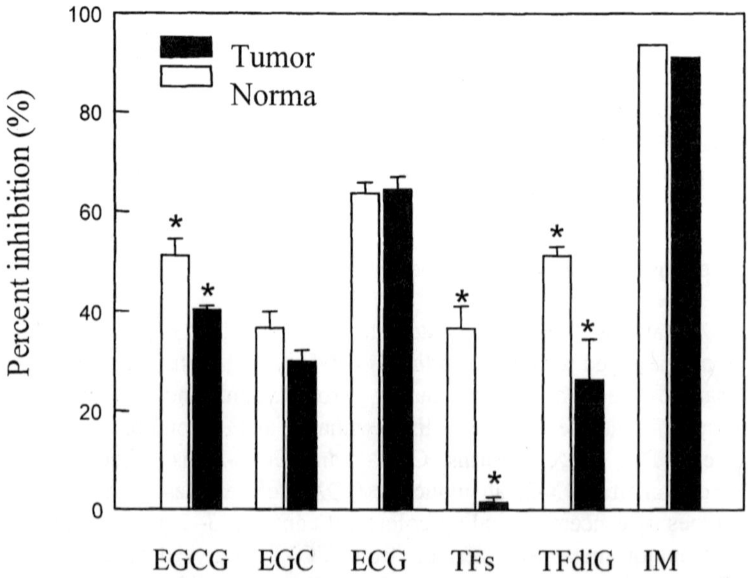

Figure 3. The effects of tea polyphenols and Indomethacin (IM) on COX-dependent metabolism of arachdonic acid in human colon. Products were analyzed from the reaction with 0.1 mg microsomal protein, 20 μM (0.22 μCi) arachidonic acid, and 1 mM glutathione, 1 mM epinephrine and 10 mM EDTA with or without 30 μg/mL tea polyphenols or 5 μM IM in 100 mM Tris-HCl buffer, pH 7.4. The reaction was carried out at 37 °C for 30 min. Percent inhibition was calculated based on the sum of the total metabolites. The data are the mean ± S.E. from 4 or 5 independent experiments. The result of indomethacin is the mean of duplicate experiments.

* *Significantly different effects ($p<0.02$) in between tumor and normal samples (Data from reference 13)*

of the major carcinogenic eicosanoids, by TFs may contribute to the weaker inhibitory effect of black tea.

Metz et al. reported that green tea administration decreased COX-2 activity without altering COX-1 activity in azoxymethane- induced preneoplastic lesion of rat colon (*33*). In the current study, green tea polyphenols such as EGCG do not seem to inhibit COX-2 preferentially. We also observed that the PGE_2 level in human rectal mucosa biopsy tissue was significantly decreased at 4 and 8 hour after the ingestion of green tea (*34*). Other mechanisms may also be involved in the inhibition of COX and PGE_2 formation in colorectum, which remain to be investigated.

Effects on Phospholipase A_2

Arachidonic acid is normally released from membrane phospholipids by the action of phospholipase A_2s (PLA_2). There are three major PLA_2 types that are involved in the release of arachidonic acid (*35*): the secretory PLA_2 ($sPLA_2$), the intracellular Ca^{2+}-independent PLA_2 ($iPLA_2$), and the cytosolic Ca^{2+}-dependent PLA_2 ($cPLA_2$). Among several types of PLA_2s, $cPLA_2$ is most importantly involved in releasing arachidonic acid in most tissues. $cPLA_2$ is an enzyme normally found in the cytosolic fraction in many tissues (reviewed in 36). In the presence of micromolar levels of calcium ion, the enzyme is translocated into membrane fractions, mainly the nuclear envelop or the endoplasmic reticulum. It shows a preference for arachidonic acid located at *sn*-2 site of phospholipids. $cPLA_2$ activity is up-regulated by the phosphorylation on Ser^{505} site by mitogen-activated protein kinases (MAPKs) (*37*). The binding of phosphatidylinositol 4,5-bisphosphate (PIP_2) to $cPLA_2$ increases the activity of the enzyme by increasing the affinity of the enzyme to membrane. (*38*).

PLA_2 has been reported to be elevated in certain types of cancers. It was found that human colon tumors have more arachidonic acid and increased levels of PLA_2 than in normal colon tissues (*39*). $cPLA_2$ was reported to play a key role in the development of polyps in the small intestine of the APC knockout mouse, a model for human familial adenomatous polyposis (*40*). The release of arachidonic acid by PLA_2 from membrane phospholipids is frequently the rate-limiting step for further arachidonic acid metabolism. Accordingly, inhibition of $cPLA_2$ and arachidonic acid release may be effective targets for cancer chemoprevention.

In order to evaluate the potential of tea polyphenols for the inhibition of $cPLA_2$, an assay system for $cPLA_2$ using microsomal fraction from HT-29 human colon adenocarcinoma cells was developed. In this system, the microsomal fraction showed 7.7 fold increase of PLA_2 activity in the presence of 5 μg/mL phosphoinositides and fully activated below 100 μM calcium concentration, whereas 1 μM bromoenol lactone (a specific $iPLA_2$ inhibitor) and 2 mM DTT (a $sPLA_2$ inhibitor) did not inhibit the PLA_2 activity, but 95% of activity was disappeared with 2mM EGTA, a calcium ion chelator, indicating that the almost all PLA_2 activity in the microsomes was from $cPLA_2$ (Data not shown). A mixture of green tea polyphenols displayed a more potent inhibition on $cPLA_2$ activity than a mixture of black tea polyphenols, whereas caffeine showed weak effect (Figure 4). In terms of individual polyphenols, TFs showed relatively higher inhibitory effects than green tea catechins (Figure 5). EGCG and ECG (50 μM) inhibited $cPLA_2$ activity by 15 and 30%, respectively. EC and EGC were less effective. TF mono- and di-gallates (50 μM) inhibited $cPLA_2$ activity by 30 - 45%, whereas TF was less potent. ECG inhibited $cPLA_2$ from HT-29 cell in a non-competitive manner with a K*i* of 147.6±10.1 μM (Figure 6).

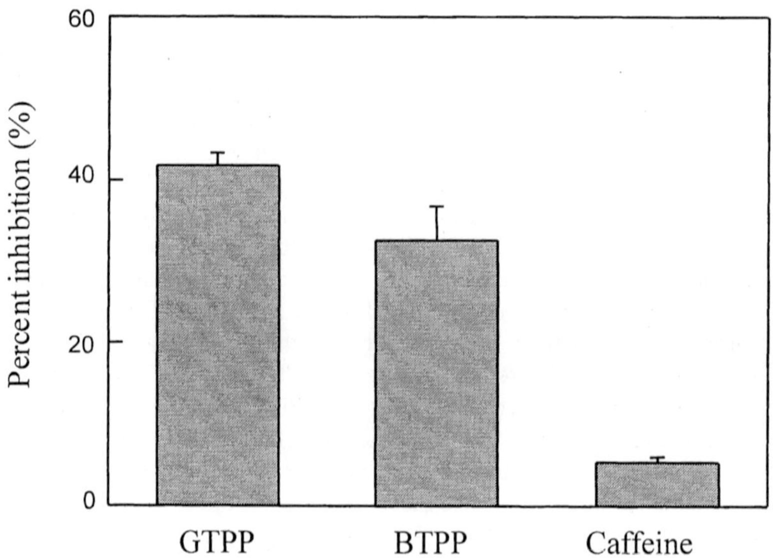

Figure 4*. The effects of mixture of green (GTPP) and black tea (BTPP) polyphenols and caffeine in $cPLA_2$ activity from HT-29 cells. The reaction mixture (100 μl) for $cPLA_2$ activity contained 20 μg microsomal protein from HT-29 cells, 40 μM substrate 1-palmitoyl 2-[1-^{14}C]arachidonyl sn-glycero-3-phosphorylcholine (hot:cold, 1:3), 5 μg/mL phosphoinositides, 100 μM $CaCl_2$ in 100 mM Tris-HCl buffer, pH 7.4 with or without tea polyphenols (50 μg/mL) or caffeine (50 μM). The reaction was carried out at 37 °C for 30 min. The data are the mean ±S.E. from 3 independent experiments.*

Currently, we are investigating the effect tea polyphenols on arachidonic acid release in intact cell system. This inhibitory effects are much more potent than on the inhibition of $cPLA_2$. In addition to the inhibition of the catalytic activity of $cPLA_2$, the tea polyphenols may inhibit arachidonic acid release in

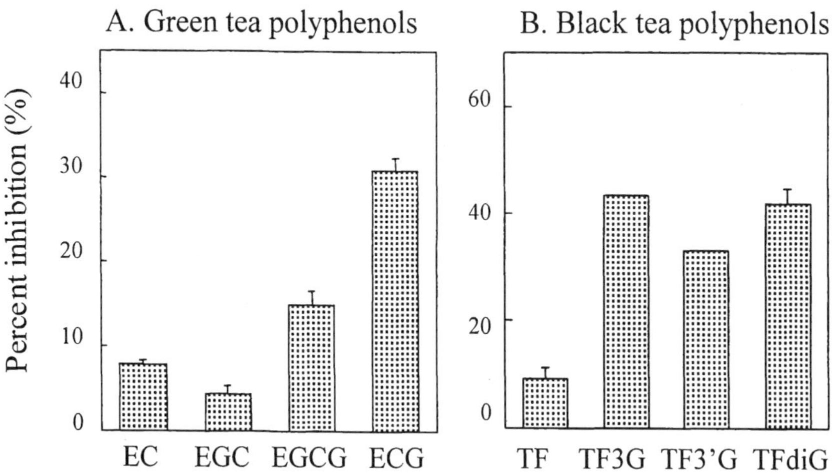

***Figure 5**. The effects of purified green and black tea polyphenols on $cPLA_2$ activity from HT-29 cells. The reaction mixture (100 μL) consisted of 20 μg microsomal protein from HT-29 cells, 40 μM substrate 1-palmitoyl 2-[1-^{14}C]arachidonyl sn-glycero-3-phosphorylcholine (hot:cold, 1:3), 5 μg/mL phosphoinositides, 100 μM $CaCl_2$ in 100 mM Tris-HCl buffer, pH 7.4 with or without 50 μM tea polyphenols. The reaction were carried out at 37 °C for 30 min. The data are the mean ± S.E. from 3 independent experiments. The results of TF3-G and TF3'-G are mean of duplicate.*

intact cell through other mechanisms such as the inhibition of the up-regulation and/or translocation of $cPLA_2$.

Conclusion

One of the serious obstacles in using food constituents for cancer prevention is their poor absorption. The effective concentrations of tea polyphenols required for inhibiting key enzymes for cancer prevention are generally higher than the concentrations observed in plasma and tissues. Colon, however, is considered as a place where significant portion of unabsorbed tea polyphenols such as EGCG can be reached and their inhibitory action in colonic mucosa may be achieved even without systemic absorption. Arachidonic acid metabolism is a complex cascade where many of metabolites are mutually regulated. Many evidences have been reported regarding the positive feed-back action of arachidonic acid metabolites (e.g. PGE_2). As inhibitors affecting several steps of arachidonic acid metabolism, tea polyphenols may inhibit the carcinogenic process and reduce the risk for colon in humans.

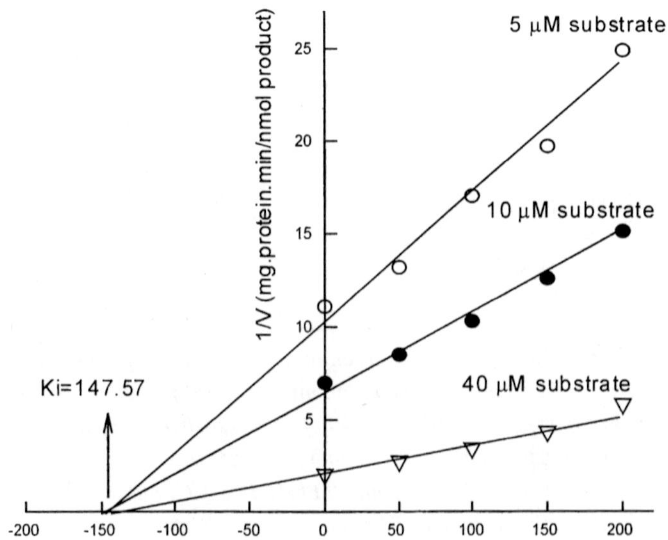

Figure 6. Inhibitory mechanism of ECG on $cPLA_2$ from HT-29 cell. The reaction was carried out at 37°C for 30 min. The incubation mixture consisted of 20 μg microsomal protein from HT-29 cells, substrate and ECG as indicated, 5 μg/mL phosphoinositides, 100 μM $CaCl_2$ in 100 mM Tris-HCl buffer, pH 7.4.

References

1. Ames B.N.; Gold L.S.; Willett W.C. *Proc Natl Acad Sci* **1995,** *92*, 5258-5265.
2. Balentine, D.A.; Wiseman, S.A.; Bouwens, L.C. *Crit Rev Food Sci Nutr* **1997,** *37*, 693-704.
3. Yang, C.S.; Wang, Z-Y. *J Natl Cancer Inst* **1993,** *85*, 1038-1049.
4. Yang, C.S.; Chen, L.; Lee, M-J.; Laudau, J.M. Effects of tea on carcinogenesis in animal models and humans. Vol. 401, pp. 51-61. New York: Plenum Press, 1996.

5. Yang, C.S.; Kim, S.; Yang, G-Y; Lee, M-J.; Liao, J.; Chung, J.Y.; Ho, C.-T. *Proc. Soc. Exp. Biol. Med.* **1999**, *220*, 213-217.
6. Conney, A.H.; Lu, Y-P.; Lou, Y-R.; Xie, J-G.; Huang, M-T. *Proc. Soc. Exp. Bio.l Med.* **1999**, *220*, 229-233.
7. Yamane, T.; Takahashi, T.; Kuwata, K.; Oya, K.; Inagake, M.; Kaito, Y.; Suganuma, M.; Fujiki, H. *Cancer Res* **1995**, *55*, 2081-2084.
8. Yang, C.S.; Landau, J.M. *J. Nutr.* **2000**, *130*, 2409-2412.
9. Kohlmeier, L.; Weterings, K.G.G.; Steck, S.; Kok, F.J. *Nutr. Cancer* **1997**, *27*, 1-13.
10. Huang, M.T.; Ho, C.-T.; Wang, Z.Y.; Ferraro, T.; Finnegan-Olive, T.; Lou, Y.R.; Mitchell, J.M.; Laskin, J.D.; Newark, H.; Yang, C.S.; Conney, A.H. *Carcinogenesis* **1992**, *13*, 947-954.
11. Katiyar, S. K.; Agarwal, R.; Wood, G.S.; Mukhtar, H. *Cancer Res.* **1992**, *52*, 6890-6897.
12. Katiyar, S. K.; Muhktar, H. *Carcinogenesis* **1997,** *18*, 1911-1916.
13. Hong, J.; Smith, T.J.; Ho, C-T.; August D.A.; Yang C.S. *Biochem Pharmacol.* **2001,** *62*, 1175-1183
14. Dong, Z.; Ma, W-Y.; Huang, C.; Yang, C.S. *Cancer Res.* **1997**, 57, 4414-4419.
15. Cao, Y.; Cao, R. *Nature* **1999**, *398*, 381.
16. Boring, C. C.; Squires, T.S.; Tong, T.; Montgomery, S. *CA Cancer J.Clin.* **1994**, *44*, 7-26.
17. Levy, G. N. *FASEB J.* **1997,** *11*, 234-247.
18. Ghosh J.; Myers C.E. *Biochem. Biophys. Res. Commun.* **1997,** *235*, 418-423.
19. Kamitani H, Geller M, and Eling T. *J Biol Chem* **1998**, 273, 21569-21577.
20. Tang DG, Chen YQ, and Honn KV, *Proc Natl Acad Sci USA* **1996,** 93, 5241-5246.
21. Shureiqi, I., Chen, D., Lotan, R., Yang, P., Newman R.A., Fischer S.M., and Lippman S.M. *Cancer Res* **2000**, 60, 6846-6850.
22. Steele, V.E., Holmes, C.A., Hawk, E.T., Kepelovich, L., Lubet, R.A., Crowell, J.A., Sigman, C.C., and Kelloff, G.J. *Cancer Epidemiol Biomark Prev* **1999**, 8, 467-483.
23. Eberhart, C.E., Coffey, R. J., Radhika, A., Giardiello, F.M., Ferrenbach, S., and DuBois, R.N. *Gastroenterology* **1994**, 107, 1183-1188.
24. Sano, H., Kawahito, Y., Wilder, R.L., Hashiramoto, A., Mukai, S., Asai, K., Kimura, S., Kato, H., Kondo, M., and Hla, T. *Cancer Res* **1995**, 55, 3785-3789.
25. Fujita, T., Matsui, M., Takaku, K., Uetake, H., Ichikawa, W., Taketo, M.M., and Sugihara, K. *Cancer Res* **1998**, 58, 4823-4826.
26. Wolff, H., Saukkonen, K., Anttila, S., Karjalainen A., Vainio, H., and Ristimaki, A. *Cancer Res* **1998,** 58, 4997-5001.

27. Zimmermann, K.C., Sarbia, M., Weber, A-A., Borchard, F., Gabbert, H.E., and Schror, K. *Cancer Res* **1999**, 59, 198-204.
28. Tsujii, M., and DuBois, R.N. *Cell* **1995**, 83, 493-501.
29. Tsujii, M., Kawano, S., and DuBois, R.N. *Proc Nat. Acad Sci USA* **1997**, 94, 3336-3340.
30. Sheng, H., Shao, J., Morrow, J.D., Beauchamp, R.D., and DuBois, R.N. *Cancer Res* **1998**, 58, 362-366.
31. Tsujii, M., Kawano, S., Tsuji, S., Sawaoka, H., Hori, M., and DuBois, R.N. *Cell* 1998, 93, 705-716.
32. Weisburger, J.H., Rivenson, A., Reinhardt, J., Aliaga, C., Braley, J., Pittman, B., and Zang, E. *Carcinogenesis* **1998**, 19, 229-232.
33. Metz, N., Lobstein, A., Schneider, Y., Gosse, F., Schleiffer R., Anton, R., and Raul, F. *Nutr Cancer*, **2000**, 38, 60-64.
34. August, D. A., Landau, J., Caputo, D., Hong, J., Lee, M-J., and Yang, C.S. *Cancer Epidemiol Biomark Prev* **1999**, 8, 709-713.
35. Balsinde J., Balboa M., Insel P., and Dennis E.A. *Annu Rev Pharmacol Toxicol*, **1999**, 39, 175-189.
36. Leslie C.C. *J Biol Chem* **1997**, 272, 16709-16712.
37. Lin L-L., Wartmann M., Lin A.Y., Knopf J.L., Seth A., and Davis R.J. *Cell* **1993**, 72, 269-278.
38. Mosior M., Six D., and Dennis E. *J Biol Chem* **1998**, 273, 2184-2191.
39. Soydan A.S., Tavares I.A., Weech P.K., Temblay N.M., and Bennett A., *Eur J Cancer* **1996**, 32, 1781-7.
40. Takaku, K.; Sonoshita, M.; Sasaki, N.; Uozumi, N.; Doi, Y.; Shimizu, T.; Taketo, M.M. *J. Biol. Chem.* **2000** *275*, 34013-34016

Signal Transduction and Gene Modulation

Chapter 5

Prevention and Therapy of Cancer by Food Factors through p53-Dependent or -Independent Apoptosis

Zigang Dong

The Hormel Institute, University of Minnesota, 801 16th Avenue N.E., Austin, MN 55912

Consumption of plant-derived foods has been linked to decreased risk of cancer. Using a cell culture model, we found that the induction of apoptosis may be involved in the chemopreventive or therapeutic activity of these food factors. Phenethyl isothiocyanate (PEITC), which occurs as a conjugate in certain cruciferous vegetables, inhibited cell transformation corresponding with the induction of apoptosis (requiring an elevation of p53). Resveratrol, found at high levels in grapes, inhibited cell transformation through the induction of apoptosis, mediated through JNKs and p53-dependent pathways. Also, Erks and p38 kinase mediate resveratrol-induced phosphorylation of p53 at serine 15. Gingerol, isolated from ginger, inhibited cell transformation and induced apoptosis, which is p53-independent. These data suggested that food factors induced apoptosis through p53-dependent or –independent pathways and may be involved in chemopreventive or therapeutic effects on cancer. [Supported by NIH grants CA74916 and CA81064, AICR grant 99A062, and The Hormel Foundation.]

Introduction

Over the past decade, scientists have gained stunning new insights into the fundamental mechanisms of cancer development. This progress has led to a continuing decline in the incidence and death rates of many types of human cancers. However, in spite of this progress, too many patients in the United States and other parts of the world continue to suffer and die from cancer everyday. The incidence of the major cancers, including colon, breast, lung, prostate, and skin cancer is still too high and the incidence of some cancers, such as melanomas, continues to rise.

The current chemotherapy of cancer is based on the assumption that cancer is a mass of cells resulting from excessive and uncontrolled cell proliferation. Therefore, most available chemotherapeutic drugs are highly toxic and cause extensive damage to normal tissues. They have many side effects including hair loss and toxicity specific to bone marrow and the gastrointestinal tract and cause extensive illness.

From the number of published scientific papers, interest in the concept and practice of chemoprevention as an approach to the control of cancer has increased greatly in the past few years. Many very recent (1999-2001) review articles focus on the issues, rationale, progress, and promise of chemoprevention as a new anticancer strategy *(1-9)*.

Mechanism-based Chemoprevention: Lessons From Recent Clinical Trials

The renewed focus on chemoprevention as a credible and practical approach to the control of carcinogenesis is attributed partially to the positive results of two important randomized clinical trials in breast cancer. These two trials used three different agents, tamoxifen, raloxifene, or 4-hydroxyphenylfenretinide *(3, 4)*. Tamoxifen and raloxifene can bind to the estrogen receptor and block endogenous estrogen-induced biological effects. An abundance of evidence is available in animal models and human tissues regarding the mechanisms of action of these agents in chemoprevention *(3,4)*. 4-Hydroxyphenylfenretinide is a synthetic retinoid and a great deal of evidence suggests that retinoids are effective in preventing cancer in different animal models and the mechanisms are well studied *(4)*. At the same time, the alarming negative results obtained for β-carotene supplementation on development of lung cancer *(5,6)* emphasize the need for caution in prescribing a potential chemopreventive substance before its mechanism of action is completely understood *(7)*.

p53, Cancer Development and Chemotherapeutic Drug Resistance

p53 is one of the most frequently mutated tumor suppressor genes in human cancer and loss of p53 function is related to more than half of all human cancers *(10-12)*. Normally, p53 is a short-lived protein. However, many signals can activate p53 by causing stabilization and accumulation of the protein within the cells. Recent studies have shown that phosphorylation of p53 may play a critical role in its stabilization, up-regulation and functional activation *(13-20)*. p53 has been clearly linked to pathways leading to apoptosis and lack of p53 protein expression is associated with an increased risk of tumor formation *(21,22)*. p53 knockout mice or transgenic mice expressing a mutant p53 are prone to both spontaneous and induced tumors *(21,22)*. More importantly, nearly all current chemotherapeutic drugs used for cancer treatment cause DNA damage and kill cancer cells mainly by activating signaling pathways leading to apoptosis *(23)*. Chemotherapeutic agents such as cisplatin, mitoxantrone, doxorubicin, methotrexate, mitomycin and bleomycin lead to an up-regulation of the CD95 receptor and p53 *(24)*. p53 inactivation is therefore related to the development of drug resistance associated with anti-cancer chemotherapy *(24,25)*.

Prevention and Therapy of Cancer by Food Factors Through p53-dependent or -independent Apoptosis

Consumption of plant derived-foods, especially fruits and vegetables, has been linked to a decreased risk of human cancer *(9,26)*. Using cell culture and animal models, many active chemopreventive compounds isolated from soy, tea, rice, ginger, garlic, pepper, and many other fruits and vegetables have been identified *(1-4,7-9,26)*. These "natural products" from foods are considered to have little or no toxicity. This review is not intended to be an extensive, comprehensive critique of chemopreventive agents, but rather a brief overview of recent work from our laboratory focusing on chemopreventive agents with the ability to induce apoptosis through p53-dependent or -independent mechanisms as illustrated in Figure 1.

Resveratrol and Its Derivatives

Resveratrol (3,5,4′-trihydroxystilbene), which occurs naturally in grapes and other foods, has chemopreventive effects in different systems, based on its striking inhibition of diverse cellular events associated with tumor initiation, promotion, and progression *(27)*. We found that resveratrol suppressed tumor-

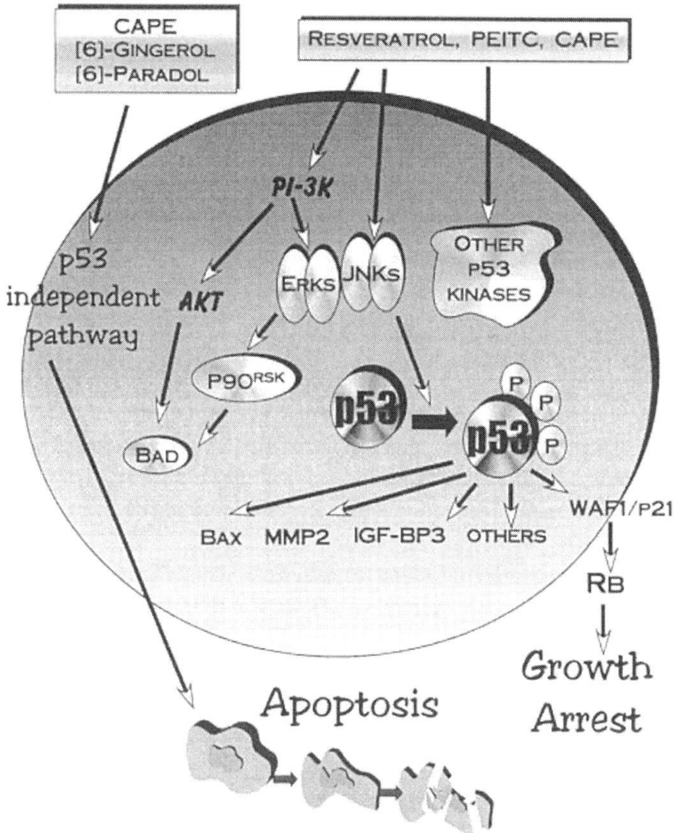

Figure 1. Chemopreventive agents induce apoptosis through p53-dependent and –independent pathways.

promoter-induced cell transformation and strongly induced apoptosis, transactivation of p53, and expression of the p53 protein in the same cell line and at the same dose *(28)*. Activation of p53 resulting in apoptosis can suppress tumor development. We found that resveratrol induced apoptosis only in cells expressing wild-type p53 ($p53^{+/+}$) and not in p53-deficient ($p53^{-/-}$) cells, thus causing apoptosis through activation of p53 *(29)*. Additionally, in a mouse JB6 epidermal cell line, resveratrol activated extracellular-signal-regulated protein kinases (ERKs), c-Jun NH_2-terminal kinases (JNKs), and p38 kinase and induced serine 15 phosphorylation of p53 *(29)*. Stable expression of a dominant negative mutant of ERK2 or p38 kinase or their respective inhibitor, PD98059 or SB202190, repressed the phosphorylation of p53 at serine 15. In contrast, overexpression of a dominant negative mutant of JNK1 had no effect on the phosphorylation. Most importantly, ERKs and p38 kinase formed a complex with p53 after treatment with resveratrol *(29)*. Strikingly, resveratrol phosphorylated p53 at serine 15 *in vitro*. Furthermore, pretreatment of the cells with PD98059 or SB202190 or stable expression of a dominant negative mutant of ERK2 or p38 kinase impaired resveratrol-induced p53-dependent transcriptional activation and apoptosis, whereas constitutively active MEK1 increased the transcriptional activation of p53. These data strongly suggest that both ERKs and p38 kinase mediate resveratrol-induced activation of p53 and apoptosis through phosphorylation of p53 at serine 15 *(29)*.

Phenethyl Isothiocyanate

Isothiocyanates are found in cruciferous vegetables such as broccoli and watercress *(8,9,30)*. They are released when the vegetables are crushed, for example, by chewing. Phenethyl isothiocyanate (PEITC), benzyl isothiocyanate, and sulphoraphane are all effective cancer chemopreventive agents in animal models *(30-33)*. The chemopreventive activity of PEITC is associated with its favorable modification of carcinogen metabolism and induction of apoptosis. We found that PEITC blocks tumor promoter 12-O-tetradecanoylphorbol-12-acetate (TPA)- or epidermal growth factor (EGF)-induced cell transformation in mouse epidermal JB6 cells, and this inhibitory activity on cell transformation corresponded with the induction of apoptosis *(34)*. Most importantly, apoptosis induction by PEITC occurs through a p53-dependent pathway. This was demonstrated not only by results showing that PEITC induced p53 protein expression and p53-dependent transactivation, but also by data showing that PEITC induced apoptosis in $p53^{+/+}$, but not in $p53^{-/-}$ cells. In contrast, PEITC induced apoptosis in cells with both normal or deficient sphingomyelinase activity. Our results demonstrated for the first time that p53 elevation is required for PEITC-induced apoptosis, which may be involved in its anti-cancer chemopreventive activity *(34)*. The role of isothiocyanates in MAPKs and caspase signaling events may be central to the observed anti-cancer effects. Low concentrations (<100 μmol/L) of PEITC or sulphoraphane activate the MAPKS (ERK2, JNK1, p38 kinases) in a concentration- and time-dependent manner. This activation led to the expression of survival genes including *c-fos* and *c-jun* and certain detoxifying enzymes such as quinone reductase and glutathione-S-transferase, thus promoting survival. Higher concentrations (above 100 μmol/L) apparently activate the caspase pathway, leading to apoptosis, whereas concentrations above 150 μmol/L lead to non-specific necrotic cell death. Benzyl isothiocyanate substantially increased JNKs activation and our data indicated that JNKs are required for PEITC-induced apoptosis *(34)*.

Inositol Hexaphosphate ($InsP_6$)

$InsP_6$, also known as phytic acid, is a ubiquitous compound found in the plant kingdom, especially in grains such as rice and corn *(35,36)*. However, it is also a component of mammalian cells and is found at concentrations between 10 and 100 μM in both resting and stimulated cells *(37,38)*. Previous studies elucidated the primary functions of $InsP_6$ *(39)*. $InsP_6$ is suggested to regulate heart rate and blood pressure, stimulate Ca^{2+} influx, bind to the clathrin assembly protein, and inhibit L-and P-selection function *in vitro* and inflammation *in vivo* *(39, 40)*. Other possible physiological functions and intracellular $InsP_6$ may be to serve as a natural antioxidant *(41)* or neurotransmitter *(42)*. Studies by Shamsuddin *et al* *(39)* and others *(43,44)* demonstrated a striking anticarcinogenic effect of $Insp_6$ and myoinositol. $InsP_6$ was shown to be both chemopreventive and chemotherapeutic in rodent colon and mammary carcinogenesis models, as well as in transplanted fibrosarcoma models *(45)*. $InsP_6$ also significantly reduced the mitotic rate in the colon crypts of animals treated with a carcinogen and inhibited human cancer growth with induction of cell differentiation at concentrations of 1-5 mM. However, the molecular mechanism of the anti-tumor effect of $InsP_6$ is not clear. $InsP_6$ regulates expression of the tumor suppressor gene p53 *(46)*. We therefore investigated the role of $InsP_6$ in tumor-promoter-induced cell transformation and signal transduction pathways leading to AP-1 activation *(47)*. $InsP_6$ blocked EGF-induced phosphatidylinositol-3 (PI-3) kinase activity in a dose-dependent manner in JB6 cells and directly *in vitro*. In separate studies, we showed that PI-3 kinase is an important mediator of TPA-induced and EGF-induced cell transformation *(47,48)*. Blocking PI-3 kinase activity with $InsP_6$ profoundly impaired JB6 cell transformation. Because PI-3 kinase plays an important role in anti-apoptosis pathways, the inhibition of PI-3 kinase by $InsP_6$ may contribute to the induction of apoptosis by $InsP_6$.

Caffeic Acid Phenethyl Ester

Caffeic acid phenethyl ester (CAPE), an active component extracted from honeybee propolis, blocks tumorigenesis in a two-stage model of mouse skin cancer that was promoted by treatment with TPA *(49)*. The anti-cancer or anti-tumor promotion effects of CAPE may be based on their ability to induce apoptosis. We found that CAPE suppresses TPA-induced cell transformation and induced apoptosis in mouse epidermal JB6 CI 41 cells *(50)*. No difference in induction of apoptosis was observed between normal lymphoblasts and sphingomyelinase-deficient cell lines. Although CAPE treatment of two p53 mutant tumor cell lines, NCI-H358 and SK-OV-3, and $p53^{-/-}$cells caused cleavage of caspase-3 as well as DNA fragmentation, caspase-3 cleavage was seen early (at 6 h) only in cells expressing wild-type p53 and Cl 41 cells *(50)*. These results suggested that p53 might be involved in the early stages of CAPE-induced apoptosis. The p53-dependent transcription activation occurred 2 h after treatment with CAPE and reached a maximum at 6 h in Cl 41 p53 DNA-binding sequence-stable transfectant cells *(50)*. Several phosphorylation sites are present in the N-terminal activation domain and the C-terminal region of the p53 protein. Recent studies have shown that phosphorylation of p53 at serine 15 and serine 20 may be critical for its stabilization and functional activation during cell stress *(13-17)*. We also showed that phosphorylation of p53 at serine 15 regulated its activation and induction of apoptosis in JB6 cells *(19,29)*. The phosphorylation of p53 protein at serine 389, a homologue of serine 392 of the human p53 protein, has been reported to play an important role in p53-mediated transcriptional activation *in vivo (51)*. To investigate the possible role of p53 in the induction of apoptosis by CAPE, we analyzed the influence of CAPE on p53 phosphorylation in JB6 cells. We found that CAPE induced p53 phosphorylation at both serine 15 and 389 *(50)*. Therefore, CAPE appears to induce apoptosis through p53-dependent and p53-independent pathways and its anti-tumor promotion activity may occur through the induction of apoptosis.

[6]-Gingerol and [6]-Paradol

Many spices possess anti-carcinogenic activity. However, the molecular mechanisms by which they exert their anti-tumorigenic effects are unknown. Plants of the ginger (*Zingiber officinale* Roscoe, Zingiberaceae) family, one of the most heavily consumed dietary substances in the world *(52)* have been shown to inhibit tumor promotion in mouse skin *(53)*. The oil from the root of ginger contains [6]-gingerol, the major pharmacologically active component *(53)*, and lesser amounts of a structurally related vanilloid, [6]-paradol. Recent studies suggest that ginger compounds suppress proliferation of human cancer cells through the induction of apoptosis *(53,54)*. We found that [6]-gingerol and [6]-paradol significantly block EGF-induced JB6 cell transformation *(55)*. [6]-Gingerol also inhibits EGF-induced AP-1 transactivation and AP-1 DNA binding activity but has no effect on EGF-induced ERKs or p38 kinase phosphorylation. At concentrations above 25 μM, [6]-paradol induces apoptosis in JB6 cells apparently through a p53-independent mechanism because it also induced apoptosis in $p53^{-/-}$ cells *(55)*.

Conclusions

The identification and development of cancer therapeutic and chemopreventive agents with limited cytotoxicity has been receiving increased interest. The development of these agents on a mechanistic basis remains a challenge for us. The p53 tumor suppresser gene plays a critical role in cancer development, and more then half of human cancers are related to the dysfunction of the p53 protein. We have therefore focused on the investigation of the potential chemopreventive or chemotherapeutic effects of food factors on p53-dependent and –independent pathways. These mechanistic-based studies represent a promising future for development of more effective chemotherapeutic and chemopreventive agents with fewer side effects for controlling human cancers.

References

1. Sporn, M. B.; Suh, N. *Carcinog.* **2000**, *21*, 525-530.
2. Sporn, M. B. *Cancer Res.* **1991**, *51*, 6215-6218.
3. Fisher, B.; Costantino, J. P.; Wickerham, D. L.; Redmond, C. K.; Kavanah, M.; Cronin, W. M.; Vogel, V.; Robidoux, A.; Dimitrov, N.; Atkins, J.; Daly, M.; Wieand, S.; Tan-Chiu, E.; Ford, L.; Wolmark, N. *J. Natl. Cancer Inst.* **1998**, *90*, 1371-1388.
4. Veronesi, U.; De Palo, G.; Marubini, E.; Costa, A.; Formelli, F.; Mariani, L.; Decensi, A.; Camerini, T.; Del Turco, M. R.; Di Mauro, M. G.; Muraca, M. G.; Del Vecchio, M.; Pinto, C.; D'Aiuto, G.; Boni, C.; Campa, T.; Magni, A.; Miceli, R.; Perloff, M.; Malone, W. F.; Sporn, M. B. *J. Natl. Cancer Inst.* **1999**, *91*, 1847-1856.
5. Albanes, D.; Heinonen, O. P.; Huttunen, J. K.; Taylor, P. R.; Virtamo, J.; Edwards, B. K.; Haapakoski, J.; Rautalahti, M.; Hartman, A. M.; Palmgren, J. *Am. J. Clin. Nutr.* **1995**, *62*, 1427S-1430S.
6. Omenn, G. S.; Goodman, G. E.; Thornquist, M. D.; Balmes, J.; Cullen, M. R.; Glass, A.; Keogh, J. P.; Meyskens, F. L.; Valanis, B.; Williams, J. H.; Barnhart, S.; Hammar, S. *N. Engl. J. Med.* **1996**, *334*, 1150-1155.
7. Report of the Chemoprevention Working Group to the American Association for Cancer Research. *Cancer Res.* **1999**, *59*, 4743-4758.
8. Bode, A. M.; Dong, Z. *Lancet Oncol.* **2000**, *1*, 181-188.
9. Dong, Z. *Biofactors* **2000**,*12*, 17-28.
10. Hollstein, M.; Rice, K.; Greenblatt, M. S.; Soussi, T.; Fuchs, R.; Sorlie, T.; Hovig, E.; Smith-Sorensen, B.; Montesano, R.; Harris, C. C. *Nucleic Acids Res.* **1994**, *22*, 3551-3555.

11. Donehower, L. A.; Harvey, M.; Slagle, B. L.; McArthur, M. J.; Montgomery, C. A., Jr.; Butel, J. S.; Bradley, A. *Nature* **1992**, *356*, 215-221.
12. Malkin, D.; Li, F. P.; Strong, L. C.; Fraumeni, J. F., Jr.; Nelson, C. E.; Kim, D. H.; Kassel, J.; Gryka, M. A.; Bischoff, F. Z.; Tainsky, M. A. *Science.* **1990**, *250*, 1233-1238.
13. Shieh, S. Y.; Ikeda, M.; Taya, Y.; Prives, C. *Cell* **1997**, *91*, 325-334.
14. Siliciano, J. D.; Canman, C. E.; Taya, Y.; Sakaguchi, K.; Appella, E.; Kastan, M. B. *Genes Dev.* **1997**, *11*, 3471-3481.
15. Unger, T.; Sionov, R. V.; Moallem, E.; Yee, C. L.; Howley, P. M.; Oren, M.; Haupt, Y. *Oncogene* **1999**, *18*, 3205-3212.
16. Lambert, P. F.; Kashanchi, F.; Radonovich, M. F.; Shiekhattar, R.; Brady, J. N. *J. Biol. Chem.* **1998**, *273*, 33048-33053.
17. Dumaz, N.; Meek, D. W. *Embo J.* **1999**, *18*, 7002-7010.
18. Huang, C.; Ma, W. Y.; Maxiner, A.; Sun, Y.; Dong, Z. *J. Biol. Chem.* **1999**, *274*, 12229-12235.
19. She, Q. B.; Chen, N.; Dong, Z. *J. Biol. Chem.* **2000**, *275*, 20444-20449.
20. She, Q.-B.; Ma, W.-Y.; Nomura, M.; Dong, Z. *Oncogene* **2002**, *in press*.
21. Donehower, L. A.; Harvey, M.; Vogel, H.; McArthur, M. J.; Montgomery, C. A., Jr.; Park, S. H.; Thompson, T.; Ford, R. J.; Bradley, A. *Mol. Carcinog.* **1995**, *14*, 16-22.
22. Lavigueur, A.; Maltby, V.; Mock, D.; Rossant, J.; Pawson, T.; Bernstein, A. *Mol. Cell. Biol.* **1989**, *9*, 3982-3991.
23. Muller, M.; Wilder, S.; Bannasch, D.; Israeli, D.; Lehlbach, K.; Li-Weber, M.; Friedman, S. L.; Galle, P. R.; Stremmel, W.; Oren, M.; Krammer, P. H. *J. Exp. Med.* **1998**, *188*, 2033-2045.
24. Husain, A.; Rosales, N.; Schwartz, G. K.; Spriggs, D. R. *Gynecol. Oncol.* **1998**, *70*, 17-22.
25. Huang, C.; Ma, W. Y.; Li, J.; Dong, Z. *Cancer Res.* **1999**,*59*, 3053-3058.
26. Surh, Y. *Mutat. Res.* **1999**, *428*, 305-327.
27. Jang, M.; Pezzuto, J. M. *Drugs Exp. Clin. Res.* **1999**, *25*, 65-77.
28. Huang, C.; Ma, W. Y.; Goranson, A.; Dong, Z. *Carcinog.* **1999**, *20*, 237-242.
29. She, Q. B.; Bode, A. M.; Ma, W. Y.; Chen, N. Y.; Dong, Z. *Cancer Res.* **2001**, *61*, 1604-1610.
30. Morse, M. A.; Amin, S. G.; Hecht, S. S.; Chung, F. L. *Cancer Res.* **1989**, *49*, 2894-2897.
31. Chung, F. L.; Morse, M. A.; Eklind, K. I. *Cancer Res.* **1992**, *52*, 2719s-2722s.
32. Wattenberg, L. W. *J. Natl. Cancer Inst.* **1977**, *58*, 395-398.
33. Stoner, G. D.; Morrissey, D. T.; Heur, Y. H.; Daniel, E. M.; Galati, A. J.; Wagner, S. A. *Cancer Res.* **1991**, *51*, 2063-2068.

34. Huang, C.; Ma, W. Y.; Li, J.; Hecht, S. S.; Dong, Z. *Cancer Res.* **1998**, *58*, 4102-4106.
35. Theibert, A. B.; Estevez, V. A.; Mourey, R. J.; Marecek, J. F.; Barrow, R. K.; Prestwich, G. D.; Snyder, S. H. *J. Biol. Chem.* **1992**, *267*, 9071-9079.
36. Cosgrove, D. J. *Inositol Phosphates. Their Chemistry, Biochemistry and Physiology*. Elsevier Science Publishers: Amsterdam.1980.
37. Szwergold, B. S.; Graham, R. A.; Brown, T. R. *Biochem. Biophys. Res. Commun.* **1987**, *149*, 874-881.
38. Bunce, C. M.; French, P. J.; Allen, P.; Mountford, J. C.; Moor, B.; Greaves, M. F.; Michell, R. H.; Brown, G. *Biochem. J.* **1993**, *289*, 667-673.
39. Shamsuddin, A. M.; Vucenik, I.; Cole, K. E. *Life Sci.* **1997**, *61*, 343-354.
40. Vucenik, I.; Shamsuddin, A. M. *J. Nutr.* **1994**, *124*, 861-868.
41. Graf, E.; Empson, K. L.; Eaton, J. W. *J. Biol. Chem.* **1987**, *262*, 11647-11650.
42. Vallejo, M.; Jackson, T.; Lightman, S.; Hanley, M. R. *Nature* **1987**, *330*, 656-658.
43. Pretlow, T. O.; O'Riordan, M. A.; Pretlow, T. G. In: *Diet and Cancer Markers, Prevention and Treatment. Jacobs*, M. M., Ed., Plenum Press: New York, NY 1994; p. 244.
44. Estensen, R. D.; Wattenberg, L. W. *Carcinog.* **1993**, *14*, 1975-1977.
45. Vucenik, I.; Tomazic, V. J.; Fabian, D.; Shamsuddin, A. M. *Cancer Lett.* **1992**,*65*, 9-13.
46. Saied, I. T.; Shamsuddin, A. M. *Anticancer Res.* **1998**, *18*, 1479-1484.
47. Huang, C.; Ma, W. Y.; Hecht, S. S.; Dong, Z. *Cancer Res.* **1997**, *57*, 2873-2878.
48. Huang, C.; Schmid, P. C.; Ma, W. Y.; Schmid, H. H.; Dong, Z. *J. Biol. Chem.* **1997**, *272*, 4187-4194.
49. Huang, M. T.; Ma, W.; Yen, P.; Xie, J. G.; Han, J.; Frenkel, K.; Grunberger, D.; Conney, A. H. *Carcinog.* **1996**, *17*, 761-765.
50. Nomura, M.; Kaji, A.; Ma, W.; Miyamoto, K.; Dong, Z. *Mol. Carcinog.* **2001**, *31*, 83-89.
51. Kapoor, M.; Lozano, G. *Proc. Natl. Acad. Sci. U. S. A.* **1998**, *95*, 2834-2837.
52. Katiyar, S. K.; Agarwal, R.; Mukhtar, H. *Cancer Res.* **1996**, *56*, 1023-1030.
53. Lee, E.; Surh, Y. J. *Cancer Lett.* **1998**, *134*, 163-168.
54. Lee, E.; Park, K. K.; Lee, J. M.; Chun, K. S.; Kang, J. Y.; Lee, S. S.; Surh, Y. J. *Carcinog.* **1998**, *19*, 1377-1381.
55. Bode, A. M.; Ma, W. Y.; Surh, Y. J.; Dong, Z. *Cancer Res.* **2001**, *61*, 850-853.

Chapter 6

Cancer Chemoprevention by Phytopolyphenols through Modulating Mitotic and Differentiating Signal Transduction Pathways

Jen-Kun Lin[1], Min-Hsiung Pan[1], Chi-Tang Ho[2], and Shoei-Yn Lin-Shiau[3]

[1]Institute of Biochemistry, College of Medicine, National Taiwan University, Number 1, Section 1, Jen-ai Road, Taipei 10018, Taiwan
[2]Department of Food Science, Rutgers, The State University of New Jersey, 65 Dudley Road, New Brunswick, NJ 08901–8520
[3]Institutes of Pharmacology and Toxicology, College of Medicine, National Taiwan University, Taipei, Taiwan

It has been demonstrated that investigations with phytopolyphenols including flavanoids (tea catechins, theaflavins), flavonoids (apigenin, myristin) and other polyphenols (curcumin, resveratrol) have provided important insights into the signal transduction pathways modulated by these compounds and the role of this modulation in executing their cancer chemopreventive action. The induction of human cancer involves a multistep process, initiating with DNA damage, oncogene mutations, malfunctions in tumor suppressor genes and followed by alterating different signaling pathways. Risk factors for cancer include age, race, environmental insults, hormones and most importantly, dietary factors. Cell cycle arrest and apoptosis are two important end-points in the operation of cancer chemoprevention. Several transducer proteins such as cdks, cyclins, cdk inhibitors, ROS, cytochrome c, caspases, PARP, Bcl-2, Bax, p53, c-jun, c-fos, c-myc , NFκB, IKK, etc are involved in these two cellular functions. Effects of several phytopolyphenols on the activities of these transducer proteins were reviewed and discussed.

Introduction

Phytopolyphenols are widespread in the plant kingdom. The major groups of phytopolyphenolic compounds are the flavanoids and flavonoids which are important in contributing the flavor, color, and taste of many fruits and vegetables. They are also important for normal growth, development and defense of plants (*1*). Phytopolyphenols have gained recent interest because of their broad pharmacological and biochemical activities. Their daily human intake has been estimated to be more than 1 g with the primary dietary source being vegetables and fruits (*2*). They are also found in several medicinal plants thus the herbal remedies containing phytopolyphenols have been used in folk medicine around the world (*3*). It has been demonstrated that diets rich in fruits and vegetables appear to protect against cardiovascular disease and some forms of cancer (*4,5*).

The important groups of phytopolyphenols in foods are flavanoids (Figure 1) and flavonoids (Figure 2), which consist mainly of flavone, flavanones, flavonols, flavanonols, isoflavones, flavanols, and anthocyanidins and their glycosides (*6*). Flavonoids are ubiquitous in plants; almost all plant tissues are able to synthesize flavonoids. There is also a wide variety of types: at least 2000 naturally occurring flavonoids (*3*). Flavonoids are present in edible fruits, leafy vegetables, roots, tubers, bulbs, herbs, spices, legumes, tea, coffee and red wine (*6*).

Curcumin (Figure 3), a yellow ingredient from tumeric (*Curcuma longae* L.) has been extensively investigated for its cancer chemopreventive potential (*7*). 6-Gingerol (Figure 3) and 6-paradol, pungent ingredient of ginger (*Zingiber offincinale* Roscoe) also have antitumor promotional effects. Resveratrol (Figure 3) found in grapes and other dietary and medicinal plants (*8*) and tea polyphenols (Figure 1) from green, oolong and black teas exert their striking inhibitory effects on diverse cellular events associated with multi-stage carcinogenesis (*8,9*).

Although flavanols, also called catechins, seem to be widely distributed in plants, they are rich only in tea leaves, where catechins may contribute up to 30% of dry leaf weight. The antioxidative and antitumor properties of green and black teas and their tea polyphenols are extensively studied, since it seems that phytopolyphenols are important not only for plants but also for humans. Therefore this brief review will discuss the current data with a particular emphasis on the effects of phytopolyphenols on cellular oxidative stress and cancer chemopreventive properties. The action mechanisms of phytopolyphenols on cancer chemoprevention will be elucidated.

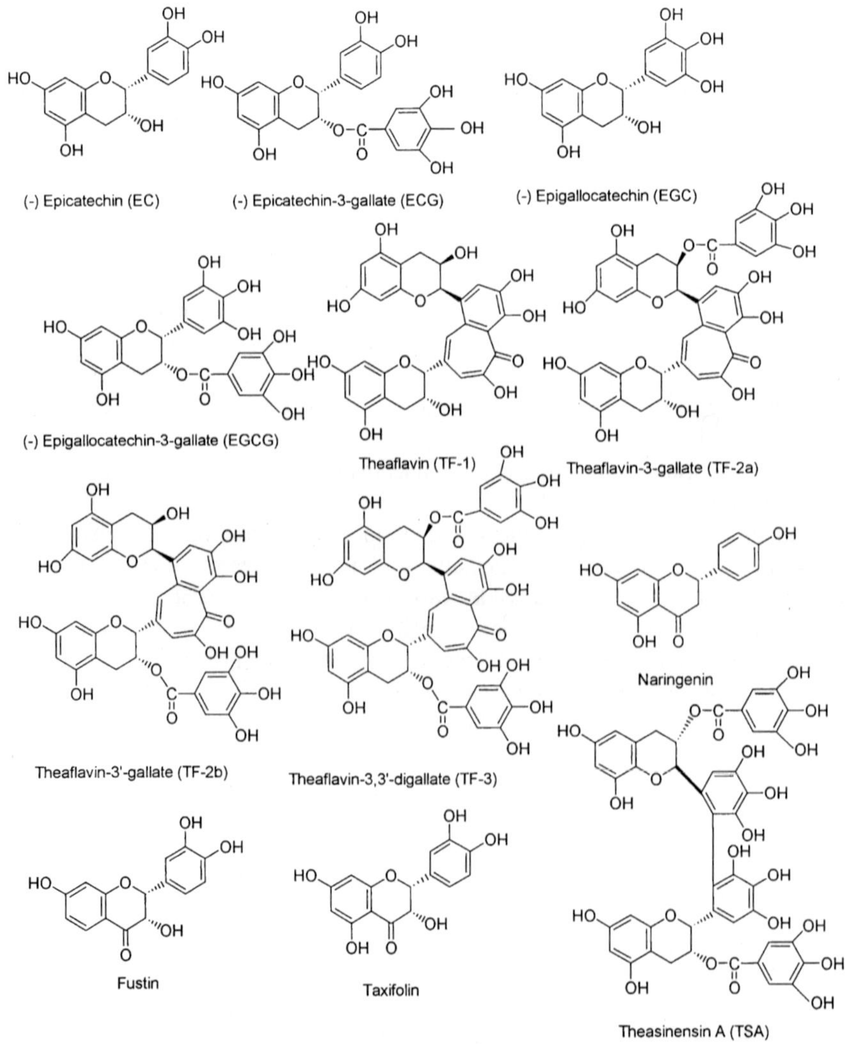

Figure 1. Chemical structures of representative flavanoids. These flavanoids comprise two major groups: Flavanones including naringenin, taxifolin and fustin and flavanols including green tea polyphenols (EC, ECG, EGC, EGCG), black tea polyphenols (TF-1, TF-2a, TF-2b, TF-3) and oolong tea polyphenol (TSA).

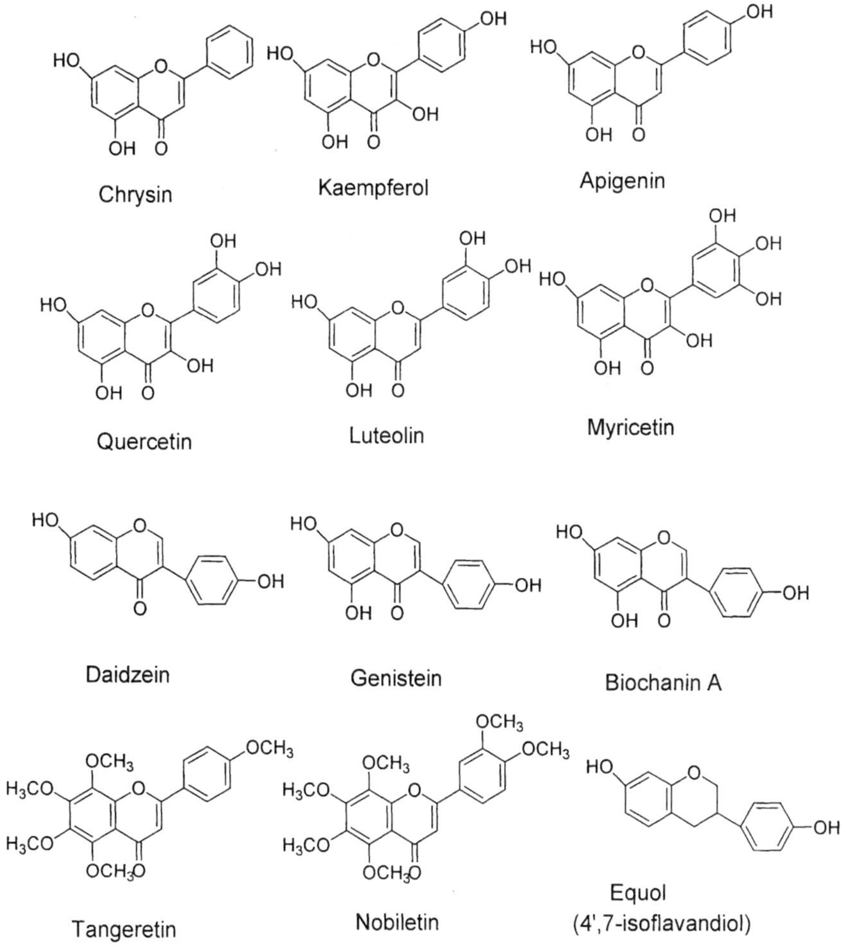

Figure 2. Chemical structures of representative flavonoids. These flavonoids are classified into three groups: flavone (apigenin, lutolin), flavonols (flavonol, kaempferol, quercetin, myricetin, tangeretin and nobiletin) and isoflavones (daizein, genistein biochanin A and equol).

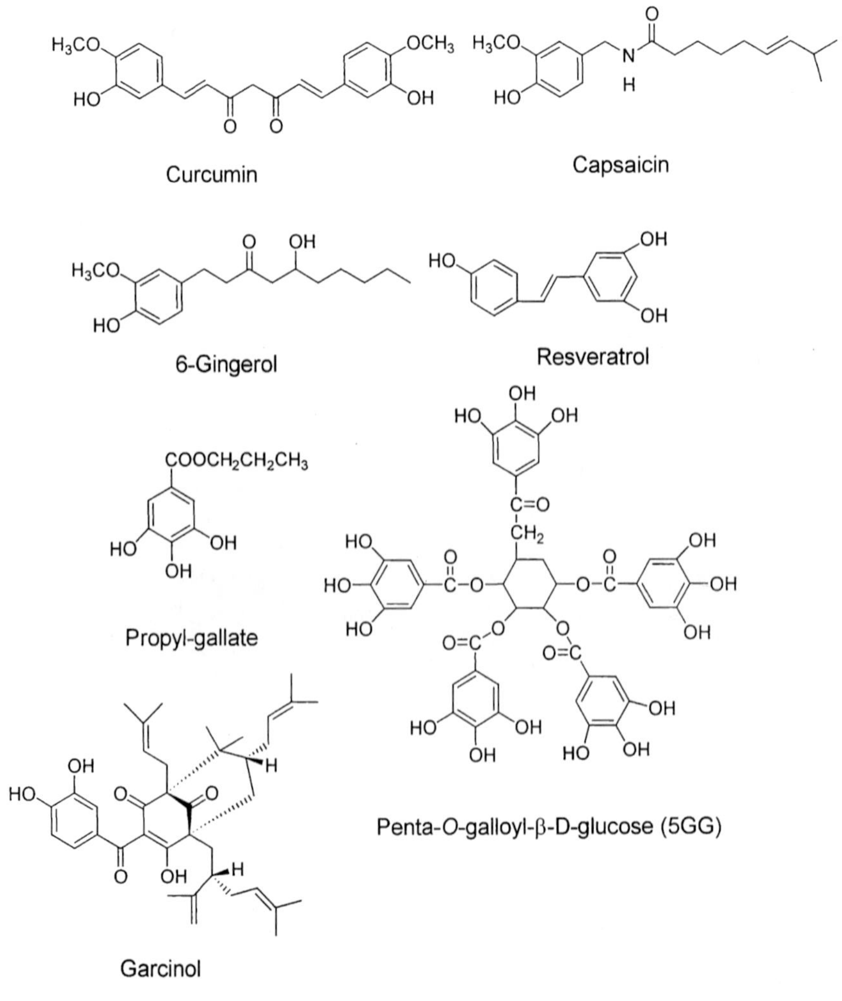

Figure 3. Chemical structures of curcuminoids and gallates.

Cancer Chemopreventive Effects of Phytopolyphenols

Tea Polyphenols

Tea polyphenols are a group of flavanoids, including catechins, from green tea, theaflavins from black tea and theasinensin A from oolong tea (Figure 1). Chemically, catechins may be regarded as monomeric skeletons of theaflavins and theasinensin A. The biochemical and pharmacological activities of these polyphenols varied in different cell systems. Among many polyphenolic compounds isolated from green tea, (-)-epigallocatechin-3-gallate (EGCG) (Figure 1) is believed to be a key active principle in terms of cancer chemopreventive activity (*10*).

The strong antioxidative activity retained in EGCG has been confirmed in numerous studies (*11,12*), and appears to contribute in part to the antimutagenic and anticarcinogenic effects of green tea. EGCG and other catechins were found to be stronger inhibitors of lipid peroxidation in rat liver homogenates than such antioxidants as ascorbic acid, tocopherol, glutathione, butylated hydroxytoluene (BHT) and butylated hydroxyanisole (BHA) (*13*). The antioxidant activities of thearubigin purified from black tea leaves were lower than those of green tea polyphenols although the total lyophilized infusion products of green tea and black tea leaves were equally active under this *in vitro* liver homogenate system (*13*). Our recent results indicate that theaflavin-3-gallate and theaflavin-3,3′-digallate were more effective than EGCG in inhibiting the activity of xanthine oxidase (*12*).

EGCG and theaflavins were found to inhibit xanthine oxidase (*12,14*) and suppress the production of ROS in HL-60 cells (*12*). EGCG and theaflavins inhibit nitric oxide production, which appears to be mediated through suppression of inducible nitric oxide synthase (iNOS), as demonstrated by its mRNA and protein levels (*15,16*). Electrophoretic mobility shift assay revealed that theaflavins and EGCG blunted activation of NFκB responsible for iNOS induction (*15*). These results indicate that these tea polyphenols inhibit the binding of NF κ B to iNOS promoter, thereby suppressing the transcription of iNOS gene.

The chemopreventive actions of tea polyphenols have been investigated using diverse rodent tumor models as reviewed by Kuroda *et al.* (*17*). EGCG exhibited protective effects against the chemical carcinogen induced murine duodenum, rat gastric, rat hepatic, mouse skin and mouse pulmonary tumorigenesis. One of the most plausible mechanisms underlying the chemopreventive activity of EGCG is suppression of promotion of carcinogenesis examined in animals and also in cultured cells (*18,19*). EGCG has been reported to influence some biochemical events related to tumor promotion, such as suppression of mouse epidermal ODC activity induced by TPA (*20*), or okadaic acid (*21*).

EGCG abrogated TPA-induced activation of protein kinase C, c-jun expression and transformation in cultured mouse fibroblasts in culture (*22*). EGCG and theaflavins inhibited EGF- or TPA- induced transformation of JB6 mouse epidermal cell line which was associated with their expression of AP-1-dependent transcriptional activity and its DNA binding activity (*23*). The inhibition of AP-1 activation by these substances appears to be mediated via down-regulation of JNK, but not the ERK pathway.

The growth inhibitory effects of EGCG in cancer cells appears, in part, to be mediated via apoptosis. EGCG induced apoptosis of human epidermoid carcinoma cell line (A431), human carcinoma keratinocyte cell line (HaCaT), human prostate carcinoma cell line (DU 145), and mouse lymphoma cell line (L5178Y) and its apoptosis inducing activity was related to the cell cycle arrest in the G0-G1 phase (*24*). Antiproliferative activity of EGCG against A431 cells has been attributed to its suppression of EGF binding to its receptor and subsequent autophosphorylation of the EGF-receptor required for EGF signaling (*25*). It has been demonstrated that inhibition of cyclin-dependent kinases 2 and 4 activities, as well as induction of Cdk inhibitors p21 and p27, arrest the growth of human breast carcinoma (MCF-7) cells by EGCG (*26*). These results suggest that EGCG either exerts its growth inhibitory effect through modulation of the activities of several key G1 regulatory proteins such as cdk 2 and cdk 4 or mediates the induction of Cdk inhibitors p21 and p27.

EGCG also possesses a potential antimetastatic activity as revealed by inhibition of matrix metalloproteinase activity in mouse B16 melanoma cells (*27*).

Our recent studies demonstrated that theasinensin A (TSA) (Figure 1), theaflavin and theaflavin-monogallates (a mixture of theaflavin-3-gallate and theaflavin-3′-gallate) displayed strong growth inhibitory effects against human histolytic lymphoma U937 cells with estimated IC_{50} values of 12 μM (*28*). The molecular mechanisms of TSA-induced apoptosis as, determined by annexin V apoptosis assay, DNA fragmentation and caspase activation were further elucidated. Loss of membrane potential and ROS generation were also detected by flow cytometry. It was found that TSA induced loss of mitochondrial transmembrane potential, elevation of ROS production, release of mitochondrial cytochrome c into the cytosol, and subsequent induction of caspase 9 activity. These results indicate that TSA allows caspase-activated deoxyribonuclease to enter the nucleus and degrade chromosomal DNA. Induction of apoptosis by TSA and other tea polyphenols may provide a pivotal mechanism for their cancer chemopreventive function (*28*).

The inhibitions of IκB kinase (IKK) activity in lipopolysaccharide (LPS)-

activated murine macrophages (RAW 264.7 cells) by EGCG, theaflavins (TF-1, TF-2a, TF-2b and TF-3) (Figure 1) and penta-*O*-galloyl-β-D-glucose (5GG) (Figure 3) were investigated (*29*). TF-3 inhibited IKK activity in activated macrophages more strongly than did the other polyphenols. TF-3 strongly inhibited both IKK1 and IKK2 activity and prevented the degradation of IκBα and IκBβ in the activated macrophages. These results suggest that TF-3 may exert its anti-inflammatory and cancer chemopreventive actions by suppressing the activation of NF κ B through inhibiting IKK activity (*29*).

Curcumin and Curcuminoids

In 1991 we found that the phorbol ester TPA induced transcriptional factor c-Jun/AP-1 in mouse fibroblast cells is suppressed by curcumin (Figure 2) (*30*). Elevated expression of gene transcriptionally induced by TPA is among the events required for tumor promotion. Functional activation of transcriptional factor c-Jun/AP-1 is believed to play an important role in signal transduction of TPA-induced tumor promotion. Suppression of the c-jun/AP-1 activation by curcumin (10 μM) is observed in mouse fibroblast cells (*30*). Curcumin also inhibits the TPA- and UVB light-induced expression of c-jun and c-fos in JB6 cells and in mouse epidermis (*31*).

Treatment of NIH3T3 cells with 15 or 20 μM curcumin for 15 min inhibited TPA-induced PKC activity in particulate fraction by 26 or 60% and did not affect the level of PKC protein (*32*). Curcumin (10 μM) inhibits EGF receptor kinase activity up to 90% in a dose- and time-dependent manner and also inhibits EGF-induced tyrosine phosphorylation of EGF-receptors in A431 cells (*33*).

Curcumin has been shown to suppress the expression of inducible nitric oxide synthase (iNOS) *in vivo* (*34*). Recent studies in our laboratory demonstrated that curcumin blocks the formation of iNOS through suppressing NF κ B activity in macrophages; Furthermore, curcumin can suppress the NFκB activation through down-regulating IκB kinase activity in macrophages (*35*). It has been demonstrated that iNOS is overexpressed in colonic tumors of humans and also in rats treated with colon carcinogens. iNOS appear to regulate COX-2 expression and production of pro-inflammatory prostaglandins, which is known to play a key role in colon tumor development. Both iNOS activity and colonic aberrant crypt foci formation in male F344 treated with azoxymethane (AOM) were significantly inhibited by curcumin (*36*).

The TPA-induced conversion of xanthine dehydrogenase to xanthine oxidase is reduced by curcumin to the basal level noted in untreated cells. Activity of xanthine oxidase is remarkably inhibited by curcumin *in vitro*, but not by its structurally related compounds; caffeic acids, chlorogenic acid and ferulic acid (*37*). When Colo205 colorectal carcinoma cells were treated with curcumin (60 μM), the appearance of apoptotic DNA ladders was delayed about 5 hr and G1 arrest was detected. The reduction of p53 gene expression was accompanied by the induction of HSP70 gene expression in curcumin-treated cells (*38*). It is interesting to note that curcumin induces apoptosis in immortalized NIH3T3 and malignant cancer cells, but not in normal embryonic fibroblast cells (*39*). Curcumin also induces apoptosis in human leukemia cells HL-60 through suppressing Bcl-2 expression. Transfection of Bcl-2 gene into HL-60 cells was found to inhibit the apoptotic effects of curcumin (*40*). Furthermore, curcumin exhibited synergistic effects on the induction of differentiation in HL-60 cells when it combined with all-trans-retinoic acid or 1α-25-dihydroxy-vitamin D_3 (*10*).

Curcumin at 10 μM inhibited 17.4 and 70.6% of cellular migration and invasion of SK-Hep-1 cells, respectively. Compared with less invasive human cellular carcinoma cell line Huh 7, SK-Hep-1 showed much higher MMP-9 secretion. Furthermore, parallel with its anti-invasion activity, curcumin inhibited MMP-9 secretion in SK-Hep-1 in a dose-dependent fashion. It seems that curcumin has a significant anti-invasion activity in SK-Hep-1 cells and this effect is associated with its inhibitory action on MMP-9 secretion (*41*).

The rhizomes of ginger contain 6-gingerol (Figure 3) and its homologs as pungent ingredients that have been found to possess many pharmacological and physiological activities, such as anti-inflammatory, analgesic and antipyretic effects (*42,43*). Gingerol inhibited the phospholipid peroxidation induced by the $FeCl_3$-ascorbate system (*44*). Gingerol protects TPA-induced ear edema, epidermal ODC activity and skin tumor promotion in Female ICR mice (*45*). Topical application of the ginger extract prior to TPA led to dramatic protection against DMBA-initiated skin carcinogenesis in SENCAR mice and suppressed TPA-induced epidermal ODC, lipoxygenase and cyclooxygenase activities (*46*).

Capsaicin (Figure 3) is a principal pungent ingredient present in hot red and chili peppers that belongs to the plant genus Capsicum (Solanaceae). Although topical application of capsaicin can initially induce ear edema in mice, subsequent applications of the compound suppressed the inflammatory response (*43,47*). Capsaicin preferentially repressed the growth of some transformed cells of human origin, including HeLa, ovarian sarcoma, mammary adenocarcinoma and HL-60 cells in culture. The capsaicin-induced growth inhibition and apoptosis in these cells were correlated with inhibition of plasma membrane NADH oxidase activity (*48*). Capsaicin abrogates the activation of NFκB by TPA, as well as by TNFα, which may provide the mechanistic basis for the possible anti-tumor promoting activity of capsaicin (*49*).

Flavonoids with Chemopreventive Activities

Most flavonoids are diphenylpropanoids that occur ubiquitously in plant foods that are important constituents of human diet. The major flavonoids are apigenin, quercetin, tangeretin, nobiletin, kaempferol, myricetin, genistein, daidzein and luteolin (Figure 2). Although flavonoids are generally considered to be non-nutritive agents, interest in flavonoids has arisen because of their potential role in the prevention of human cancer (*50*).

Apigenin and other related flavonoids inhibited carcinogen-induced tumors in rats and mice (*51,52*). Apigenin suppressed TPA-induced tumor promotion of mouse skin. Apigenin also reduced the level of TPA-stimulated phosphorylation of cellular proteins and inhibited TPA-induced c-jun and c-fos expression (*53,54*).

Soy is a unique dietary source of isoflavones, namely genistein, biochanin A and daidzein (Figure 2). Heavy consumption of soy in Southeast Asian populations is associated with reduction in the rate of breast and prostate cancer and cardiovascular disease. The potential chemopreventive efficacy of genistein appears to be related to its phytoestrogenic effects (*55*). Genistein competes with estradiol for estrogen receptors and the complex translocates to the nucleus, stimulating estrogen-related cellular events and accelerating cell differentiation (*56*). Some estrogen-independent mechanisms of genistein are important for its biological action. Genistein significantly inhibits tyrosine-specific protein kinase activity (57), this may in turn inhibit cell proliferation and growth factor-stimulated responses and immune response, as well as induce cell differentiation.

Effect of soy isoflavone supplementation on markers of oxidative stress in men and women has been studied (*58*). Soy isoflavone (genistein and daidzein) supplementation decreases levels of oxidative DNA damage (5-hydroxymethyl-2′-deoxyuridine) in humans, and this may be a mechanism behind the cancer preventive effects of soy isoflavones.

On the contrary, a recent study indicated that dietary genistin resulted in increased growth of estrogen-dependent breast cancer, pS2 expression and cellular proliferation similar to that observed with genistein (*59*). Dietary genistin is capable of eliciting biological activity similar to genistein with regards to stimulation of growth of estrogen-dependent breast cancer transplanted into athymic mice. The stimulatory effect of genistin appears to be directly related to the estrogen agonist activity of the compound that results in an increase in cellular proliferation within the tumor (*59*). At concentrations as low as 200 nM genistein has been shown to act as an estrogen agonist and promote the growth of estrogen-dependent human breast cancer (MCF-7) cells *in vitro* (*60*).

Tannic acid

It has been shown that tannic acid (TA) exerts cancer chemopreventive activity in various animal models (*61*). TA induced either growth arrest or apoptotic death (*62*). TA induced apoptosis more in human oral squamous cell carcinoma and salivary gland tumor cell lines than in normal human gingival fibroblasts, whereas gallic acid, a component unit of TA, showed much weaker selective cytotoxicity (*63*). Recently, it was shown that inhibition of the proteosome of living Jurkat cells results in accumulation of two natural proteosome substrates, the cyclin-dependent kinase inhibitor $p27^{kip1}$ and the proapoptotic protein Bax, followed growth arrest in G1 and induction of apoptotic cell death (*64*).

Resveratrol

Resveratrol (3,5,4′-trihydroxystilbene) (Figure 3) is a phytoalexin present in grapes and a variety of medicinal plants. Jang *et al.* (*65*) demonstrated that resveratrol is a potent chemopreventive agent in assays representing the three major stages (e.g. tumor initiation, promotion and progression) of carcinogenesis. This effect has been attributed to the antioxidant activity, anti-inflammatory activity and inhibition of platelet aggregation by resveratrol. Resveratrol was also shown to inhibit the *in vitro* growth of a number of human cancer cell lines (*66*). Recently, resveratrol was shown to inhibit nitric oxide synthase through down-regulating the activation of NFκB in macrophages (*67*).

Carnosol

Carnosol (Figure 4), a phenolic antioxidant extracted from the herb rosemary, exhibits anticancer activity in animal model for both breast and skin tumorigenesis (*68,69*). Carnosol induced apoptosis accompanied by a disruption of the mitochondrial membrane potential (*70*). Further analysis revealed that carnosol treatment down-regulated the anti-apoptotic protein Bcl-2 in leukemia cell lines and this reduction of Bcl-2 may contribute to the apoptotic effects of carnosol. Recently we demonstrated that carnosol suppresses inducible nitric oxide synthase through down-regulating NFκB in mouse macrophages (*71*).

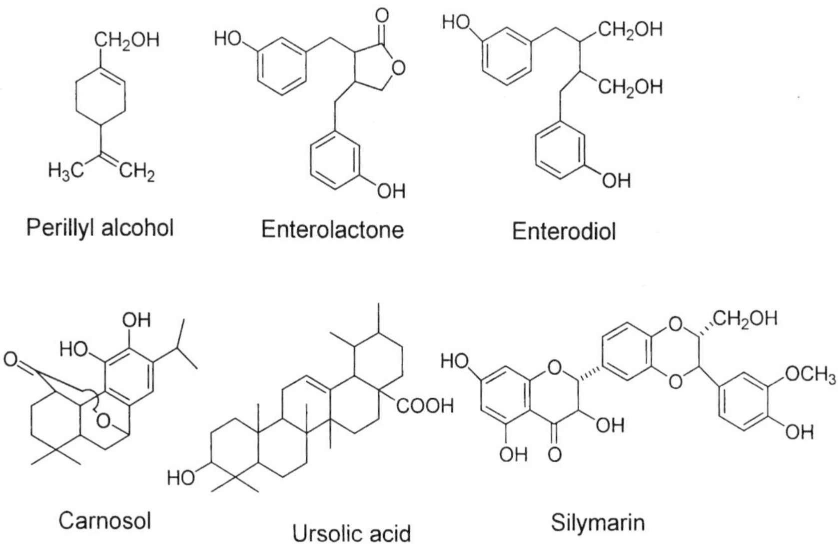

Figure 4. Chemical structures of perillyl alcohol, silymarin and other polyphenols.

Perillyl Alcohol and Silymarin

The essential oil of many plants which are commonly consumed contain a wide variety of monoterpenes such as limonene and perillyl alcohol (Figure 4). These compounds have been shown to have a wide spectrum of anticancer activities (*72*). These compounds can detoxify carcinogen via the induction of phase II enzymes.

They can also block the carcinogenic process at the promotion and progression stage. In addition to these chemopreventive activities, monoterpenes can be used to treat a variety of cancers (*73*). The inhibition of protein isoprenylation has been demonstrated in monoterpene chemoprevention target tissue; i.e. the *in situ* mammary gland epithelial cells (*74*).

Silymarin (Figure 4), a flavanoid compound isolated from milk thistle plant (*Silybum marianum* L. Gaertn) has been used clinically in Europe as an anti-hepatotoxic agent (*75*). Silymarin is a very strong antioxidant compound capable of scavenging both free radicals and ROS. Silymarin possesses strong inhibitory effects against the induction of ODC activity and mRNA expression in SENCAR mice caused by TPA and several other known tumor promoters (*76*). Silymarin inhibits activation of erbB1 signaling and induces cyclin-dependent kinase inhibitors Cip/p21 and kip/p27, G1 arrest and anticarcinogenic effects in human prostate carcinoma DU 145 cells (*77*).

General Consideration on the Action Mechanisms of Phytopolyphenols

Signal Transduction in Cell Proliferation

High cell proliferation is the common characteristic of most cancer cells. This cellular property is well reflected in the up-regulation of signal transduction, cell cycle and DNA-synthesis in the cancer cells. Cell growth is determined by extracellular conditions that act before the onset of DNA synthesis. The proliferation rate is initially determined by the probability of switching from the quiescent G0 to G1 phase of cell cycle (*78*). Two major sites of control exist between G0 and S: competence and restriction point. Much is being learned about the molecules that regulate passage through these control points. Proto-oncogenes and tumor suppressor genes are of great interest in this regard. Some of these genes code for DNA-binding proteins such as fos and jun, which form a complex and bind to specific gene-regulating DNA sequences during the competence process. Other proto-oncogenes code for growth factor receptors such as the gene that encodes the EGF receptor. Still others, such as c-raf appear to have distinct functions coding for protein kinases that act on substrates in the cascade involved in second messenger metabolism.

The cyclin proteins appear to play a major role in cell cycle regulation (*79*). Cyclins are a family of proteins that accumulate in the G1 phase (G1-cyclins), and again during late S-G2 phases before mitosis (mitotic cyclins) (*80*). After they reach a peak concentration, cyclin proteins are rapidly degraded.

Most phytopolyphenols such as tea polyphenols, genistein and silymarin can produce cell arrest at G1 phase through inhibiting cyclin dependent kinase (cdk-2 and cdk-4) activities and inducing Cdk inhibitors p21 and p27.

Signal Transduction in Cell Differentiation

Most cancer cells show abnormal differentiation patterns as compared to their normal counterparts. For years, the molecular mechanisms of differentiation have been intensively investigated, but poorly understood. Differentiation begins shortly after the first few cell divisions that follow fertilization. Throughout development, and in adult organisms, the ability of a cell to proliferate is intimately connected to its state of differentiation. Adult tissues generally express a variety of factors that act to maintain both the proliferation and differentiation status of cells. These include secreted molecules, transmembrane receptors, intracellular signaling molecules and transcription factors. For example, myoD (*81*) and c/EBP-α (*82*) are nuclear factors that activate the transcription of muscle- and adipocyte-specific genes, respectively; in addition, both proteins are potent inhibitors of cell proliferation.

Differential gene expression (differentiation) occurs extensively during embryogenesis, but some cell types differentiate throughout life. The mechanisms that regulate differential gene expression are incompletely understood, however, they most certainly entail the sequential action of cell-type-specific or cell-lineage-specific transcription factors that repress or activate the differentiation-specific genes. Programs of gene expression are generally instituted early in embryogenesis and subsequently altered or modified by some expgenoue stimuli as development proceeds (*83,84*).

A number of compound known to induce differentiation in various model systems have been used clinically. For example, estrogens and androgens have been useful in treating some breast and prostate tumors, providing that tumor cells express the appropriate nuclear receptor. Other differentiation-inducing drugs have been more widely studied. For example, high dose of retinoic acid or 5-azacytidine can induce differentiation and inhibit the growth of several type of tumors in laboratory models (*85*). It is worthy to note that some phytopolyphenols such as curcumin, and genistein may induce differentiation in cancer cell lines (*10,57*).

Signal Transduction in Tumor Promotion

The tumor promotion stage is the rate limiting step in carcinogenesis. Elucidating the molecular mechanisms of tumor promotion is, therefore, prerequisite for cancer chemoprevention. Mitogenic stimulation for cell proliferation is likely to be an important pivotal force of tumor promotion. However, that alone is not significant for transformation, and additional changes in gene expression are required to escape from normal growth regulation or differentiation. In general, alterations in the transcription of a specific set of cellular genes are mediated by specific regulatory DNA binding proteins or transcription factors that regulate gene expression directly by binding to specific DNA sequences in promoter regions (*86*). The expression of genes induced by TPA and other tumor promoters such as UV irradiation are thought to be required in tumor promotion.

Studies conducted in the past decade, however, generated important insights into the mechanism of action of tumor promoters and led to unification of the field of tumor promotion with signal transduction. The best studied class of tumor promoters consists of phorbol esters (TPA) and related molecules. Phorbol esters were known to exert profound effects on cellular function including hormone release, blood cell activation, cell differentiation, mitogenesis and tumor promotion. PKC appears to be the target of action of TPA. More recently, two important additional links between tumor promotion and signal transduction have been established. Thapsigargin, a potent tumor promoter, acts by inhibiting calcium uptake/sequestration, thereby promoting elevation in calcium levels (*87*). Okadaic acid, another tumor promoter, appears to inhibit serine-threonine protein phosphatases (PP1 and PP2A) and results in increased phosphorylation of protein substrates (*88*). It appears that activation of calcium dependent protein kinases or inhibition of protein phosphatases results in tumor promotion.

The products of most oncogenes appear to be integral members of signal transduction pathways. An understanding of their mechanism of action must involve dissection of their impact on signal transduction during normal cell function and determining how oncogenesis is related to disruption of these processes. It appears that when any essential component of a signal transduction pathway is rendered hyperactive autonomously, it may acquire the ability to drive the cell into unchecked proliferation or abnormal differentiation and finally lead to tumor promotion. Certain phytopolyphenols may block or attenuate the hyperactivity of these components of signal transduction as discussed below.

Inhibition of Tumor Promotion Through Blocking Signal Transduction by Phytopolyphenols

The detailed dissection of signaling pathways and their precise roles in cell regulation and cell transformation will offer a unique advantage in the development of specific preventive and therapeutic modalities of malignant disorders. It is expected that detailed biochemical and molecular analysis of biopsy material from individual tumors will generate insight into the cause and pathogenesis of these tumors. This would then allow the development of specific therapeutic intervention. It is conceivable that modulation of receptors, coupling mechanisms, effectors, second messengers, protein kinases, protein phosphatases and related substrates may also have profound therapeutic effects.

Accumulate evidence has demonstrated that signal transduction events leading to the activation of the mitogen activated protein kinase (MAPK) pathways (including ERK, JNK and p38) and NFκB pathways can result in cell proliferative, survival, differentiating, or apoptotic responses (Figure 5). This proposal model illustrates the possible action mechanisms of phytopolyphenols for the inhibition of carcinogenesis (cancer chemoprevention) and induction of program cell death (apoptosis). Extracellular growth factors (EGF, TNF), cytokines (IL-1, IFN) or tumor promoter TPA binds to membrane receptors such as EGFR, TNFR1, TNFR2 or PKC, resulting in the activation of a number of serine, threonine or tyrosine kinases which include ras, NF κ B inducing kinase (NIK), mitogen-activated protein kinases (MAPKs, MKK, MEK), extracellular response kinase (ERK), p38 kinase, c-Jun N-terminal kinase (JNK) and IκB kinase (IKK). JNK is activated by MAPK kinase (MKK) and then activates the c-Jun protein which forms heterodimer with c-Fos protein and enhances the activity of transcription factor AP-1. The EGFR can be activated by binding with its ligand EGF that leads to receptor dimerization and autophosphorylation. The growth signaling was transmitted to ras, raf and MAPK (MEK cascade) through adaptor proteins GRB2 and SOS. Caspase pathways (caspases 9 and 3) are activated by polyphenols through down regulation of Bcl-2. The inhibitor of caspase activated Dnase (CAD) is cleavaged by caspase 3 and leads to DNA fragmentation. Both IKK and PKC are important for activation of NF κ B that leads to enhanced expression of c-myc, iNOS and other cellular proliferation genes. Reactive oxygen species (ROS) are considered as endogenous mitogenic factors (or apoptotic factors in certain conditions) that can activate NFκB and other transcription factors in the nucleus. Ultimately, activation of the MAPK family members causes activation of specific transcription factors such as NFκB, AP-1, serum response factor (SRF) , Bcl-2 and its family, p53, Rb, PCNA,Cdk-2, Cdk-4, cyclins, Cdk inhibitors, and others which contribute to determine cell fate including proliferation, differentiation, inflammation, carcinogenesis or apoptosis. Several polyphenols have been demonstrated to block several sites of

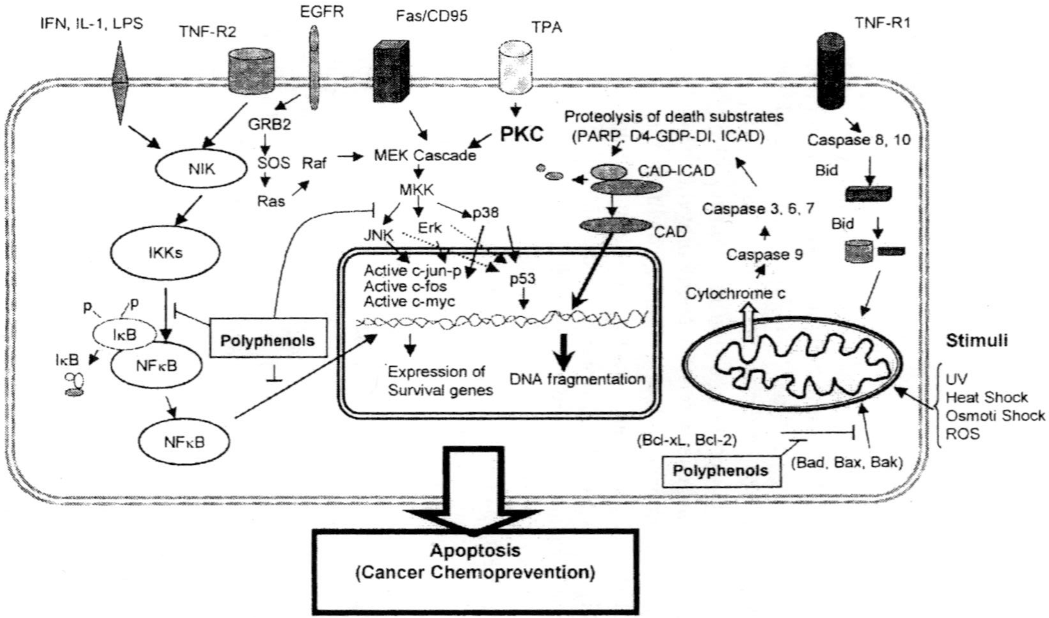

Figure 5. Possible action mechanisms of phytopolyphenols in cancer Chemoprevention. As discussed in the last paragraph of the text, most phytopolyphenols can act as cancer chemopreventive agents through either blocking multiple mitiotic and differentiating signal transduction pathways or inducing cellular apoptosis. The activation of caspase cascades and degradation of ICAD by phytopolyphenols may lead to apoptosis. Furthermore, suppression of IKK, NFκB and PKC may enhance the apoptotic pathways.

these multiple signal transduction pathways, as indicated by the blockade symbol (⊥). The main theme of this scheme is to emphasize the action mechanisms of polyphenols that lead to the inhibition of survival gene expression (c-jun, c-fos, c-myc, etc) and activation of apoptotic signal transduction pathways (caspase 8 and 9 cascades). In this scheme, we have tried to illustrate three important signaling events, namely the MAPK, NIK (NFκB inducing kinase) and caspase cascade (ICE/ced3 family proteases) pathways. Most phytopolyphenols can suppress the MAPK and NIK pathways but activate the caspase cascade pathways that lead to apoptotic response in the target cells.

Most phytopolyphenols with cancer chemopreventive activities are antioxidants. It should be emphasized that in addition to acting as ROS scavengers, these compounds can act through multiple mechanisms (*89*) to modulate the functions of receptors, effectors, protein kinases, protein phosphatases and protein substrates in the mitogenic and differentiating signal transduction pathways that link to the process of tumor promotion (Figure 5). The detailed mechanisms that phytopolyphenols see to interact with these transducers deserve further investigation.

References

1. Ho, C.-T.; Lee, C. Y.; Huang, M. T. (Eds.) *Phenolic Compounds in Food and Their Effects on Health I. Analysis, Occurrence & Chemistry.* ACS Symp. Ser. 506, American Chemical Society: Washington DC, **1992**.
2. Das, D. K. *Method Enzymol.* **1994**, *234*, 410-420.
3. Huang, M. T.; Ho, C.-T.; Lee, C. Y. (Eds.) *Phenolic Compounds in Food and Their Effects on Health II. Antioxidants and Cancer Prevention.* ACS Symp. Ser. 507, American Chemical Society: Washington DC, **1992**
4. Block, G. A. *Nutr. Rev.* **1992**, *50*, 207-213.
5. Hertog, M. G. L.; Fesken, E. J. M.; Hollman, P. C. H.; Katan, M. B.; Kromhout, D. *Lancet* **1993**, *342*, 1007-1011.
6. Ho, C.-T. In *Food Factors for Cancer Prevention*, Ohigashi, H.; Osawa, T.; Terao, J.; Watanabe, S.; Yoshikawa, T. (Eds.) Springer-Verlag: Tokyo, **1997**, 593-594.
7. Lin, J. K., Lin-Shiau, S. Y. *Proc. Natl. Sci. Council (B),* **2001**, *25(2)*, 59-67.
8. Lin, J. K.; Tsai, S. H. *Proc. Natl. Sci. Council (B),* **1999**, *23(3)*, 99-106.
9. Lin, J. K., Liang, Y. C. *Proc. Natl. Sci. Council (B)*, **2000**, *24(1)*, 1-13.
10. Conney, A. H.; Lou, Y. R.; Xie, J. G.; Osawa, T.; Newmark, H. L.; Lin, Y.; Chang. R. L.; Huang, M. T. *Proc. Soc. Exp. Biol. Med.* **1997**, *216*, 234-245.
11. Ho, C.-T., Chen, Q.; Shi, H.; Zhang, K. Q.; Rosen, R. T. *Prev. Med.* **1992**, *21*, 520-525.

12. Lin, J. K.; Chen, P. C.; Ho, C.-T., Lin-Shiau, S. Y. *J. Agric. Food Chem.* **2000**, *48*, 2736-2743.
13. Yoshino, K.; Hara, Y.; Sano, M.; Tomita, I. *Biol. Pharm. Bull.* **1994**, *17*, 146-149.
14. Aucamp, J.; Gaspar, A.; Hara, Y. *Anticancer Res.* **1997**, *17*, 4381-4385.
15. Lin, I. L.; Lin, J. K. *Mol. Pharmacol.* **1997**, *52*, 465-472.
16. Lin, I. L.; Tai, S. H.; Lin-Shiau, S. Y.; Ho, C.-T., Lin, J. K. *Eur. J. Pharmacol.* **1999,** 367, 379-388.
17. Kuroda, Y.; Hara, Y., *Mutat. Res.* **1999**, *436*, 69-97.
18. Huang, M. T.; Ho, C.-T., Wang, Z. Y.; Ferrano, T.; Finnegan-Olive, T.; Lou, Y. R.; Mitchell, J. M.; Laskin, J. D.; Newmark, H.; Yang, C. S. *Carcinogenesis* **1992**, *13*, 947-954.
19. Komatsu, K.; Tauchi, H.; Yano, N.; Endo, S.; Matsuura, S.; Shoji, S. *Cancer Lett.* **1997**, *112*, 135-139.
20. Katiyar, S. K.; Agarwal, R.; Wang, Z. Y.; Bhatia, A. K.; Mukhtar, H. *Nutr. Cancer* **1992**, *18*, 73-83.
21. Fujiki, H.; Yoshizawa, S.; Horiuchi, T.; Suganuma, M.; Yatsunami, J.; Nishiwaki, S.; Okabe, S.; Nishiwaki-Matsushima, R.; Okuda, T.; Sugimura, T. *Prev. Med.* **1992**, *21*, 503-509.
22. Lee, S. F.; Lin, J. K. *Nutr. Cancer* **1997**, *28*, 177-183.
23. Dong, Z.; Ma, W.; Huang, C.; Yang, C. S. *Cancer Res.* **1997**, *57*, 414-419.
24. Ahmad, N.; Feyes, D. K.; Nieminen, A. L.; Agarwal, R.; Mukhtar, H. *J. Natl. Cancer Inst.* **1997**, *89*, 1881-1886.
25. Liang, Y. C.; Lin-Shiau, S. Y.; Chen, C. F.; Lin, J. K. *J. Cell. Biochem.* **1997**, *67*, 55-65.
26. Liang, Y. C.; Lin-Shiau, S. Y.; Chen, C. F.; Lin, J. K. *J. Cell Biochem.* **1999**, *75*, 1-12.
27. Sazuka, M.; Imazwa, H.; Shoji, Y.; Mita, Y.; Hara, M. *Biosci Biotechnol. Biochem.* **1997**, *61*, 1504-1506.
28. Pan, M. H.; Lin-Shiau, S. Y.; Ho, C.-T., Lin, J. K. *J. Agric. Food Chem.* **2000**, *48*, 6337-6346.
29. Pan, M. H.; Lin-Shiau, S. Y.; Ho, C.-T., *Biochem. Pharmacol.* **2000**, *59*, 357-367.
30. Huang, T. S.; Lee, S. C.; Lin, J. K. *Proc. Natl. Acad. Sci. USA* **1991**, *88*, 5292-5296.
31. Lu, Y. P.; Chang, R. L.; Lou, Y. R.; Huang, M. T.; Newmark, H. L.; Reuhl, K. R.; Conney, A. H. *Carcinogenesis* **1994**, *65*, 1363-2370.
32. Liu, J. Y.; Lin, S. J.; Lin, J. K. *Carcinogenesis* **1993,** *14*, 857-861.
33. Korutla, L.; Kumar, R. *Biochim. Biophys. Acta* **1994**, *1224*, 597-600.
34. Chan, M. M. Y.; Huang, H. I.; Fenton, M. R.; Fong, D. *Biochem. Pharmacol.* **1998**, *55*, 1955-1962.

35. Pan, M. H.; Lin-Shiau, S. Y.; Lin, J. K. *Biochem. Pharmacol.* **2000**, *60*, 1665-1676.
36. Rao, C. V.; Kawamori, T.; Hamid, R.; Reddy, B. S. *Carcinogenesis* **1999**, *20*, 641-644.
37. Lin, J. K.; Shih, C. A. *Carcinogenesis* **1994**, *15*, 1717-1721.
38. Chen, Y. C.; Kuo, T. C.; Lin-Shiau, S. Y.; Lin, J. K. *Mol. Carcinogenesis* **1996**, *17*, 224-234.
39. Jiang, M. C.; Yen, H. F.; Yen, J. J.; Lin, J. K. *Nutr. Cancer* **1996**, *26*, 111-120.
40. Kuo, M. L.; Huang, T. S.; Lin, J. K. *Biochim. Biophys. Acta* **1996**, *1317*, 95-100.
41. Lin, L.I.; Ke, Y. F.; Ko, Y. C.; Lin, J. K. *Oncology*, **1998**, *55*, 349-353.
42. Nascolo, N.; Jain, R.; Jain, S. C.; Capasso, F. *Ethanopharmacol.* **1989**, *27*, 129-140.
43. Surh, Y. J. *Mutat. Res.* **1999**, *428*, 305-327.
44. Aeschbach, R.; Löliger, J.; Scott, B. C.; Murcia, J.; Halliwell, B.; Aruoma, O. I. *Food Chem. Toxicol.* **1994**, *32*, 31-36.
45. Park, K. K.; Chun, K. S.; Lee, J. M.; Lee, Surh, Y. J. *Cancer Lett.* **1998**, *129*, 139-144.
46. Katiyar, S. K.; Agarwal, R.; Mukhtar, H. *Cancer Res.* **1996**, *56*, 1032-1030
47. Inoue, H.; Nagata, N.; Koshihara, Y. *Inflammation Res.* **1995**, *44*, 470-474.
48. Morre, D. J.; Chueh, P. J.; Morre, D. M. *Proc. Natl. Acad. Sci USA*, **1995**, *22*, 1831-1835.
49. Singh, S.; Natarajan, N.; Aggarwal, B. B. *J. Immunol.* **1996**, *157*, 4412-4420.
50. Hertog, M. G. L.; Hallman, P. C.; Katan, M. B.; Kromhout,D. *Nutr. Cancer* **1993**, *20*, 21-29.
51. Wei, N.; Tye, L.; Bresnick, E.; Birt, D. F. *Cancer Res.* **1990**, *50*, 499-502.
52. Verma, A. K.; Johnson, J. A.; Gould, M. N.; Tanner, M. A. *Cancer Res.* **1988,** *48*, 5754-5758.
53. Lin, J. K.; Chen, Y. C.; Huang, Y. T.; Lin-Shiau, S. Y. *J. Cell Biochem.* **1997,** Suppl.*28/29*, 39-48.
54. Huang, Y. T.; Kuo, M. L.; Lin, J. Y.; Lin, J. K. *Eur. J. Cancer* **1996**, *32A*, 146-151.
55. Fritz, W. A.; Coward, L.; Wang, J.; Lamartiniere, C. A. *Carcinogenesis* **1998**, *19*, 2151-2158.
56. Folman, Y.; Pope, G. S. *J. Endocrinol.* **1996**, *34*, 215-225.
57. Akiyama, T.; Ishida, J.; Nakayama, O.; Ogawara, H.; Watanabe, S.; Itoh, N.; Shibaya, M.; Fukami, Y. *J. Biol. Chem.* **1987**, *262*, 5592-5595.
58. Diuric, Z.; Chen,G.; Doerge, D. R.; et al. *Cancer Lett.* **2001**,*172*, 1-6
59. Allred, C. D.; Ju, Y. H.; Allred, K. F.; Chang, J.; Helferich, W. G.; *Carcinogenesis* **2001**, *22*, 1667-1673.

60. Hsieh, C. Y.; Santell, R. C.; Haslam, S. Z.; Helferich, W. G. *Cancer Res.* **1998**, *58*, 3833-3838.
61. Nepka, C.; Asprodini, E.; Kouretas, D. *Eur. J. Drug Metab. Pharmacokinet.* **1999**, *24*, 183-189.
62. Yang, L. L.; Lee, C. Y.; Yen. K. Y. *Cancer Lett.* **2000,** *157*, 65-75
63. Sakagami, H.; Jiang, Y.; Kusama, K.; Atsumi, T.; Ueha, T.; Toguchi, M.; Iwakura, I.; Satoh, K.; Ito, H.; Hatano, T.; Yoshida, T. *Phytomedicine* **2000,** *7*, 39-47.
64. Nam, S.; Smith, D. M.; Dou, Q. P. *Cancer Epidemiol. Biomark. Prevent.* **2001**, *10*, 1083-1088.
65. Jang, M.; Cai, L.; Udeani, G. D.; Slowing, K. V.; Thomas, C. F.; Beecher, C. W.; Fong, H. H.; Farnsworth, N. R.; Kinghorn, A. D.; Mehta, R. G.; Moon, R. C.; Pezzuto, J. M.; *Science* **1997**, *275*, 218-220.
66. Mabonyebi, O. P.; Russo, J.; Russo, I. H. *Int. J. Oncol.* **1998**, *12*, 865-869.
67. Tsai, S. H.; Lin-Shiau, S. Y.; Lin, J. K. *Br. J. Pharmacol.* **1999**, 126, 673-680.
68. Singletary, K.; MacDonald, C.; Wallig, M. *Cancer Lett.* **1996**, *104*, 43-48.
69. Huang, M. T.; Ho, C.-T.; Wang, Z. Y.; Ferraro, T.; Lou, Y.R.; Stauber, K.; Ma, W.; Georgiadis, C.; Laskin, J.D.; Conney, A.H. *Cancer Res.* **1994**, *54*, 701-708.
70. Dorrie, J.; Sapala, K.; Zunino, S. J. *Cancer Lett.* **2001**, *170*, 33-39.
71. Lo, A. H.; Liang, Y. C.; Lin-Shiau, S. Y.; Ho, C.-T.; Lin, J. K. Carcinogenesis 2002, *23*, in press.
72. Gould, M. N. *Environm. Health Persp.* **1997**, *105(suppl.4),* 977-979.
73. Jirtle, R. L.; Haag, J. D.; Ariazi, E. A.; Gould, M. *Cancer Res.* **1993**, *53*, 3849-3852.
74. Zhibin, R.; Gould M. *Carcinogenesis* **1998**, *19*, 827-832.
75. Mourelle, M.; Muriel, P.; Favari, L.; Franco, T. *Fundam. Clin. Pharmacol.* **1989**, *3*, 183-191.
76. Agarwal, R.; Katiyar, S. K.; Lundgren, D. W.; Mukhtar, H. *Carcinogenesis* **1994**, *15*, 1099-1103.
77. Zi, X.; Grasso, A. W.; Kung, H. J.; Agarwal, R. *Cancer Res.* **1998**, *58*, 1920-1929.
78. Pardee, A. B. *Science* **1989**, *246*, 603-8.
79. Keyomarsi, K.; Pardee, A. B. *Proc. Natl. Acad. Sci.* USA **1993**, *90*, 1112-1116.
80. Lewis, B. *Cell* **1990**, *61*, 743-748.
81. Sorrentino, V.; Pepperkok, R.; Davis, R. L.; Ansorge, W.; Philipson, L. *Nature* **1990**, *345*, 813-816.
82. Umek, R. M.; Friedman, A. D.; Mcknight, S. L. *Science* **1991**, *251*, 288-291.
83. Gurdon, J. B. *Development* **1987**, *99*, 285.
84. Jan, Y. N.; Jan, L. Y. *Cell* **1993**, *75*, 827-833.

85. Warrell, R. P.; Frankel, S. R.; Miller, W. H. Jr.; Scheiberg, D. A.; Jtri, L. M.; Hittelman, W. N.; Vyas, R.; Andreeff, M.; Tafuri, Y.; Jakubowski, A. *N. Engl. J. Med.* **1991**, *324*, 1385-1388.
86. Angel, P.; Baumann, I.; Stein, B.; Delius, H.; Rahmsdorf, H. J.; Herrlich, P. *Mol. Cell Biol.* **1987**, *7*, 2256-2266.
87. Thastrup, O.; Cullen, P. J.; Drobak, B. K.; Hanley, M. R.; Dawson, A. P. *Proc. Natl. Acad. Sci. USA*, **1990**, *87*, 2466-2470.
88. Haystead, T. A.; Sim, A. T.; Carling, D.; Honner, R. C.; Tsukitani, Y.; Cohen, P.; Hardie, D. G. *Nature* **1989**, *337*, 78-81.
89. Lin, J. K.; Liang, Y. C.; Lin-Shiau, S. Y. *Biochem. Pharmacol.* **1999**, *58*, 911-915.

Chapter 7

Significance of Bcl-2 Protein Phosphorylation in Cancer Cells for Pharmaceutical and Nutraceutical Discovery

Mohamed M. Rafi

Department of Food Science, Cook College, Rutgers, The State University of New Jersey, 65 Dudley Road, New Brunswick, NJ 08901–8520

Isolation and identification of Bcl-2 phosphorylating compounds from Nutraceuticals has been accomplished using this novel bioassay. The understanding of apoptotic pathways provides new insights into development of new anticancer compounds from nutraceuticals. Nutraceuticals that modulate these pathways may induce apoptosis or sensitize tumor cells to other chemodrugs by synergistic mechanisms. Bcl-2 phosphorylating compounds from nutraceuticals may be one of the promising candidates for the future development of anticancer pharmaceutical drugs.

The overexpression of the anti-apoptotic protein Bcl-2 in cancer has been associated with resistance to chemotherapeutic agents. The phosphorylation of Bcl-2 is one mechanism by which antimicrotubule agents in clinic such as paclitaxel, taxotere and vinblastine inactivate the Bcl-2 proteins. Many natural products and semi-synthetic molecules are used in clinic for anticancer activity. In this chapter, the importance of the Bcl-2 phosphorylating molecule from nutraceuticals that shed light on the future development of molecules for chemoprevention and anticancer drugs will be discussed. The roots of Licorice (*Glycyrrhiza glabra*) have been used in traditional medicine for a variety of therapeutic purposes. In the present studies, Licorice roots extracts were assessed for effects on Bcl-2 to identify novel cytotoxic agents. The root extract isolated from Licorice induces Bcl-2 phosphorylation, which are assayed by immunoblots. By bioassay directed fractionation, we identified the active fraction in 70:30 water methanol extract. Further fractionation and HPLC analysis identified a pure novel molecule responsible for its activity. This article emphasizes the importance of novel bioassays to further understand and elucidate the ways in which specific nutraceuticals work to block pathways that lead to certain cancers, specifically the impact of these phytochemicals on the anti-apoptotic protein Bcl-2 in cancer cells.

Nutraceuticals and Health

Herbs and medicinal plants have been used for centuries to treat many diseases throughout Asia and Europe, particularly in Germany, France and Italy. An estimated 25% of all modern pharmaceutical drugs are derived from herbs, including aspirin (from white willow bark); the heart medication digitalis (foxglove); and the cancer treatment drug, Taxol (Pacific yew tree). Approximately 15 million Americans take herbs at the same time as prescription medications (*1*). Many of the herbs, foods and spices contain phytoestrogens (*2,3*). Health promoting properties of common herbs containing specific nutraceutical compound has been identified (*4*). Chemoprevention through the consumption of nutraceuticals eg. resveratrol from grapes (*5*), lycopene from tomato (*6*), genistein from soy (*7*) may reduce both morbidity and mortality in cancer. Many diet-rich plant foods have been reported to contain nutraceuticals that have health promoting, disease preventing or medicinal properties (*8,4*). The foods and herbs that possess the anticancer activity include garlic, soybeans, cabbage, ginger, licorice, onions, flax, turmeric, cruciferous vegetables, tomatoes, peppers, brown rice, wheat and the umbelliferous vegetables like carrot, celery, cilantro, parsley, and parsnips (*9*). Natural products and their isolated constituents have been shown to possess strong chemopreventive activity in animal models (*10,11,12*). The effect of Nutraceuticals on different pathways, different targets will be helpful to design and develop novel targets for cancer prevention and treatment of cancer.

Programmed Cell Death (Apoptosis) and Bcl-2

Apoptosis or programmed cell death is a genetically controlled process of cell suicide that plays a pivotal role in maintaining homeostatsis and preventing disease (*13,14*). Apoptosis is a tightly controlled mechanism and its disregulation has been shown to play a key role in a number of human diseases including cancer, neurodegenerative diseases and autoimmune diseases. Currently all chemotherapeutic drugs kill tumor cells by activating an endogenous biochemical pathway for cell suicide, known as programmed cell death (PCD) or apoptosis. However, tumor cells develop defects in the regulation of genes that control apoptosis, rendering them resistant to the induction of apoptosis by a wide variety of stimuli, including chemotherapeutic drugs and radiotherapy. The Bcl-2 families of proto-oncogenes are one of the critical regulators of apoptosis whose expression frequently becomes altered in human cancers, including some of the most common types of lymphomas and leukemia. Bcl-2 was first discovered as the gene on chromosome 18q21 at the breakpoint of the t(14;18) chromosomal translocation found in B-cell follicular lymphomas (*15*). This translocation places the bcl-2 gene next to the immunoglobulin heavy chain enhancer, leading to the overexpression of Bcl-2. Over expression of Bcl-2 also occurs in many other types of human tumors, including cancers of the prostate, colon, and lung, and has been associated with chemoresistance and radioresistance in some types of malignancy (*16*) Since the discovery of Bcl-2 a few decades ago, several other cellular and viral genes encoding homologous proteins have been identified, some of which suppress cell death akin to Bcl-2 (Bcl-XL, Mcl-1, A1/Bfl-1, Nr13, Ced-9, BHRF-1) and others, which promote apoptosis (Bax, Bcl-Xs, Bak, Bik, Bad). Several of these Bcl-2 family proteins are capable of physically interacting with each other through a complex network of homo- and heterodimers. The interactions of apoptotic and anti-apoptotic proteins and signaling events leading to apoptosis are shown in Figure 1. The Bcl-2 family regulates apoptosis through a cascade of reactions as shown in the pathway and altering the mitochondrial function. Phosphorylation of Bcl-2 releases cytochrome c release from mitochondria, which induced the activation of caspases (cysteine proteases that cleave after aspartic acid). Mutiple proteases have been identified as caspases. A *Caenorhabditis elegans* ced-4 homologue Apaf-1 was identified that interact with cytochrome c to activate caspases. Multiple proteins regulate the process of cytochrome c release. Bcl-2 and Bcl-X_L regulate the pore opening by inhibiting Bax mediated release of cytochrome c. When activated, caspases induce a protease cascade that can result in a pattern of programmed cell death or apoptosis, including the cleavage of PARP (Poly ADP-ribose polymearse). Understanding pathways responsible for the progression of cancer can help select targets for drug discovery. Although many potential targets exists, the focus here is on targeting Bcl-2 proteins.

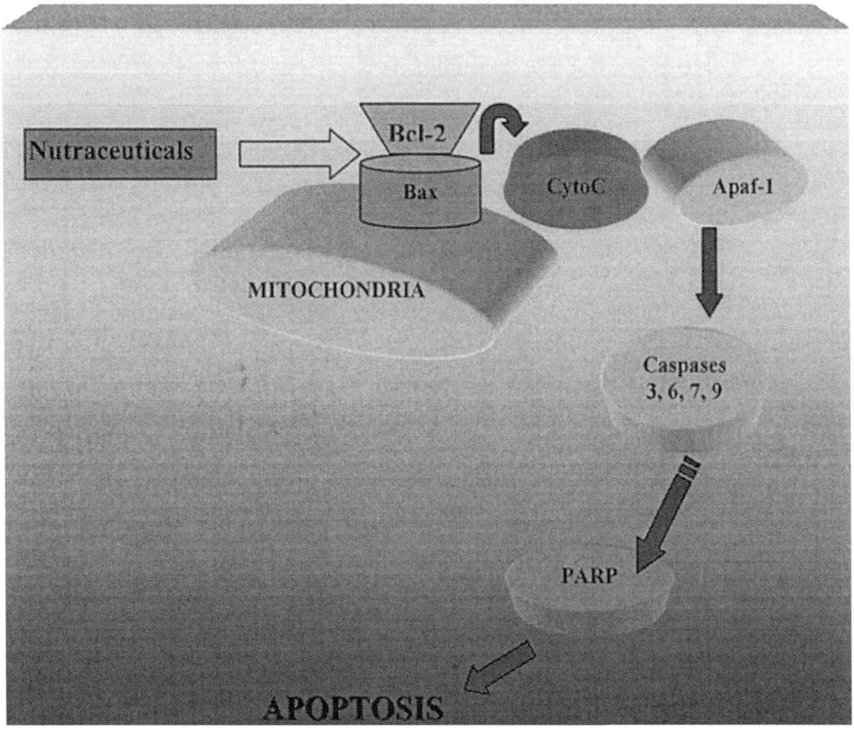

Figure 1. Molecular pathways involved in programmed cell death.

Over Expression of Bcl-2 and Resistance to Chemotherapy

Over expression of tumor suppressor gene bcl-2 plays an important role in cellular resistance to apoptosis caused by various factors (*17*). Lin et al have shown that over expression of anti-apoptotic Bcl-2 and Bcl-X_L proteins may play a role in the development of resistance to cancer therapy (*18*). Functional over expression of Bcl-2 has been reported to confer an anti-apoptotic potential in a variety of cell types. The role of Bcl-2 in epithelial cell-cycle control and in interactions with other cell-cycle regulators is not clearly understood. Its expression has been correlated with the hormone- and chemo-resistant phenotype in advanced prostate cancer (*19*). Granville et al have shown that overexpression of Bcl-2 in HL-60 cells prevented apoptosis-related events including caspase 3 and 6 activation, poly (ADP-ribose) polymerase cleavage by photodynamic therapy (*20*). Over expression of HER2 in estrogen receptor (ER)-positive human breast tumors has been associated with resistance to endocrine therapy.

HER2 over expression in MCF-7 cells is accompanied by up-regulation of antiapoptotic Bcl-2 and Bcl-X_L proteins were also reported (*21*). Transgenic mouse generated with the proto-oncogene Bcl-2 protects cells of the hematolymphoid system from the consequences of ionizing radiation and increase the radioresistance (*22*). Raffo et al have shown that overexpression of Bcl-2 can protect human prostate cancer cells from apoptotic stimuli *in vitro* and *in vivo* (*23*).

Modulators of Bcl-2

An et al have shown that novel dipeptidyl proteasome inhibitors overcome Bcl-2 protective function and selectively accumulate the cyclin-dependent kinase inhibitor p27 and induce apoptosis in transformed, but not normal, human fibroblasts (*24*).

We have shown that Licochalcone-A isolated from Licorice root extract, represses the antiapoptotic protein Bcl-2 in breast and leukemic cell lines (25). DiPaola et al have shown that 13-cis retinoic acid and interferon can down regulate Bcl-2 protein in peripheral blood mononuclear cells of patients (26). A clinical study with 18-base fully phosporothioated Bcl-2 antisense oligonucleotide administrated in patients represses the Bcl-2 level in non-Hodgkin lymphoma patients (*27*).

Bcl-2 Phosphorylation

Phosphorylation of Bcl-2 protein is a post-translational modification and is an important event in apoptosis (*28*). Exposure of most of the tumor cell lines to cytotoxic agents phosphorylates Bcl-2 and induces apoptosis (*29,30,31*). Recent evidence indicates that anti-apoptotic functions of Bcl-2 can be regulated by its phosphorylation (*32*). According to the 'mitotic arrest-induced' model, multi-site phosphorylation of the Bcl-2 loop domain is followed by cell death. Blagosklonny's review article (*30*) discussed that these models are not mutually exclusive but reflect different cellular contexts. During mitotic arrest, signal transduction is unique and is fundamentally different from classical mitogenic signaling, since the nucleus membrane is dissolved, gene expression is reduced, and numerous kinases and regulatory proteins are hyperphosphorylated. Hyperphosphorylation of Bcl-2 mediated by paclitaxel and other microtubule-active drugs are strictly dependent on targeting microtubules that in turn cause mitotic arrest. In addition to serine-70 (S70), microtubule-active agents promote phosphorylation of S87 and threonine-69 (T69), inactivating Bcl-2 (*32*). Recently, Pathan et al (*33*) have shown that phosphorylated Bcl-2 protein was discovered to associate in M-phase-arrested cells with Pin1, a mitotic peptidyl prolyl isomerase (PPIase) known to interact with substrates of Cdc2 during mitosis. Since the region in Bcl-2 containing serine 70 and serine 87 represents a proline-rich loop that has been associated with autorepression of its antiapoptotic activity, the discovery of Pin1 interactions with phosphorylated Bcl-2 raises the possibility that Pin1alters the conformation of Bcl-2 and thereby modulates its function in cells arrested with antimicrotubule drugs (*33*). Thomas et al have reported that p53 mediates Bcl-2 phosphorylation in BRK cells and apoptosis via activation of the small G family protein Cdc42/JNK1 pathway (*34*). Furukawa et al have shown that Bcl-2 is phosphorylated by CDC-2 kinase, a master regulator in G2/M phase of cell cycle (*35*). Pratesi et al have shown that in addition to antimicrotubule agents, effective DNA-damaging agents were also able to induce Bcl-2 phosphorylation (*36*). Srivastava et al have shown that deletion of the loop region of Bcl-2 and mutation in the phosphorylation sites completely blocks paclitaxel induced apoptosis and shown that Bcl-2 phosphorylation is important in inducing apoptosis (*37*). Wang et al have shown the involvement of signaling pathways JNK/SAPK in association with Bcl-2 phosphorylation and the effect of antimitotic agents in signaling pathways and Bcl-2 phosphorylation (*38*). Yamamoto et al have shown that signal transduction enzymes ASKI/JNK is involved in Bcl-2 phosphorylation (*39*). Ling et al have shown that Bcl-2 phosphorylation is tightly associated with mitotic arrest and fail to demonstrate that it is a determinant of progression into apoptosis after mitotic arrest induced by anti-tubulin agents (*40*). Attalla et al have shown that the natural estrogen metabolite 2-methoxyestradiol (2ME) is anti- angiogenic *in vivo*, and it phosphorylates Bcl-2 and a strong growth inhibitor *in vitro*. Earlier reports indicate that Raf-1 and JNK/SAPK kinases, both of which have been reported to be involved in Bcl-2 inactivation. Attalla's study has shown that both of them are not directly involved in Bcl-2 phosphorylation (*41*). The pathway of Bcl-2 phosphorylation leading to apoptosis is shown in Figure 2.

Bcl-2 Phosphorylating Molecule from Natural Products

Genistein, which is isolated from soy, inactivates Bcl-2 by phosphorylation, delays the G2/M phase of the cell cycle, and induces apoptosis of human breast adenocarcinoma MCF-7 cells and it is also an inhibitor of protein tyrosine kinase and topoisomerase II (*42*). The natural estrogen metabolite 2-methoxyestradiol (2ME) is anti- angiogenic *in vivo*, can phosphorylate Bcl-2 and its mechanism of action is independent of the signaling enzymes JNK/SAPK (*41*). The dolastatins are natural peptides, which inhibit microtubule assembly and induce apoptosis and phosphorylate Bcl-2 in small cell lung cancer (SCLC) (*43*). Beta-Lapachone,

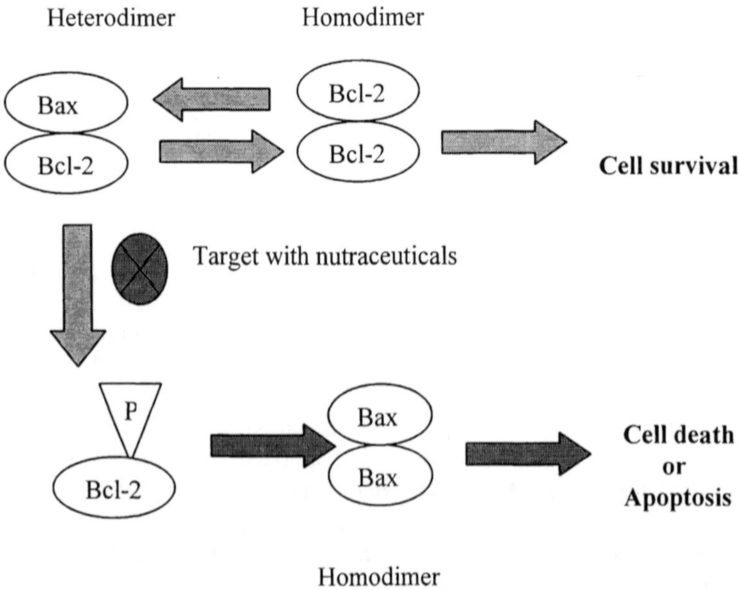

Figure 2. The mechanism of Bcl-2 phosphorylation.

a plant product, has been shown to be a novel inhibitor of DNA topoisomerase I, with a mode of action different from camptothecin and a chemical structure distinct from those of current anti-cancer drugs (*44*).

Taxol, isolated from *Taxus brevefolia*, Vincristine and Vinblastine isolated from *Vinca rosea*, and Taxotere, a semisynthetic form of Taxol, can induce Bcl-2 phosphorylation in tumor cell lines. The antiapoptotic potential of Bcl-2 has now been well established. But the biochemical mechanism of Bcl-2 action is still poorly understood (*45*). Haldar et al have shown that phosphorylated Bcl-2 can no longer prevent lipid peroxidation as required to protect cells from apoptosis (*46*). We have isolated and identified a novel polyphenol from Licorice that induces apoptosis, phosphorylating anti-apoptotic protein Bcl-2, causes G2/M cell cycle arrest in breast and prostate cancer cell lines (*31*).

Need for Novel Bcl-2 Molecules from Nutraceuticals

Bcl-2 has been described as a factor that can protect cancer cells from apoptosis (*47,48*). The protective effect of Bcl-2 may be lost if the protein is phosphorylated or by repressing its expression (*26,31,46,49*). Agents that affect microtubule depolymerization or prevent microtubule assembly can induce Bcl-2 phosphorylation. Currently all available Bcl-2 phosphorylating molecules in clinics are highly toxic with side effects. In conclusion, several molecular mechanisms involved in the progression of cancer and the development of resistance to chemotherapy is associated with overexpression of Bcl-2. Therefore, the need for discovery of novel Bcl-2 phosphorylating molecules from Nutraceutical or herbal products or medicinal plants is warranted.

Bioassay Directed Fractionation of Bcl-2 Phosphorylating Molecule from Licorice

Licorice

The beneficial effect of Licorice has been well documented due to its wide – range of therapeutic properties which includes antibacterial, antimutagenic, antiulcer, anti-inflammatory, use for liver dysfunction, cough and cancer (*10*). The major compononent of licorice is Glycyrrhizin, which is well studied and is used in treating hepatitis patients in Japan (*50*). Glycyrrhzin is also shown to have anti-inflammatory and anti-viral properties (*51*). A variety of chalcones and flavonoids were isolated from Licorice root and shown to exhibit anti-tumorgenic activity, anti-mitotic activity very similar to the vinca alkaloids, which are anti-oxidant, estrogenic and which represses the expression of anti-apoptotic protein Bcl-2 (*52,39,25*). Many of the known constituents of licorice were tested for Bcl-2 phosphorylation and none turned out to be active. Surprisingly, whole licorice extract can induce Bcl-2 phosphorylation and this observation lead us to fractionate and identify the active Bcl-2 phosphorylating molecule from Licorice. The only compound which induces Bcl-2 phosphorylation (Figure 3) in prostate and breast cancer cell line is DHP- β from Licorice root (*31*). A clinical trial has been initiated at the Cancer Institute of New Jersey for prostate cancer patients with Licorice capsules. The various fractions of root extract were tested for Bcl-2 phosphorylation in breast cancer cell lines by western blot using Bcl-2 monoclonal antibodies (Figure 4). Further fractionation was accomplished using bioassay directed fractionation with western blots as the assay for detecting Bcl-2 phosphorylating molecule. During each step individual peaks were collected and analyzed for Bcl-2 phosphorylation (*31*). Bcl-2 phosphorylation in breast cancer cells and prostate cancer cells using DHP-β is shown in Figure 5. In contrast, DHP-α did not induce Bcl-2 phosphorylation in breast cancer cell lines (Figure 6). Previously it has been shown that Bcl-2 phosphorylation is associated with G2/M cell cycle arrest and we have shown that Bcl-2 phosphorylation fractions from licorice also induce G2/M arrest by cell cycle analysis (Figure 7). In conclusion, it was demonstrated that Licorice root has a biological activity of inducing Bcl-2 phosphorylation and G2/M cell cycle arrest. Using bioassay directed fractination a novel polyphenols DHP-β was identified that can induce Bcl-2 phosphorylation, apoptosis and G2/M cell cycle arrest (*31*).

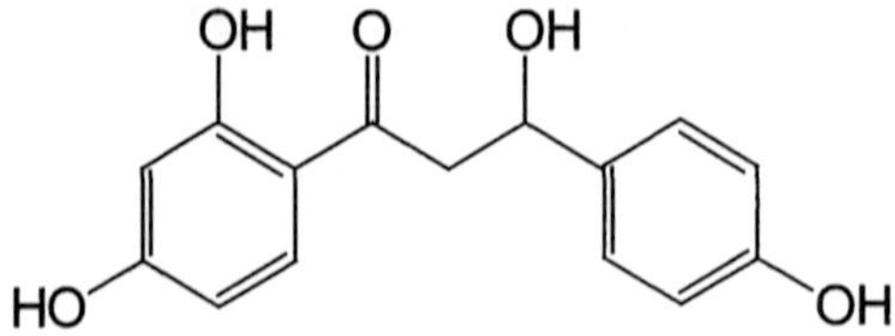

Figure 3. Structure of novel molecule DHP-β isolated from licorice root.

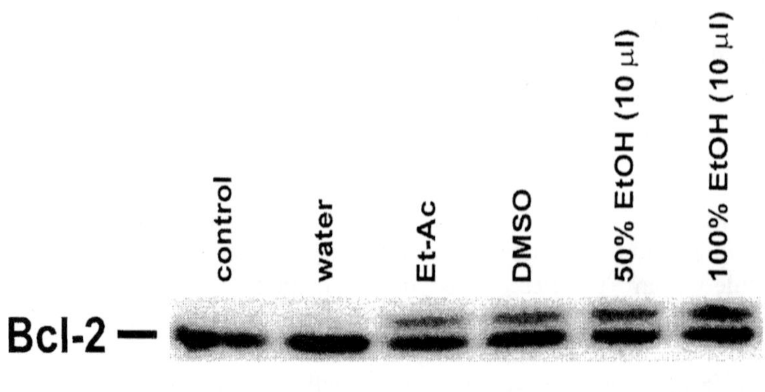

Figure 4. Immunoblot of Bcl-2 phosphorylation. Breast cancer cells treated with different extracts of licorice root. Cells were lyzed and assayed with monoclonal Bcl-2 antibody.

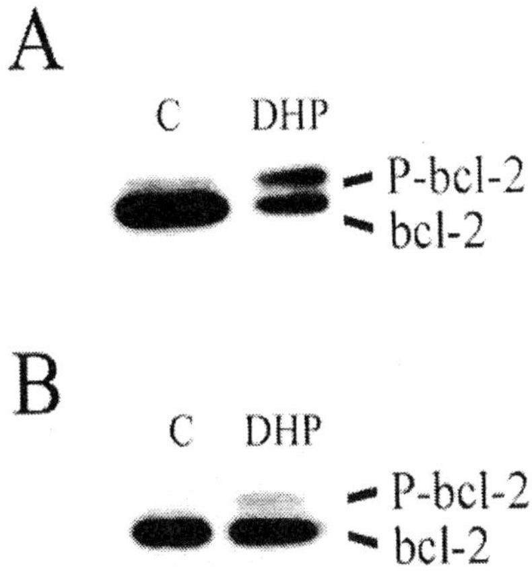

Figure 5. Immunoblot of Bcl-2 phosphorylation. Breast (A) and prostate (B) cancer cell lines were treated with DHP-β for 12 hours.

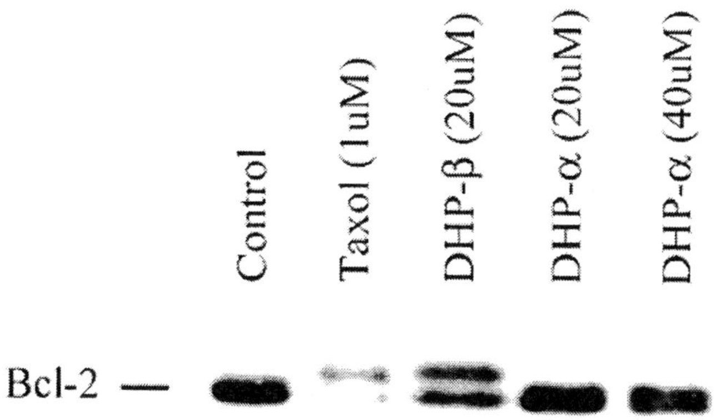

Figure 6. Immunoblot showing the structure specificity of DHP-β and DHP-α for Bcl-2 phosphorylation. Breast cancer cells treated with 20-40 μM concentration of DHP isomers and compared with known Bcl-2 phosphorylating molecule (Taxol).

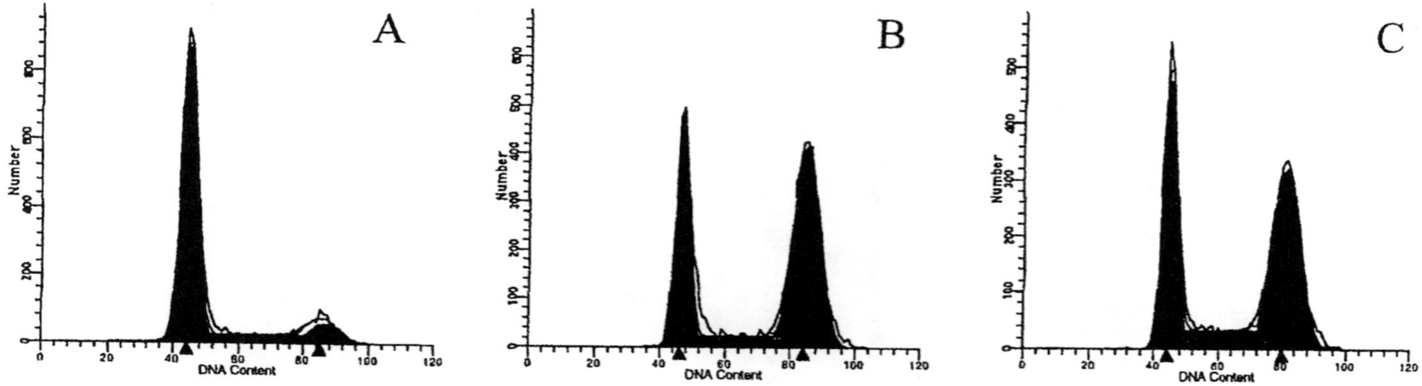

Figure 7. Effect of DHP-β on cell cycle analysis showing G2/M arrest. Breast cancer cells treated with alcohol control(A), 10 μM Taxol(B) and 10 μM DHP-β(C) for 12 hours.

References

1. Eisenberg, D.M.; Davis, R.B.; Ettner S.L.; Appel, S.L.; Wilkey, S.; Van Rombay, M.; Kessler, R.C. *JAMA* **1998**, *280*, 1569-1575.
2. Zava, D.T.; Dollbaum, C..M.; Blen, M. *Proc. Soc. Exp. Biol. Med.* **1998**, *217*, 369-378.
3. DiPaola, R.S.; Zhang, H.; Lambert, G.H.; Licitra, E.; Rafi, M.M.; Zhu, B.T.; Splauding , H.; Goodin, S.; Toledano, M.B.; Hait, W.N.; Gallo, M.A. *N. Eng. J. Med.* **1998**, *339*, 785-791.
4. Craig, W.J. Am. *J. Clin. Nutr.* **1999**, *70*, 491-499.
5. Jang, M.; Cai, L.; Udeani, G.O.; Slowing, K.V.; Thomas, C.F.; Beecher, C.W.; Fong, H.H.; Fornsworth, N.R.; Kinghorn, A.D.; Mehta, R.G.; Moon, R.C.; Pezzuto, J.M. *Science* **1997**, *275*, 218-220.
6. Heber, D.; Lu, Q.Y.; Go, V.L. *Adv. Exp. Med. Biol.* **2001**, *492*, 29-37.
7. Bergan, R.C.; Waggle, D.H.; Carter, S.K. Horak, I.; Slichenmyer, W.; Meyers, M. *Urology* **2001**, *57*, 77-80.
8. Lachance, P.A. *Nutr. Rev.* **1998**, *56*, 34-39.
9. Craig W.J. J. Amer. Diet. Assoc. **1997**, 97, 199-204.
10. Mehta, R.G.; Steele, V.; Pierson, H. et al. In *Nutraceuticals: Designer Foods III Garlic, soy and Licorice*, **1997**, pp. 265-278.
11. Nishino, H. In *Nutraceuticals: Designer Foods III Garlic, Soy and Licorice*, **1997**, pp. 279-283.
12. Shibata, S.; Inoue, H.; Iwata, S.; Ma, R.D.; Yu, L.J.; Uleyama, H.; Takayasu, J.; Hasegawa, T.; Tokuda, H.; Nishino, A. *Planta Med.* **1991**, *57*, 221-224.
13. Jacobson, M.D.; Weil, M.; Raff, M.C. *Cell* **1997**, *88*, 347-354.
14. White, E. *Genes. Dev.* **1996**, *10*, 1-15.
15. Tsujimoto, Y.; Croce, C.M. *Proc. Natl. Acad. Sci.* **1986**, *83*, 5214-5218
16. Reed, J.C. *Semin. Haematol.* **1997**, *34*, 9-19.
17. Revskoi, S.I. *Vopr. Onkol.* **2001**, *47*, 224-229
18. Lin, J.; Page, C.; Jin, X.; Sethi, A.O. et al. *Anticancer Res.* **2001**, *21*, 831-839.
19. Chaudhary, K.S.; Abel, P.D.; Lalani, E.N. *Environ. Health Perspect.* **1999**, *107*, 49-57.
20. Granville, D. J.; Jiang, H.; An, M.T.; levy, J.G.; McManus, B.M.; Hunt, D.W. *Br. J. Cancer* **1999**, *79(1)*. 95-100.
21. Kumar, R.; Mandal, M.; Lipton, A.; Harvey, H.; Thompson, C.B. *Clin. Cancer Res.* **1996**,.*2*, 1215-1219.
22. Domen, J.; Gandy, K.L; Weissman, I.L. *Blood* **1998**, *91*, 2272-82.
23. Raffo, A.J.; Perlman, H.; Chen, M.W. Streitman, J.S.; Buttyan, R. *Cancer Res.* **1995**, *55*, 4438-4445.

24. An, B.; Goldfarb, R. H.; Siman, R.; Dou, Q.P. *Cell Death Differ* **1998**, *5*, 1062-1075.
25. Rafi, M.M.; Rosen, R.T.; Vassil, A.; Ho, C.-T.; Zhang, H.; Ghai, G.; Lambert, G.; DiPaola, R. S. *Anticancer Res.* **2000**, *20*,, 2653-2658.
26. DiPaola, R.S.; Rafi, M.M.; Vyas, V.; Toppmeyer, D.; Rubin, E.; Patel, J.; Goodin, S.; Medina, M.; Medina, P.; Zamek, R.; Zhang, C.; White, E.; Gupta, E.; Hait, W.N. *J. Clin. Oncol.* **1999**, *17,* 2213-2218.
27. Webb, A.; Cunningham, D.; Cotter, F., Clarke, P.A.; di Stefano, F.; Ross, P.; Corbo, M.; Dziewanowska, Z. *Lancet* **1997**, *349* 1137-1141.
28. Srivastava, R. K.; Mi, Q. S.; Hardwick, J. M.; Longo, D.L. *Proc. Natl. Acad. Sci. U S A* **1999**, *96*, 3775-3780.
29. Haldar, S.; Chintapalli, J.; Croce, C.M. *Cancer Res.* **1996**, *56*, 1253-1255.
30. Blagosklonney, M.V.; Ginnakakou, P.; El-Diery, W.S.; Kingston, D.G.; Higgs, P.I.; Neckers, L.; Fojo, T. *Cancer Res.* **1997**, *57*, 130-135.
31. Rafi, M.M.; Vastano B.C.; Rosen R.T.; Ho, C.T.; Rosen, R.T.; Gallo, M.A.; DiPaola, R.S. *J. Agric. Food Chem.* **2002**, *50*, 677-684.
32. Blagosklonney, M.V. *Leukemia* **2001**, *15*, 869-74.
33. Pathan, N.; Aime-Sempe, C.; Kitada, S.; Haldar, S.; Reed, J.C. *Neoplasia* **2001**, *3,* 70-79.
34. Thomas, A.; Giesler,T.; White E. *Oncogene* **2001**,*19*, 5259-5269.
35. Furukawa, Y.; Iwase, S.; Kikuchi, J.; Terui, Y.; Nakamura, M.; Yamada, H.; Kano, Y.; Matsuda, M. *J. Biol. Chem.* **2000**, *275*, 21661-21667.
36. Pratesi, G.; Polizzi, D.; Perego, P.; Dal Bo, L.; Zunini, F. *Biochem. Pharmacol.* **2000**, *60*, 77-82.
37. Srivastava, R. K.; Mi, Q.S.; Hardwick, J.M.; Longo, D.L. *Proc. Natl. Acad. Sci. USA* **1999**, *96*, 3775-3780.
38. Wang, T.H.; Popp, D.M.; Wang, H.S.; Saitoh, M.; Mutal, J.G.; Henley, D.C.; Ichijo, H.; Wimalasena, J. *J. Biol. Chem.* **1999**, *274*, 8208-8216.
39. Yamamoto, K.; Ichijo, H.; Korsmeyer S.J. *Mol. Cell. Biol.* **1999** 19:8469-8478.
40. Ling, Y.H.; Tornos, C.; Perez-Soler, R. *J. Biol. Chem.* **1998**, *273*, 18984-18991.
41. Attalla, H;, Westberg, J.A.; Andersson, L.C.; Adlercreutz, H.; Makela, T.P. *Biochem. Biophys. Res. Commun.* **1998**, *247*, 616-619.
42. Constantinou, A.I.; Kamath, N.; Murley, J. S. *Eur J Cancer* **1998**, *34*, 1927-1934.
43. Ali, M.A.; Rosati, R.; Pettit, G.R. Kalemkerian, G.P. *Anticancer Res.* **1998**, *18*, 1021-1026.
44. Li, C. J.; Wang, C.; Pardee, A. B. *Cancer Res.* **1995**, *55*, 3712-3725.
45. Haldar, S.; Jena, N.; Croce, C.M. *Biochem. Cell Biol.* **1994**, *72*, 455-462

46. Haldar, S.; Jena, N.; Croce, C.M. *Proc. Natl. Acad. Sci.* **1995**, *92*, 4507-4511.
47. Yang ,J.; Liu, X.; Bhalla, K; Kim, C.N.; Ibrado, A.M.; Cai, J.; Peng, T.I.; Jones, D.P.; Wang, X. *Science* **1997**, *257*, 1129-1133.
48. DiPaola, R.S.; Patel, J. Rafi M..M. *Hematology Oncology Clinics of North America* **2001**, *15*, 509-524.
49. Haldar, S.; Basu, A.; Croce C.M. *Cancer Res.* **1997**, *57*, 229-233.
50. Suzuki, H.; Ozha, Y.; Takino, T. Fujusawa, K.; Hirayama, C. *Asian Med. J.* **1983**, *23*, 423-438.
51. Poempi, R.; Pani, A; Flore, O.Marcialis, M.A.; Loddo, B.L. *Experientia* **1980**, *3*, 304.
52. Edwards, M.L.; Stemerick, D.M.; Sunkara, P.S. *J Med. Chem* **1990**, 33, 1948-1954.

Chapter 8

Modulation of Cytokine Gene Expression by Curcumin

Marion Man-Ying Chan[1,2], Hsing-I Huang[3], John A. Mattiacci[4], and Dunne Fong[2]

[1]Department of Microbiology and Immunology, Temple University School of Medicine, Philadelphia, PA 19140
[2]Department of Cell Biology and Neuroscience, Rutgers, The State University of New Jersey, Piscataway, NJ 08854
[3]Laboratory of Oncology and Experimental Immunology, Cathay Medical Research Institute, Taiwan
[4]School of Podiatric Medicine, Temple University, Philadelphia, PA 19107

Curcumin, a phytochemical with antioxidant and anti-inflammatory properties, is valued as a cancer chemopreventive agent. Previously, we have shown that curcumin reduces the gene expression of inducible nitric oxide synthase (iNOS) in murine macrophages, *in vitro,* and in the liver, *in vivo.* Here, we continued to examine its effect on iNOS expression in other organs. Curcumin inhibited lipopolysaccharide (LPS)-induced iNOS gene expression in the spleen, mesenteric lymph nodes, small intestine and colon. Furthermore, it inhibited gene expression of three cytokines that enhance iNOS production. *In vitro*, curcumin reduced the gene expression of tumor necrosis factor α (TNFα) and interleukin-1β (IL-1β) by LPS-stimulated peritoneal cells. *In vivo*, it reduced the gene expression of TNFα and IL-1β in the liver and spleen, and reduced the gene expression of interferon γ (IFNγ) in the spleen and lymph nodes. Nitric oxide (NO) enhances the activity of cyclooxygenase-2 (COX-2); we found that curcumin also reduced COX-2 gene expression in RAW 264.7 macrophages.

INTRODUCTION

There are ample precedents that constituents of terrestrial plants are effective as treatments for human ailments. Curcumin (Figure 1), difeuroylmethane, one of the active principles in the plant *Curcuma longa* Linn, the rhizome of which is ground into powder, called turmeric, is used as food and medicine in Asia. Turmeric is used as a food colorant and spice, and medicinally to promote wound healing, to treat liver disorders, diabetes, and inflammatory conditions such as rheumatism, arthritis, and sinusitis. It is also used as a quick household topical remedy for insect bites, minor wounds, swellings, burns and sprains (*1, 2*). Currently, curcumin in the form of 70% curcumin, and 30% demethoxycurcumin and bisdemethoxycurcumin, is in clinical trials for prevention of colon cancer and leukoplakia, as curcumin has been shown to prevent cancers of the skin and digestive tract in animals. Its mode of action in carcinogenesis includes inhibition of the production of inflammation-induced growth factors and free radicals (*3, 4*). In this report, we will show that the anti-inflammatory properties of curcumin include the inhibition of gene expression of iNOS, iNOS activating cytokines, and an iNOS activated enzyme.

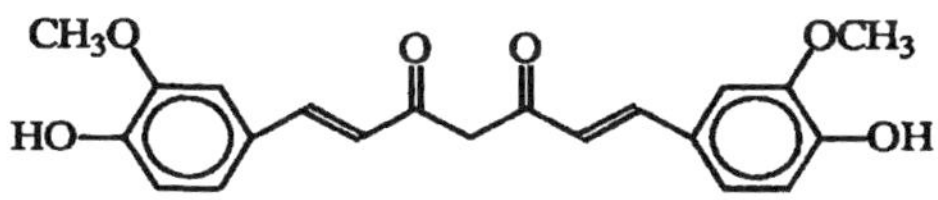

Figure 1. Chemical structure of curcumin

Over-production of nitrogen and oxygen free radicals, inflammatory cytokines, prostaglandins and leukotrienes has been implicated in the etiology of many inflammatory diseases, such as arthritis and ulcerative colitis. For joint destruction in osteoarthritis, nitric oxide (NO), TNFα, IL-1β and COX-2, have been regarded as targets for therapeutics (*5*).

Our laboratory has been investigating the impact of minor nutrients, specifically, phytochemicals, on gene expression in the inflammation pathways. In a murine model, we have reported that treatment with curcumin reduces the gene expression of iNOS in macrophages *in vitro*, and in the liver *in vivo* (*6*). Transcription of the iNOS gene is controlled by a number of inflammatory mediators during infection and inflammation. Cytokines and LPS can induce the gene expression of iNOS in macrophages and other cells (*7, 8*).

Here, we extended the study by examining, at the gene expression level, the effect of curcumin on three cytokines that enhance the production of NO, namely, TNFα, IL-1β and IFNγ, as well as the efficacy of curcumin in organs besides the liver.

NO enhances COX-2 activity through a direct interaction with the COX-2 enzyme, and oxidative stress and inflammatory stimuli, including LPS, TNFα and IL-1β induce COX-2 gene expression in macrophages (*9*). During inflammation, activation of COX-2 leads to metabolism of arachidonic acid to prostaglandins and leukotrienes, which induce vasodilation of the microcirculation, nociception, vascular permeability, and chemotaxis of neutrophils. Consequently, it leads to exacerbated inflammation and enhanced tissue degradation. It has previously been shown that curcumin inhibits transcription of the COX-2 gene in colon cancer cells and in the rat colon (*10-12*). However, the signal transduction pathways might be different in various cell types (*8*). An enhancer of iNOS expression in one cell type may be an inhibitor in another. Thus, the effect of curcumin on COX-2 gene transcription in murine macrophages was also examined.

MATERIALS AND METHODS

Materials

Curcumin was purchased from Kalsec and Fluka. This extract contained 70% curcumin, 30% demethoxycurcumin and bisdemethoxycurcumin.

In vitro studies

The non-elicited peritoneal exudate cells (PEC) from BALB/c mice and the murine macrophage line RAW264.7 were cultured and treated with curcumin as described (*6, 13, 14*). Total RNA of cultured cells was extracted with the Purescript RNA isolation kit (Gentra), and reverse transcription-polymerase chain reaction (RT-PCR) was performed (*6*). Primers for cytokines were purchased from Clontech except those for COX-2 were from Ambion. Their sequences (5' to 3') are as follows: sense CCC TTC CGA AGT TTC TGG CAG CAG C and antisense GGC TGT CAG AGC CTC GTG GCT TTG G for iNOS; sense TTC TGT CTA CTG AAC TTC GGG GTG ATC GGT CC and antisense GTA TGA GAT AGC AAA TCG GCT GAC GGT GTG GG for

TNF-α; sense ATG GCA ACT GTT CCT GAA CTC AAC T and antisense CAG GAC AGG TAT AGA TTC TTT CCT TT for IL-1β; sense TGC ATC TTG GCT TTG CAG CTC TTC CTC ATG GC and antisense TCG ACC TGT GGG TTG TTG ACC TCA AAC TTG GC for IFN-γ; sense GTC TGA TGA TGT ATG CCA CAA TCT G and antisense GAT GCC AGT GAT AGA GGG TGT TAA A for COX-2; and sense TGA AGG TCC GTG TGA ACG GAT TTG GC and antisense CAT GTA GGC CAT GAG GTC CAC CAC for glyceraldehydes-3-phosphate dehydrogenase (GAPDH). After hot start at 94°C for 3 minutes, the thermal cycling was 94°C for 45 seconds, 60°C for 45 seconds, and 72°C for 1 minute, for a total 23 to 40 cycles. For iNOS, a 65°C annealing temperature was used instead. The appropriate number for cycles of amplification was determined by analyzing the PCR products at the end of different cycle numbers. A 10 μl aliquot from each PCR reaction was electrophoresed in 1.6% agarose gel and stained with SYBR Green I dye (Molecular Probes). The gel was analyzed using a Molecular Dynamics Storm fluorescence scanning system (*6*). Signals from iNOS, TNFα, IL-1β, and COX-2 were normalized relative to their corresponding GAPDH signal from the same RNA sample.

In vivo studies

BALB/c mice (Jackson Laboratory) were housed in microisolator cages with filter tops and maintained in a temperature-controlled room with 12 hour light/12 hour dark periods and fed with water and standard diet *ad libitum*. The animals were divided into three groups: treatment with LPS alone, with curcumin plus LPS, and with curcumin alone, as reported previously (*6*). Curcumin solutions were prepared fresh for each feeding. The compound was dissolved in 0.5 N NaOH for making 100 mM solution, then immediately diluted with phosphate buffered saline (PBS) to make a 10 μM curcumin solution, and given to the animals by gavage. The vehicle group received PBS instead of curcumin. To enhance absorption and avoid loss of compound due to binding by food matrix, food was removed for 20 hours before the first feeding of curcumin. Five hours after administration of curcumin, food was returned for 2 hours and then removed again for 12 hours before the second feeding of curcumin. An hour after the second feeding, 0.5 mg/kg LPS was injected i.v. to induce the inflammation reaction of the experimental animals. The animals were sacrificed 5 hours after LPS challenge. Their organs were removed and preserved in a -70°C freezer until use. TriReagent (Sigma) was used for RNA isolation from tissue samples; and RT-PCR was performed as *in vitro* studies. The feeding schedule is shown below.

Feeding Schedule

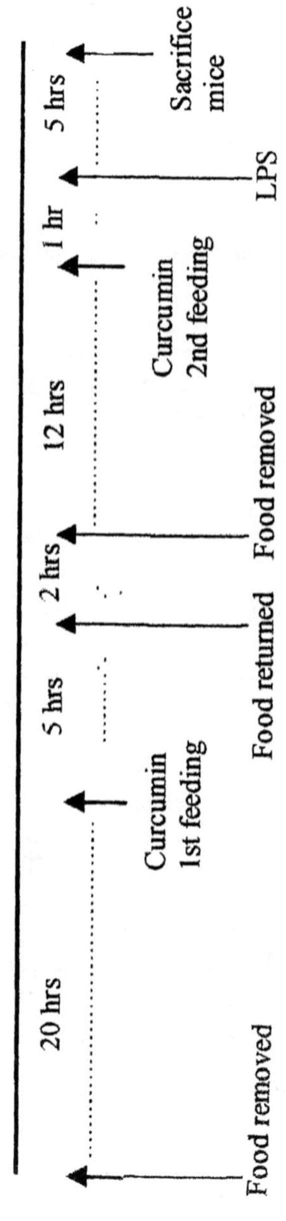

RESULTS

In vivo effect on iNOS gene expression in lymphoid and gastrointestinal organs

NO has been thought to play an important role in the mortality due to septic shock, hypotension and death caused by endotoxin (*15*). Therefore, administration of low level of LPS was used to cause endotoxemia, sepsis and trigger the expression of iNOS. At 5 hours after i.v. injection, iNOS mRNA was induced in the liver, spleen, mesenteric lymph nodes, small intestine, and colon, organs of the gastrointestinal tracts. Comparison was made in mice that had been treated with LPS alone, with LPS and curcumin, and with curcumin alone (for each organ, as shown in three lanes, see Figure 2). The curcumin given orally at 184 ng/g body weight inhibited the expression of iNOS in these organs, and the inhibition of iNOS was specific since the mRNA levels of GAPDH, a housekeeping gene, were unaffected. This result is consistent with our previous report that oral administration of curcumin has bioefficacy in the murine liver (*6*). Interestingly, in the colon, iNOS gene expression was strongly induced by intravenous injection of LPS and almost totally (over 90%) suppressed by curcumin. Similarly, the compound also had efficacy in the mesenteric lymph nodes, spleen and liver. Moreover, we also observed that iNOS expression was independent of LPS injection in the brain, heart, kidney, and lung, and curcumin treatment did not reduce the mRNA levels in these organs (not all data shown). In the stomach, we were unable to detect iNOS expression. Nonetheless, this observation is consistent with a previous report that shows intraperitoneal administration of LPS causes the expression of iNOS mRNA in esophagus, duodenum, jejunum, ileum, and colon but not in stomach in the rat (*16*).

Effect on mRNA levels of TNF-α and IL-1β in PEC

The pro-inflammation mediators, TNF-α and IL-1β, play important roles in inflammation as initiators and regulators of the inflammatory reaction. These two cytokines induce the production of other mediators further downstream, including the gene expression of iNOS in many cell types. We examined, *in vitro*, the effect of curcumin on gene expression of TNF-α and IL-1β by primary macrophages, using non-solicited PEC collected from BALB/c mice. RT-PCR analyses showed that, at 4 hours after activation, curcumin

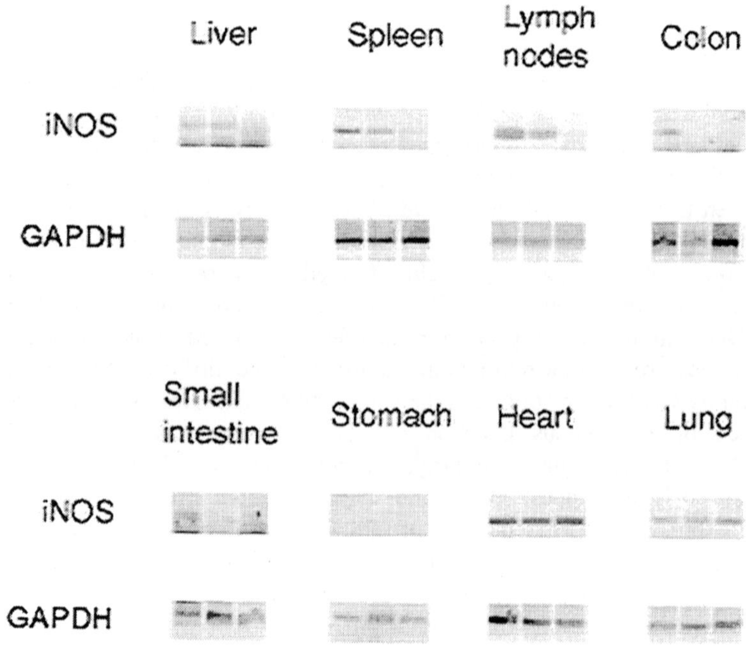

Figure 2. Effect of curcumin on iNOS mRNA expression in vivo. BALB/c mice were treated as described in Materials and Methods. The organs were collected and the induction of iNOS mRNA was evaluate d by applying RT-PCR. GAPDH was used to normalize the iNOS mRNA levels. Several organs were tested to evaluate the effects of LPS and curcumin treatment on iNOS mRNA induction. For each organ, the three lanes, from left to right, show LPS, LPS plus curcumin, and curcumin treatment of mice.

reduced the steady state RNA level for TNF-α in a dose-dependent manner. At concentrations of 1 μM, 2.5 μM, 5 μM and 10 μM, the degrees of reduction were 17%, 23%, 26% and 35%, respectively (Figure 3). IL-1β was affected similarly. At 1 μM, 2.5 μM, 5 μM and 10 μM of curcumin, the percentages of suppression on IL-1β were 12%, 15%, 21% and 31%, respectively (Figure 4).

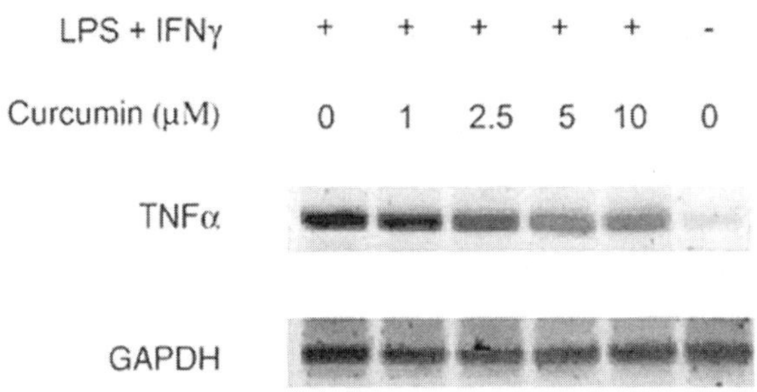

Figure 3. Effect of curcumin on TNFα mRNA expression in murine PEC. Peritoneal exudate cells were collected from BALB/c mice. They were exposed to medium only, LPS (0.01 μg/ml) and IFNγ (10 units/ml), and graded concentrations of curcumin with LPS and IFNγ. Total RNA was extracted from PEC after an incubation of 4 hours, and the mRNA levels of TNFa and GAPDH were determined by RT-PCR.

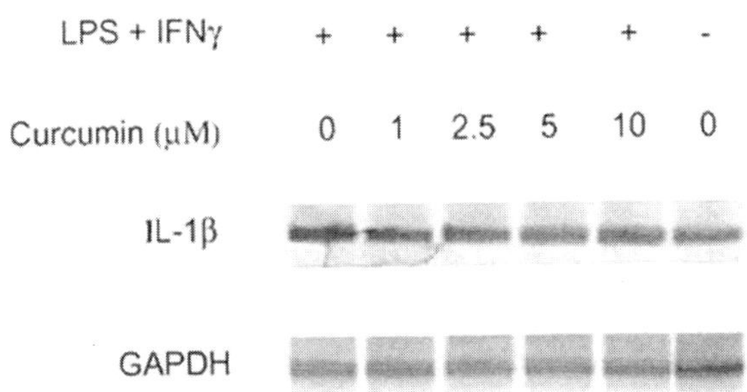

Figure 4. Effect of curcumin on IL-1β mRNA expression in murine PEC. Peritoneal exudate cells were collected from BALB/c mice. They were exposed to medium only, LPS (0.01 μg/ml) and IFNγ (10 units/ml), and graded concentrations of curcumin with LPS and IFNγ. Total RNA was extracted from PEC after an incubation of 4 hours, and the mRNA levels of IL-1β and GAPDH were determined by RT-PCR.

In vivo effect on mRNA levels of iNOS-inducing cytokines, TNF-α, IL-1β and IFNγ

In vivo, the gene expression of TNFα and IL-1β was also inhibited by curcumin. The levels of steady state mRNA in the liver, spleen and mesenteric lymph nodes of mice treated with LPS alone, LPS and curcumin, and curcumin alone, were compared (Figure 5). In a typical experiment, curcumin inhibited the induction of TNFα mRNA by 55%, 27%, and 60% in the liver, spleen and mesenteric lymph nodes, respectively. The production of IL-1β mRNA was also decreased by 40-50% in the liver and spleen. IFNγ, a cytokine that is produced by T helper-1 cells, plays an essential role in the induction of NO production in murine macrophages. Thus, the effect of curcumin on its gene expression was determined in the lymphoid organs. The induction of IFNγ was inhibited by curcumin. IFNγ mRNA was reduced, in a typical experiment, by 25% in the spleen and by over 90% in the mesenteric lymph nodes (Figure 6).

Effect on expression of COX-2 mRNA in RAW264.7 cells

COX-2 is an enzyme that is crucial for the synthesis of prostaglandins during inflammation, and is expressed in macrophages upon stimulation with LPS, TNFα, and IL-1β. The effect of curcumin on the gene expression of COX-2 was examined. Unfortunately, unlike TNFα and IL-1β, COX-2 mRNA could

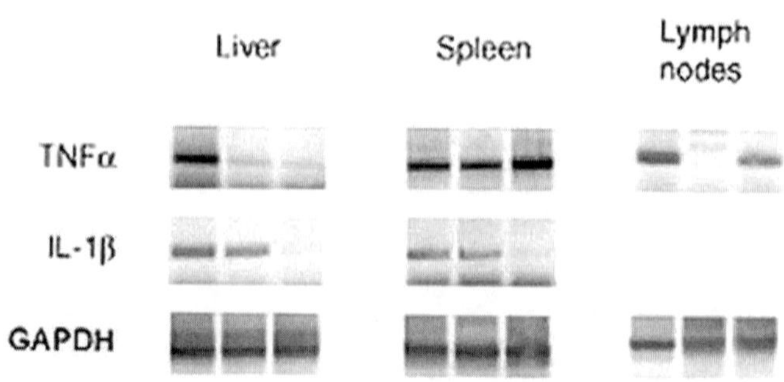

Figure 5. Effect of curcumin on TNFα and IL-1β mRNA expression in vivo. The liver, spleen and lymph nodes of BALB/c mice were collected and the induction of TNFα and IL-1β mRNA was evaluated by applying RT-PCR. GAPDH was used to normalize the cytokine mRNA level. For each organ, the three lanes, from left to right, show LPS, LPS plus curcumin, and curcumin treatment of mice.

not be detected by RT-PCR in the murine PEC. Nonetheless, the murine macrophage cell line, RAW264.7, produced quantifiable amount of COX-2 mRNA after stimulation with 0.01 μg/ml LPS and 10 units of IFNγ. After 5 hours of incubation, the induction of COX-2 mRNA was inhibited by curcumin in a concentration-dependent manner (Figure 7). At concentration of 1 μM, 2.5 μM, 5 μM and 10 μM, the inhibitory percentage was 0%, 5%, 13% and 23%.

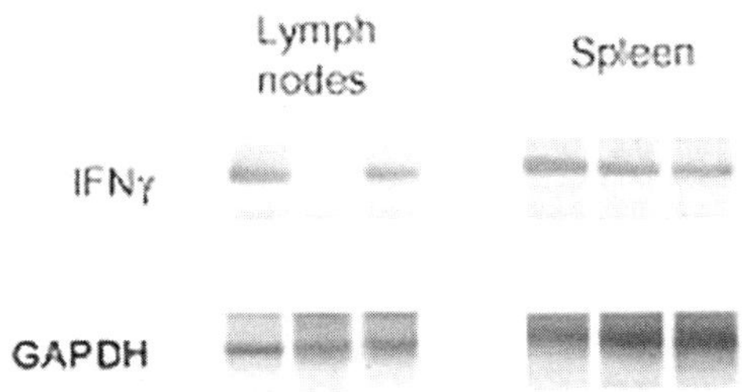

Figure 6. Effect of curcumin on IFNγ mRNA expression in vivo. The spleen and lymph nodes of BALB/c mice were collected and the induction of IFNγ mRNA was evaluated by applying RT-PCR. GAPDH was used to normalize the cytokine mRNA level. The three lanes, from left to right, show LPS, LPS plus curcumin, and curcumin treatment of mice.

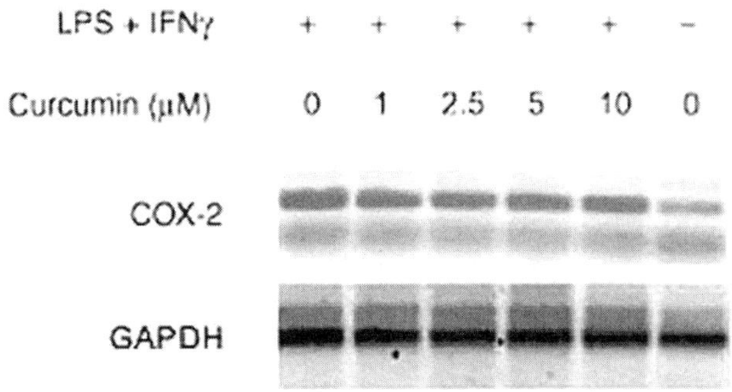

Figure 7. Effect of curcumin on COX-2 mRNA expression in murine macrophages. RAW264.7 cells were stimulated with LPS (0.01 μg/ml) and IFNγ (10 units/ml) in the presence of increasing concentrations of curcumin. Total RNA was extracted after an incubation of 4 hours, and the mRNA levels of COX-2 and GAPDH were determined by RT-PCR.

DISCUSSION

This report describes our study on the anti-inflammatory actions of curcumin in a murine system, in terms of the induction of iNOS, TNFα, IL-1β, IFNγ and COX-2 gene expression, *in vitro* and *in vivo*. We have found that its action on murine and human macrophages may be similar with respect to the production of TNFα and IL-1β, for we have previously shown that they are both suppressed in the human macrophage cell line, MonoMac 6, at the protein level (*13*). The inhibition can result from blocking the activation of the free radical-activated transcription factors, nuclear factor kappa B (NFκB) and activator protein-1 (AP-1). We have found that curcumin reduces LPS-induced NFκB nuclear translocation in human macrophages (*13*), and this finding has been confirmed by others using TNFα (*17*). Huang et al. (1991) have found that it inhibits the activation of AP-1 (*18*). NFκB and AP-1 are master switches that regulate the gene expression of a growing list of cytokines intrinsically linked to coordinate inflammatory response and tissue destruction, including TNFα, IL-1β, iNOS and COX-2.

Curcumin inhibits the production of many cytokines that are under the control of the NFκB pathway as shown in various cell types. Besides IL-1β and TNF-α, it inhibits the production of IL-2, IL-4, IL-5 and IL-8 by human monocytes and macrophages (*19, 20*). Curcumin also inhibits IL-12 production, though not IL-10, in murine macrophages. It may bias the T-helper 1/T helper 2 balance by decreasing the production of IFNγ and increasing the production of IL-4 (*21, 22*). For chemotaxis, in rat and human intestinal epithelial cells, IL-1β-mediated expression of IL-8 is suppressed by curcumin (*23*). In human osteoblasts, epinephrine-induced expression of IL-6 and IL-12 is also inhibited by curcumin though it is via the AP-1 pathway, rather than the NF-κB pathway (*24*).

The molecular mechanism by which curcumin can inhibit these transcription factors is complex. Since they are redox-regulated, curcumin may suppress their activation by removing free radicals. At another level, curcumin may block activation by blocking signal transduction. Curcumin inhibits activation of protein kinase C and phosphorylase kinase (*25, 26*). It also inhibits inhibitor kappa B (IκB) kinases 1 and 2 (IKK1 and 2), blocks phosphorylation of IκB, and suppresses IκB dissociation from the p65 subunit of NFκB (*23, 27*).

The action of curcumin includes those of the commonly used non-steroidal anti-inflammatory drugs (NSAIDs). The anti-inflammatory action of aspirin and sodium salicylate is through the inhibition of prostaglandin synthesis, via a direct inhibition of the COX enzymes. Curcumin inhibits COX-2 at both the gene expression and the enzyme activity levels. At a concentration of 100 μM, it substantially inhibits the enzyme activity of lipoxygenase and cyclooxygenase, each by about 79%, as measured by a decrease in the formation of metabolic products (*28*). At the gene level, here we have shown that curcumin inhibits COX-2 gene expression in murine macrophages, which corroborates a previous observation in colon cancer cells (*12*). In addition, both curcumin and aspirin inhibit the activation of NF-κB (*13, 17, 29*).

We have previously reported that curcumin down-regulated iNOS expression in the liver of mice when fed at dietary attainable quantity. This report confirmed that finding and further established its *in vivo* efficacy (*6*). Here, we show that curcumin was also effective in other organs along the alimentary tract, namely, small intestine and colon, as well as in lymphoid organs in the area, namely, spleen and mesenteric lymph nodes. This is in agreement with the results from the rat models. Curcumin can be detected in the plasma, liver and the colon mucosa when administered by gavage (500 mg/kg) (*30*). In another rat model using spontaneous tumor regression, curcumin decreases iNOS of peritoneal macrophages, increases iNOS of natural killer (NK) cells, and decreases the levels of TNFα and IL-12 in the serum (*31*). In humans, a recent clinical trial has found that curcumin, ingested at 440 mg of *Curcuma* extract (containing 36 mg curcumin) per day for 29 days, is accompanied by a 59% decrease in lymphocytic glutathione-S-transferase activity; and curcumin and its metabolites have been recovered from the feces, though not from blood or urine (*32*).

In conclusion, curcumin has been widely used in Asia for centuries as an anti-inflammation treatment. Currently, the dietary supplement industry in the U.S is marketing this phytochemical for the prevention of arthritis, and the National Cancer Institute (NCI) is examining its potential as a chemopreventive agent against colon and oral cancer. Studies in our laboratory, in conjunction with those from other investigators, have unraveled part of the molecular mechanisms of the compound, and have shown that it has *in vivo* anti-inflammatory activities in the digestive tract and the associated lymphoid tissues. Hence, the prospect for using curcumin for prevention of inflammation-associated tumorigenesis, such as colon cancer, and chronic inflammation of the gut, such as colitis, is very good.

Acknowledgment

We thank Drs. Mou-Tuan Huang and Chi-Tang Ho for sharing their knowledge and compounds with us throughout our studies on phytochemcials. We thank Dr. Robert Herman for his helpful comments on the manuscript. This work was supported in part by the National Institutes of Health grant AI-45555 to Marion Chan.

References

1. Ammon, H.P.T.; Wahl, M.A. *Planta Med.* **1990,** 57, 1-7.
2. Araujo, C.A.C.; Leon, L.L. *Mem. Inst. Oswaldo Cruz.* **2001,** 96, 723-728.
3. Kelloff, G.J.; Crowell, J.A.; Hawk, E.T.; Steele, V.E.; Lubet, R.A.; Boone, C.W.; Covey, J.M.; Doody, L.A.; Omenn, G.S.; Greenwald, P.; Hong, W.K.; Parkinson, D.R.; Bagheri, D.; Baxter, G.T.; Blunden, M.; Doeltz, M.K.; Eisenhauer, K.M.; Johnson, K.; Knapp, G.G.; Longfellow, D.G.; Malone, W.F.; Nayfield, S.G.; Seifried, H.E.; Swall, L.M.; Sigman, C.C. *J. Cell. Biochem. Suppl.* **1996,** 26, 54-71.
4. Huang, M.T.; Newmark, H.L.; Frenkel, K. *J. Cell. Biochem. Suppl.* **1997,** 27, 26-34.
5. Goldring, M.B. *Conn. Tissue Res.* **1999,** 40, 1-11.
6. Chan, M.M.; Huang, H.; Fenton, M.R.; Fong, D. *Biochem. Pharmcol.* **1998,** 55, 1955-1962.
7. Lorsbach, R.B.; Murphy, W.J.; Lowenstein, C.J.; Snyder, S.H.; Russell, S.W. *J. Biol. Chem.* **1993,** 268, 1908-1913.
8. Rao, K.M. *J. Toxicol. Environ. Health B. Crit. Rev.* **2000,** 3, 27-58.
9. Salvemini, D.; Seibert, K.; Masferrer, J.L.; Settle, S.L.; Misko, T.P.; Currie, M.G.; Needleman, P. *Adv. Prostaglandin Thromboxane Leukot. Res.* **1995,** 23, 491-493.
10. Zhang, F.; Altorki, N.K.; Mestre, J.R.; Subbaramaiah, K.; Dannenberg, A.J. *Carcinogenesis* **1999,** 20, 45-451.
11. Rao, C.V.; Kawamori, T.; Hamid, R.; Reddy, B.S. *Carcinogenesis* **1999,** 20, 641-644.
12. Goel, A.; Boland, C.R.; Chauhan, D.P. *Cancer Lett.* **2001,** 172, 111-118.
13. Chan, M.M. *Biochem. Pharmacol.* **1995,** 49, 1551-1556.
14. Chan, M.M.; Mattiacci, J.A.; Hwang, H.S.; Shah, A.; Fong, D. *Biochem. Pharmacol.* **2000,** 60, 1539-1548.
15. MacMicking, J.D.; Nathan, C.; Hom, G.; Chartrain, N.; Fletcher, D.S.; Trumbauer, M.; Stevens, K.; Xie, Q.W.; Sokol, K.; Hutchinson, N. *Cell* **1995,** 81, 641-650.
16. Chen, K.; Inoue, M.; Okada, A. *Biochem. Biophys. Res. Commun.* **1996,** 224, 703-708.
17. Singh, S.; Aggarwal, B.B. *J. Biol. Chem.* **1995,** 270, 24995-5000.

18. Huang, T.S.; Lee, S.C.; Lin, J.K. *Proc. Natl. Acad. Sci. USA* **1991, 88,** 5292-5296.
19. Kobayashi T, Hashimoto S, Horie T. *Biochem. Pharmacol.* **1997,** 54, 819-824.
20. Abe, Y.; Hashimoto, S.; Horie, T. *Pharmacol. Res.* **1999,** 39, 41-47.
21. Kang, B.Y.; Song, Y.J.; Kim, K.M.; Choe, Y.K.; Hwang, S.Y.; Kim, T.S. *Br. J. Pharmacol.* **1999,** 128, 380-384.
22. Kang, B.Y.; Chung, S.W.; Chung, W.; Im, S.; Hwang, S.Y.; Kim, T.S. *Eur. J. Pharmacol.* **1999,** 384, 191-195.
23. Jobin, C.; Bradham, C.A.; Russo, M.P.; Juma, B.; Narula, A.S.; Brenner, D.A.; Sartor, R.B. *J Immunol.* **1999,** 163, 3474-3483.
24. Kondo, A.; Mogi, M.; Koshihara, Y.; Togari, A. *Biochem. Pharmacol.* **2001,** 61, 319-326.
25. Liu, J.Y.; Lin, S.J.; Lin, J.K. *Carcinogenesis* **1993,** 14, 857-861.
26. Reddy, S.; Aggarwal, B.B. *FEBS Letters* **1994,** 341, 19-22.
27. Pan, M.H.; Lin-Shiau, S.Y.; Lin, J.K. *Biochem Pharmacol.* **2000,** 60, 1665-1676.
28. Huang, M.T.; Lysz, T.; Ferraro, T.; Conney, A.H. *Cancer Res.* **1991,** 51, 813-819.
29. Kopp, E.; Ghosh, S. *Science* **1994,** 265, 956-959.
30. Sharma, R.A.; Ireson, C.R.; Verschoyle, R.D.; Hill, K.A.; Williams, M.L.; Leuratti, C.; Manson, M.M.; Marnett, L.J.; Steward, W.P.; Gescher, A. Clin *Cancer Res.* **2001,** 7, 1452-1458.
31. Bhaumik, S.; Jyothi, M.D.; Khar, A. FEBS Lett. **2000,** 483, 78-82.
32. Sharma, R.A.; McLelland, H.R.; Hill, K.A.; Ireson, C.R.; Euden, S.A.; Manson, M.M.; Pirmohamed, M.; Marnett, L.J.; Gescher, A.J.; Steward, W.P. *Clin. Cancer Res.* **2001,** 7, 1894-1900.

Chapter 9

Suppression of Transcriptional Activity of Gene Promoter for Cyclooxygenase-2 and Inducible Nitric Oxide Synthase in Colon Cancer Cells

Michihiro Mutoh[1,2], Hirofumi Matsui[1], Mami Takahashi[2], Takeji Takamura-Enya[2], and Keiji Wakabayashi[2]

[1]**Department of Gastroenterology, Institute of Clinical Medicine, University of Tsukuba, Tennoudai 1–1–1, Ibaraki 305–0006, Japan**
[2]**Cancer Prevention Division, National Cancer Center Research Institute, 1–1 Tsukiji 5-chome, Chuo-ku, Tokyo 104–0045, Japan**

Expression levels of cyclooxygenase (COX)-2 and/or inducible nitric oxid synthase (iNOS) were elevated in colon tumors; their suppression may be an effective approach for prevention of colon cancer. Using a reporter gene assay system, various potential chemopreventive agents including some flavonoids were tested for their effects on COX-2 and/or iNOS transcriptional activity. The results of intensive examination of the relationships between flavonoid structures and suppression of COX-2 transcriptional activities suggest that low electron density of oxygen atom bonded to the 5,7-positions of the A ring, the number of hydroxyl groups on the B ring, and an oxo group at the 4-position of the C ring are important. Furthermore, sodium butyrate was found to inhibit iNOS transcriptional activity. These findings offer clues to effective preventive approaches for colon cancer, targeting multiple signal pathways, and provide novel insights into the molecular mechanisms of COX-2 and iNOS regulations.

Much evidence suggests that chronic inflammation is closely related to colon carcinogenesis. Thus, factors involved in chronic inflammation are of great interest as targets of cancer chemopreventive agents. Cyclooxygenase-2 (COX-2) and inducible nitric oxide synthase (iNOS) are abundantly expressed in the epithelium of colitis and colon cancer cells and appear to play an important role in colon carcinogenesis (*1-4*).

The COX isozymes are prostaglandin (PG) synthases which catalyze sequential synthesis of PGG_2 and PGH_2 from arachidonic acid by virtue of intrinsic cyclooxygenase and peroxidase activities. Two forms have been reported, COX-1 and COX-2, the first being constitutively expressed, while COX-2 is upregulated in response to stimulation with growth factors, tumor promoters and cytokines. The COX-2 gene is also responsive to several oncogenes such as *v-H-ras, v-src*, and members of the *Wnt* pathway. Nitric oxide is endogenously produced by a family of three distinctive NOS isoforms. Two, nNOS and eNOS, are constitutive and calcium-dependent, nNOS being present in neurons of the nervous system and eNOS in vascular endothelial cells. The third, iNOS, is inducible and calcium-independent and provides sustained release of NO in response to many agents such as cytokines. Overproduction of NO by iNOS has been reported to give rise to N-nitroso compounds and also cause DNA damage. In addition, NO induces COX-2 expression, angiogenesis and vasodilation, which enhances blood flow to the tumor tissues supporting their growth. It has been reported that inhibition of COX-2 and/or iNOS enzyme activity can prevent colon carcinogenesis (*5-7*). From results with a COX-2 knockout mouse, it is likely that agents that can suppress COX-2 expression at the gene level may be equally advantageous (*8*). This is also likely to be the case for compounds suppressing iNOS expression at the gene level.

Improvement of the dietary lifestyle to reduce the risk of colon cancer has attracted a great deal of interest. In extensive studies, risk has been found to be elevated by high consumption of dietary fat and a low intake of cereal grains, fruits, vegetables and dietary fiber (*9*). Thus, constituents of fruits and vegetables such as flavonids are of great interest as candidate chemopreventive agents against colon carcinogenesis.

Reporter Gene Assay for COX-2 and/or iNOS Promoter-dependent Transcriptional Activity

To test for the effects of chemopreventive agents on COX-2 and/or iNOS transcriptional activity, we constructed a β-galactosidase (β-gal) reporter gene system in human colon cancer DLD-1 cells.

The basic vector β-gal-blasticidin S deaminase fusion plasmid pB2-βGal-BSD was constructed from the pSV-β-gal vector (Promega, Madison, WI) by insertion of the blasticidin S deaminase (BSD) gene. The p/B2-βGal-BSD, pCOX-2/B2-βGal-BSD or piNOS/B2-βGal-BSD plamid DNAs were transfected into DLD-1 cells and cells were designed as DLD-1/ B2-βGal-BSD, DLD-1/COX-2-B2-βGal-BSD or DLD-1/iNOS-B2-βGal-BSD, respectively (*10-12*). From heterogeneous population of DLD-1/COX2-B2-βGal-BSD cells and DLD-1/iNOS-B2-βGal-BSD, a subclone containing intact DNA fragment of the 2078-base pair COX-2 promoter region or the 1123-base pair iNOS promoter region with the *lacZ* gene downstream in the genome DNA was obtained by the limiting dilution method. Cells were seeded at a density of $2x10^4$ cells per well in 96-well microtiter plates, treated with test reagents and the total β-gal activities of DLD-1 cells in each well were determined by a colorimetric assay using o-nitrophenyl-β-D-galactopyranoside (ONPG). The background β-gal activity of DLD-1 cells was determined in control non-treated culture of DLD-1/B2-βGal-BSD cells, and the value was set as zero. Basal β-gal activity of non-treated DLD-1/COX2-B2-βGal-BSD or DLD-1/iNOS-B2-βGal-BSD was set as 100 %. The percentage β-gal activity with each treatment was then calculated using data from triplicate wells. The values for β-gal activity were normalized for viable cell number and assessed by the MTT assay (*10*). All assays were carried out in triplicate and each experiment repeated at least three times.

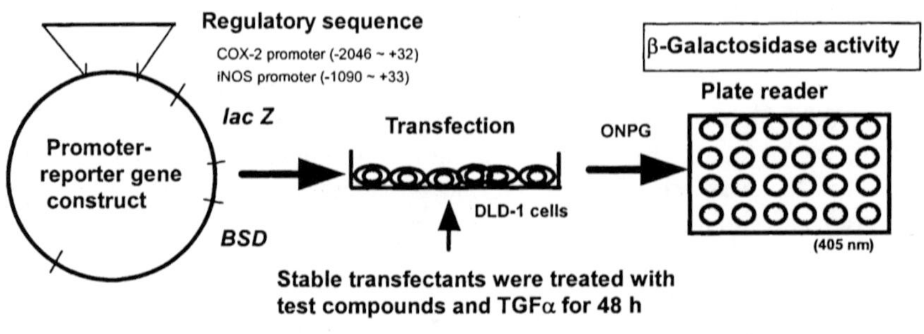

Figure 1. Schematic flow chart of the β-galactosidase reporter gene system for assessment of COX-2 and/or iNOS transcriptional activity

Suppressive Effects of Chemopreventive Agents on COX-2 Transcriptional Activity

Suppression of COX-2 Transcriptional Activity by Polyphenols

Treatment of cells with 100 ng/ml TGFα for 48 h increased COX-2 transcriptional activity to 2.1-times the value in untreated DLD-1/COX2-B2-βGal-BSD cells. The effects of 24 compounds (in Table I) known to have chemopreventive and antioxidative properties were examined. Among these, quercetin, rhamnetin, genistein, eriodictyol, luteolin, kaempferol, resveratrol, fisetin, phloretine, epicatechin, catechin, and resorcinol, all suppressed TGFα-stimulated COX-2 transcriptional activity in a dose-dependent fashion (*10, 11*). Values for their ability to induce a 50% decrease in TGFα-stimulated COX-2 transcriptional activity (IC_{50} values) are shown in Table I. In addition, these compounds also suppressed COX-2 transcriptional activity below the basal level (*10*) (see Figure 2).

Based on the IC_{50} values, the flavonoids could be classified into three groups of potent, weak, and no suppression. Eriodictyol, fisetin, genistein, keampherol, luteolin, quercetin, phloretine and rhamnetin were potent suppressors of COX-2 transcriptional activity, with IC_{50} values of 18.6-52.5 μM. In contrast, catechin and epicatechin showed only very weak suppression (IC_{50}=415.3 μM) and epigallocatechin, epigallocatechin gallate (EGCG) and myricetin exhibited no suppression (*11*).

Relationship between Suppression of COX-2 Transcriptional Activity and Structures of Flavonoids

Ten of the twelve chemopreventive agents which suppressed COX-2 transcriptional activity (quercetin, kaempferol, genistein, resveratrol, eriodictyol, luteolin, phloretine, catechin, epicatechin and resorcinol) had a common resorcinol moiety in their structure, as indicated by the box in Figure 3 (*11*). Structures of quercetin, kaempherol, eriodictyol, luteolin and epicatechin are shown in Figure 4. Daidzein, an analogue of genistein, but not having a resorcinol moiety in its structure, did not inhibit COX-2 transcriptional activity. Therefore, the resorcinol moiety may play a critical role. However, myricetin

Table I. Effects of Chemopreventive Agents on COX-2 Transcriptional Activity

Compounds[a]		IC_{50} (μM)
Polyphenols	Quercetin	10.5±0.7
	Rhamnetin	18.6±2.1
	Genistein	20.7±1.4
	Eriodictyol	22.0±0.2
	Luteolin	22.0±0.4
	Kaempferol	39.3±2.1
	Resveratrol	44.0±5.6
	Fisetin	47.9±2.9
	Phloretine	52.5±3.4
	Epicatechin	415.3±17.0
	Catechin	415.3±25.4
	Resorcinol	463.2±27.1
	Daidzein	>500
	EGCG	>500
	Myricetin	>500
	Genistin	>500
	Tannic acid	>100
Vitamins	Ascorbic acid	>100
	Alpha-tocopherol	>100
	Beta-carotene	>100
Others	Sodium butyrate	>1000
	Curcumin	>10
	DHA	>10
	Glutathione	>5000

[a] Abbreviations are: EGCG, epigallocatechin gallate; and DHA, docosahexaenoic acid.

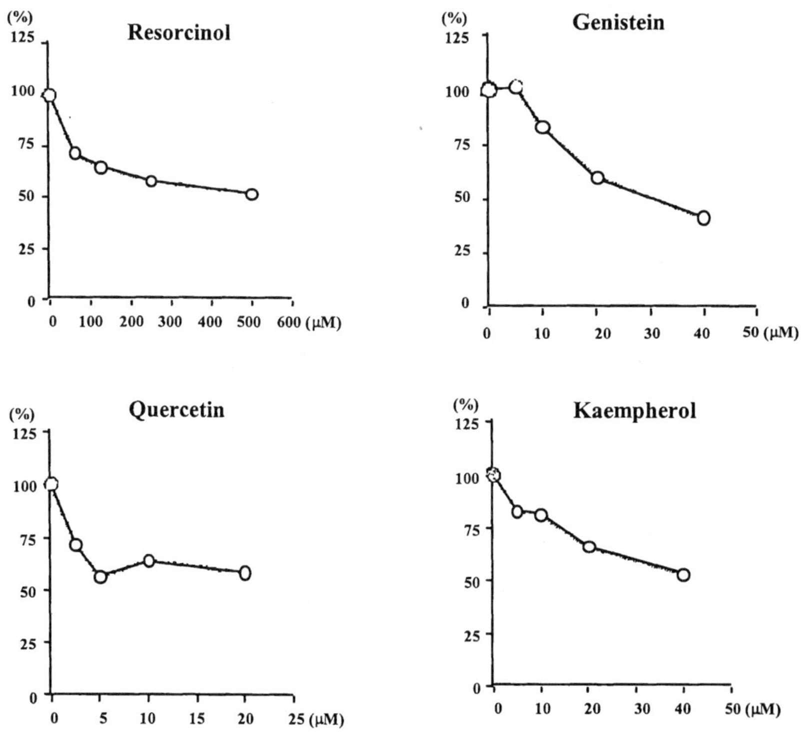

Figure 2. Suppression of the level of COX-2 transcriptional activity in DLD-1 cells by chemopreventive agents. COX-2 transcriptional activity was normalized for viable cell numbers assessed by MTT assay and plotted as the percentage of the unstimulated control culture value.

showed no inhibitory effect on COX-2 transcriptional activity, even though it contains a resorcinol moiety. Other elements may thus be also involved.

Flavonoids are ubiquitously present in foods of plant origin and have long been recognized to possess many properties such as anti-inflammatory, antiviral, antiproliferative, and anticarcinogenic potencial (*13, 14*). Physically, they are characterized by two phenyl rings connected by a pyran ring or a similar structure of three carbons. These rings are referred to as A, B, and C, respectively, as indicated for quercetin in Figure 4. Subclasses of flavonoids are categorized based on variation in the heterocyclic C ring.

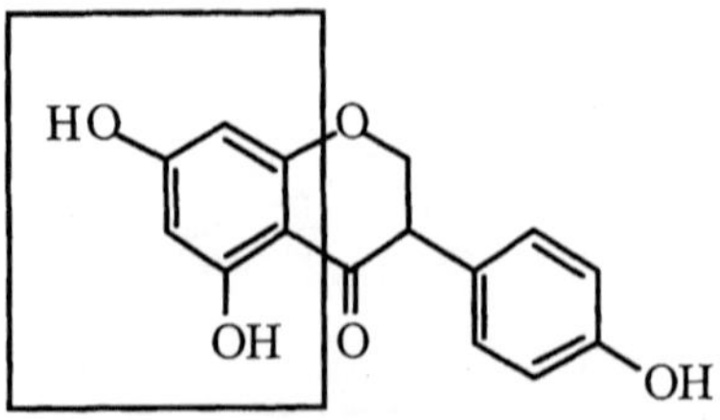

Genistein

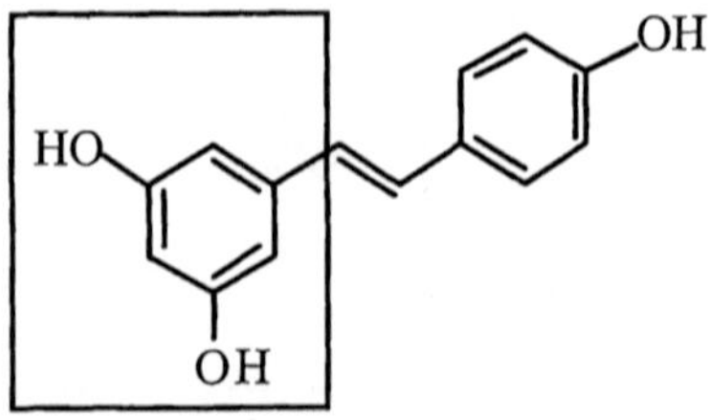

Resveratrol

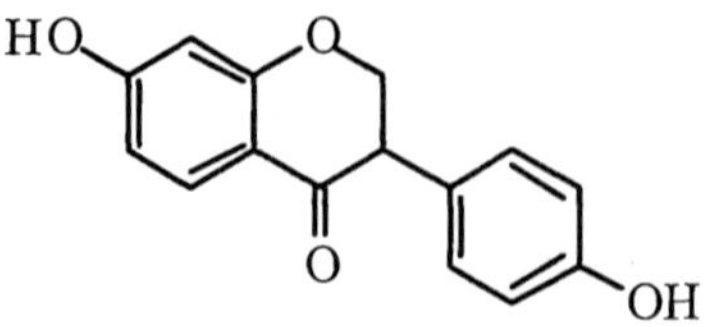

Daidzein

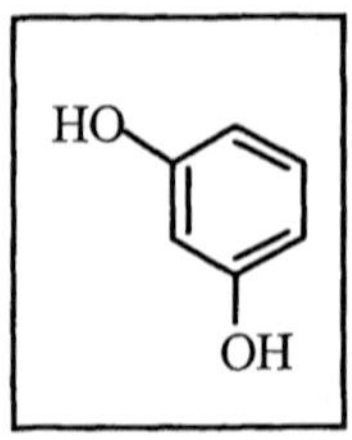

Resorcinol

Figure 3. Chemical structures of daidzein, genistein, resorcinol and resveratrol. All agents have a common resorcin moiety, except for daidzein, indicated by the box.

Structure-activity analysis (see Figure 4) of quercetin, a flavonol, and epicatechin, a flavanol, indicated that these compounds differ with regard to the state of saturation of the C2-C3 bond and the presence of a 4-oxo group. The structure-activity analysis of eriodictyol and luteolin suggested that the molecular conformation caused by the 2,3-double bond of the C ring has little effect on COX-2 transcriptional activity. Thus, these results suggest that the presence of the 4-oxo group plays an important role in suppressing COX-2 transcriptional activity. Furthermore, all flavonoids with a 4-oxo group, except for myricetin, were found to be potent suppressors. On the other hand, compounds that lacked a 4-oxo group, catechin, epicatechin, epigallocatechin and EGCG exhibited a weak or no activity. The potent COX-2 suppressors, eriodictyol, fisetin, luteolin, quercetin and rhamnetin, also have 3', 4'-OH groups in their B ring. Compounds, such as epigallocatechin, EGCG and myricetin, with three hydroxyl groups on the B ring did not suppress COX-2 transcriptional activity (*11*). Therefore, the number of hydroxyl groups on the B ring may be related to a molecular conformation that influences the interactions between flavonoids and enzymes such as protein-tyrosine kinases (PTKs) and protein kinase C (PKC), which are involved in the induction of COX-2 expression (*15*).

Several recent studies have demonstrated that flavonoids may be potent inhibitors of enzymes, including PTKs, PKC and phosphatidylinositol 3-kinase (PI3-kinase) (*16, 17*). It has been reported that flavonoids which inhibit PTKs and PKC have 3', 4'-OH groups on the B ring, and 5,7-OH groups on the A ring (*16, 17*). These results suggest that flavonoid structures required for the inhibition of PTKs and PKC are involved in suppressing COX-2 expression.

Crystallography has demonstrated that there is an intramolecular hydrogen bond between the 5-hydroxy group and the 4-oxo group in quercetin (*18*). Since, a free 7-hydroxy group in the A ring may be able to attack enzymes such as PTKs and PKC, the electron density of the 5- and 7-oxygen to determine the relationship between the electron density of oxygen atoms in hydroxy groups of the compounds and their suppressive effects on COX-2 transcriptional activity was examined. Densities were calculated by the semi-empirical quantum mechanical method, AM-1, using MOPAC ver 6.3. With this approach, the initial geometry was constructed from standard bond lengths and angles, and then completely optimized using an algorithm in the MOPAC program (*19*). The potent suppressor, quercetin, had a lower calculated electron density for the 7-oxygen than the weak suppressors, epicatechin. Among flavonoids with the same B ring structure and a resorcinol moiety, an inverse correlation was observed between the electron density of the 7-oxygen and the suppression of COX-2 transcriptional activity (see Figure 4). A similar correlation was observed for the electron density of the 5-oxygen (*11*).

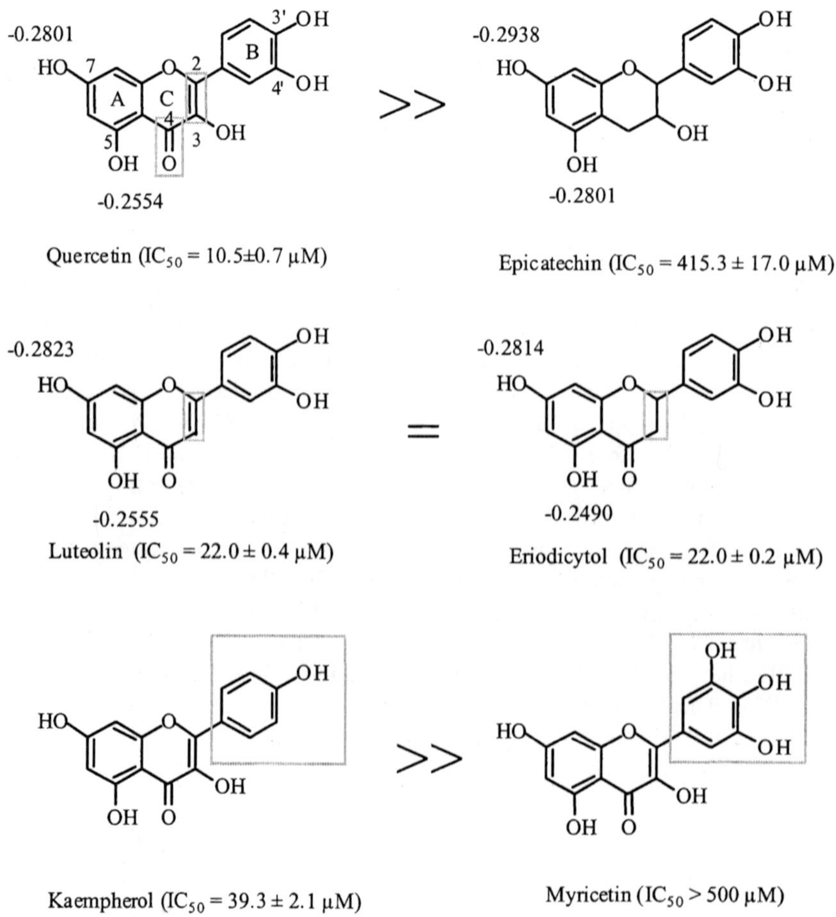

Figure 4. Structures of the flavonoids . The moieties employed for assessment of structure-activity relationships are indicated by boxes. IC_{50} values are described next to the name. Electron densities are given beside the hydroxyl groups.

To confirm that the electron density of 7-oxygen plays a role in suppression of COX-2 transcriptional activity, resacetophenone was brominated to reduce the electron density. As shown in Figure 5, 3,5-dibromo-2,4-dihydroxyacetophenone (BHAP) has a lower electron density for oxygens at positions 2 and 4 in the resorcinol moiety than resacetophenone. BHAP suppressed COX-2 transcriptional activity in a dose-dependent manner, and was 6.8-times more potent than resacetophenone (*11*).

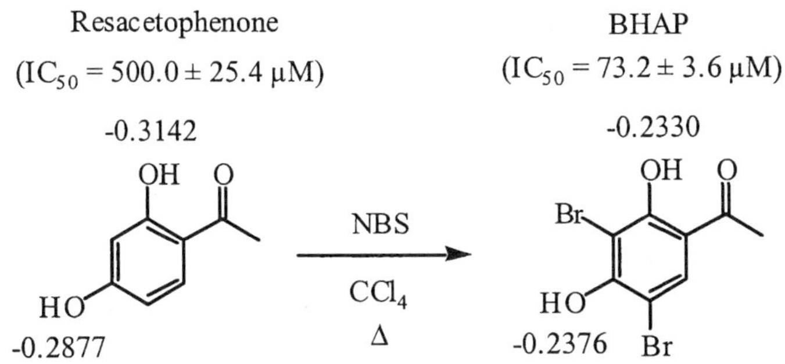

Figure 5. Synthesis of BHAP from resacetophenone. Electron densities of oxygens and IC_{50} values are also shown.

Suppression of iNOS Promoter-dependent Transcriptional Activity by Butyrate

Increased fiber intake and the consumption of fruits and vegetables are well-known chemopreventive dietary strategies against colon carcinogenesis. It is reported that fiber intake reduces colonic transit time and increases the production of short chain fatty acids such as butyric acid. The latter is produced in the mammalian colon in mM concentrations as a by-product of anaerobic bacterial fermentation of dietary fiber. Butyric acid has been recognized as one candidates chemopreventive active against colon carcinogenesis because it induces apoptosis and differentiation in colon cancer cell lines.

Sodium butyrate at 0.1-1.0 mM was tested in this reporter gene assay system for iNOS transcriptional activity, and was shown to reduced iNOS transcriptional activity dose-dependently, by 75 and 80% at 0.3 and 0.5 mM, respectively (Figure 6) (*12*). From this study, the chemopreventive activity of fiber against colon carcinogenesis could be partly attributed to the suppression of iNOS gene expression by butyrate, suggesting a novel protective effect. It is reported that butyrate inhibits inflammatory responses through inhibition of NF-κB activation (*20*). Thus, it is possible that butyrate may suppress iNOS expression via inhibiting NF-κB activity. However, this may not be enough explanation for the mechanism that sodium butyrate suppresses iNOS expression. It is known that COX-2 can also be induced by NF-κB activation. However, sodium butyrate increased COX-2 transcriptional activity, as shown in Figure 6. Thus, an alternative explanation might involve effects of butyrate on

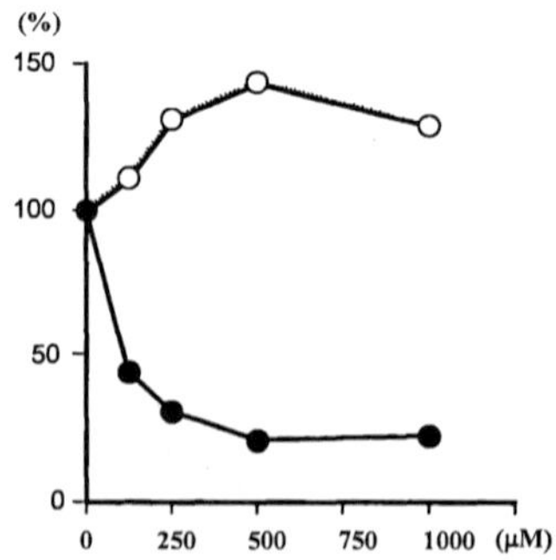

Figure 6. Effects of sodium butyrate on COX-2 and iNOS transcriptional activity in DLD-1 cells. COX-2 (open circles) and iNOS (closed circles) transcriptional activities were normalized for viable cell numbers as assessed by MTT assay and plotted as the percentage of the unstimulated control culture value.

processes such as phosphoriation of transcription factors or promoter region methylation.

Conclusions

The present method appears to have advantage in the search for novel inhibitors of COX-2 and/or iNOS expression which might be effective as anti-inflammatory and/or cancer preventive agents. From our results, we propose that the structural requirements for the suppression of COX-2 transcriptional activity by flavonoids are the presence of a 4-oxo group in the C ring, low electron density in the 7-oxygen group in the A ring, and a 3', 4'-dihydroxy structure in the B ring. We also propose that resorcinol and resacetophenon have one of the minimal essential structural features required for suppression of COX-2 transcriptional activity and may provide a basis for the design of superior compounds. Suppression of iNOS expression and resultant decrease of NO production by butyrate may be involved in the mechanisms by which dietary fiber show preventive effects against colon cancer. It is known that butyrate enemas have potent protective effects against ulcerative colitis. Elucidation of the mechanisms by which butyrate suppresses iNOS upregulation in colon cancer cells may also provide novel information for development of chemopreventive agents against colon carcinogenesis.

References

1. Eberhart, C. E.; Coffey, R. J.; Radhika, A.; Giardiello, F. M.; Ferrenbach, S.; DuBois, R. N. *Gastroenterology* **1994**, *107*, 1183-1188.
2. Singer, II; Kawka, D. W.; Schloemann, S,; Tessner, T.; Riehl, T,; Stenson, W. F. *Gastroenterology*. **1998**, *115*, 297-306.
3. Ambs, S.; Merriam, W. G.; Bennett, W. P.; Felley-Bosco, E.; Ogunfusika, M. O.; Oser, S. M.; Klein, S.; Shields, P. G.; Billiar, T. R.; Harris, C. C. *Cancer Res.* **1998**, *58*, 334-341.
4. Godkin, A. J.; De Belder, A. J.; Villa, L.; Wong, A.; Beesley, J. E.; Kane, S. P.; Martin, J. F. *Eur. J. Clin. Invest.* **1996**, *26*, 867-872.
5. Fukutake, M.; Nakatsugi, S.; Isoi, T.; Takahashi, M.; Ohta, T.; Mamiya, S.; Taniguchi, Y.; Sato, H.; Fukuda, K.; Sugimura, T.; Wakabayashi, K. *Carcinogenesis* **1998**, *19*, 1939-1942.
6. Rao, C. V.; Kawamori, T.; Hamid, R.; Reddy, B. S. *Carcinogenesis* **1999**, *20*, 641-644.
7. Kawamori, T.; Takahashi, M.; Watanabe, K.; Ohta ,T.; Nakatsugi, S.; Sugimura, T.; Wakabayashi, K. *Cancer Lett.* **2000**, *148*, 33-7.
8. Oshima, M.; Dinchuk, J. E.; Kargman, S. L.; Oshima, H.; Hancock, B.; Kwong, E.; Trzaskos, J. M.; Evans, J. F.; Taketo, M. M. *Cell* **1996**, *87*, 803-809.
9. Bruce, W. R.; Giacca, A.; Medline, A. *Cancer Epidemiol Biomarkers Prev.* **2000**, *9*, 1271-1279.
10. Mutoh, M.; Takahashi, M.; Fukuda, K.; Matsushima-Hibiya, Y.; Mutoh, H.; Sugimura, T.; Wakabayashi, K. *Carcinogenesis* **2000**, *21*, 959-63.
11. Mutoh, M.; Takahashi, M.; Fukuda, K.; Komatsu, H.; Enya, T.; Matsushima-Hibiya, Y.; Mutoh, H.; Sugimura, T.; Wakabayashi, K. *Jpn. J. Cancer Res.* **2000**, *91*, 686-691.
12. Sasahara, Y.; Mutoh, M.; Takahashi, M.; Fukuda, K.; Tanaka, N.; Sugimura, T.; Wakabayashi, K.; *Cancer Lett.* **2002**, *177*, 155-61.
13. Middleton, E. Jr.; Kandaswami, C. *Biochem. Pharmacol.* **1992**, *43*, 1167-1179.
14. Wattenberg, L. W. *Cancer Res.* **1992**, *52*, 2085S-2091S.
15. Akarasereenont, P.; Mitchell, J. A.; Appleton, I.; Thiemermann, C.; Vane, J. R. *Br. J. Pharmacol.* **1994**, *113*, 1522-1528.
16. Ferriola, P. C.; Cody, V.; Middleton, E. *Biochem. Pharmacol.* **1989**, *38*, 1617-1624.
17. Agullo, G.; Gamet-Payrastre, L.; Manenti, S.; Viala, C.; Remesy, C.; Chap, H.; Payrastre, B. *Biochem. Pharmacol.* **1997**, *53*, 1649-1657.

18. Rossi, M.; Rickles, L. F.; Halpin, W. A. *Bioorgan Chem.* **1986**, *14*, 55-69.
19. Dewar, M. J. S.; Zoebisch, E. G.; Healy, E. F.; Stewart, J. J. P. *J. Am. Chem. Soc.* **1985**, *107*, 3902-3909.
20. Segain, J. P.; Raingeard, de la Bletiere, D.; Bourreille, A.; Leray, V.; Gervois, N.; Rosales, C.; Ferrier, L.; Bonnet, C.; Blottiere, H. M.; Galmiche, J. P. *Gut.* **2000**, *47*, 397-403.

Chapter 10

Divergent Cytotoxic Effects of Conjugated Linoleic Acid Isomers on NCI-N87 Cells

Sook J. Park, Cherl W. Park, Seck J. Kim, Jung K. Kim, Young R. Kim, Young S. Kim, and Yeong L. Ha

Division of Applied Life Science, Graduate School, Institute of Agriculture and Life Sciences, Gyeongsang National University, Chinju 660–701, Korea

Cytotoxic effects of four conjugated linoleic acid (CLA) isomers (*trans*-10,*cis*-12 CLA; *cis*-9,*trans*-11 CLA; *trans*-10,*trans*-12 CLA; and *trans*-9,*trans*-11 CLA) were evaluated in NCI-N87 gastric cancer cells. NCI-N87 cells were incubated in serum-free medium with 20 μM CLA isomers and linoleic acid over a period of 6 days. All CLA isomers inhibited the proliferation of the cells, however, linoleic acid did not. Efficacy of *trans*-9,*trans*-11 CLA in inhibiting the cell proliferation was similar to that of *trans*-10,*trans*-12 CLA and was much higher than that of *trans*-10,*cis*-12 CLA or *cis*-9,*trans*-11 CLA. These results indicate that cytotoxicity of *trans*-9,*trans*-11 and *trans*-10,*trans*-12 CLA (designated *trans*/*trans* CLA) isomers for NCI-N87 cells was stronger than that of their corresponding *cis*-9,*trans*-11 CLA or *trans*-10,*cis*-12 CLA (designated *cis*/*trans* CLA) isomers.

Conjugated linoleic acid (CLA) is a collective term for positional (9,11 and 10,12) and geometric (*trans,cis*; *cis,trans*; *cis,cis*; and *trans,trans*) isomers of octadecadienoic acid (C18:2) with a conjugated double bond. Synthetic CLA, prepared from linoleic acid by alkaline isomerization, exhibits potent anticarcinogenic activities in several carcinogen-induced animal models (*1-4*) and cytotoxicities for several cancer cell lines (*5-8*). Other biological activities, such as immune stimulation (*9*), body fat reduction (*10,11*), modulation of cholesterol content (*12*) and growth stimulation (*13*) were also reported.

Predominant CLA isomers in the synthetic CLA are *trans*-10,*cis*-12 CLA and *cis*-9,*trans*-11 CLA; small amounts of *trans*-10,*trans*-12 CLA and *trans*-9,*trans*-11 CLA isomers also occur. There is evidence that CLA isomers exhibit different biological activities in an animal study; Park et al. reported that the *trans*-10,*cis*-12 CLA isomer is more effective for the reduction of mice body fat than the *cis*-9,*trans*-11 CLA isomer (*14*). However, to date, most studies were accomplished with this CLA isomer mixture, but the activity of each isomer was not well understood.

In the present study we examined the cytotoxic effects of four CLA isomers (*trans*-10,*cis*-12; *cis*-9,*trans*-11; *trans*-10,*trans*-12 and *trans*-9,*trans*-11 CLA) on NCI-N87 cells.

MATERIALS AND METHODS

Reagents

Linoleic acid and 3-(4,5-dimethylthiazol-2-yl)-2,5-diphenyltetrazolium bromide (MTT) were obtained from Sigma Chemical Co. (St. Louis, MO). Dulbeccos Modified Eagle's Medium/Hams F-12 nutrient mixture (DMEM/F12) containing 2 μM linoleic acid, fetal bovine serum (FBS), trypsin-EDTA, penicillin-streptomycin, selenium and transferrin were purchased from Gibco BRL (Rockville, MD). Other chemicals used were of reagent grade.

Synthesis of CLA Mixture

CLA, mainly composed of 47% *trans*-10,*cis*-12 CLA and 45% *cis*-9,*trans*-11 CLA, was synthesized from linoleic acid by alkaline isomerization and methylated with 4% sulfuric acid/methanol solution as described by Park et al.

(*15*). A round bottom flask (3 L) containing ethylene glycol (1 L) was maintained at 190 °C for 10 min, followed by cooling down to 165 °C. After carefully adding KOH (250 g) to the round bottom flask, the bottle was heated to 180 °C. The linoleic acid (500 mL) was slowly added and maintained at 180 °C with frequent swirling. One hour later the reactant was cooled to room temperature by a string of running tap water. All of the steps were performed under nitrogen. Methanol (500 mL) and 6N HCl (1 L) were added to the reactant in order. Synthetic CLA was extracted with hexane (500 mL x 2) and washed with distilled water (250 mL x 3). The hexane extract was dried over anhydrous Na_2SO_4. Synthetic CLA was obtained by removing the hexane solvent under vacuum.

Preparation of Individual CLA Isomers

The *trans*-10,*cis*-12 or *cis*-9,*trans*-11 CLA-Me isomer fraction was separated from the synthetic CLA-Me in acetone (100 g/1200 mL) by low-temperature precipitation at -68 °C and -71 °C. These fractions were refluxed in acetone (1200 mL) containing urea (100 g) for 2 hrs and then crystallized at 4 °C over night (*16*). The purified *trans*-10,*cis*-12 and *cis*-9,*trans*-11 CLA-Me isomer fractions were saponified by conventional method, followed by isomerizing to their corresponding *trans,trans* isomers by methylation in a boiling water bath for 30 min with 14% BF_3/methanol. The *trans*-10,*trans*-12 and *trans*-9,*trans*-11 CLA-Me fractions recovered by conventional method were further purified by both low-temperature precipitation at -68 °C and urea treatment described by Kim et al. (*16*) and Park et al. (*17*).

Analysis of CLA-Me Isomers

The purity of CLA isomers was analyzed by GC (Hewlett Packard 5890, Avondale, PA) equipped with a flame ionization detector (FID) and a Supelcowax-10 capillary column (60 m x 0.32 mm, i.d., 25 μ film thickness). The carrier gas used was N_2. The oven temperature was increased from 170 °C to 200 °C at a rate of 2 °C/min. The injector and detector temperatures were 240 °C and 260 °C, respectively. The percentage of individual CLA isomers was calculated by the peak area ratio of a given CLA-Me isomer to that of total CLA-Me isomers (Hewlett Packard 3396 Series III, Avondale, PA). CLA-Me isomers of samples were identified by comparison with the relative retention time of standard CLA-Me isomers and by the reported method of Ha et al. (*1*). The purity of *trans,trans* CLA-Me isomer fractions was analyzed by Ag^+-HPLC (Young-Lin M930 solvent delivery system; Anyang,

Korea), equipped with a UV detector (M720) and ChromSpher 5 analytical silver-impregnated column (4.6 mm i.d. x 250 mm stainless steel; 5 μ particle size; Chrompack, Bridgewater, NJ). The wavelength of the UV used was 233 nm. The mobile phase was 0.1% acetonitrile in hexane and operated isocratically at a flow rate of 1.0 mL/min by the report of Sehat et al. (*18*). Composition of *trans,trans* CLA-Me isomers was calculated by the area ratio of individual isomers.

Cytotoxicity Assay

The NCI-N87 cells were maintained in DMEM/F12 medium supplemented with 10% FBS, 100 units/ml penicillin and 100 μg/mL streptomycin in a CO_2 incubator (5% CO_2 and 95% air, 37 °C). The cells (5×104 cells/1 mL/well) were incubated in a 12-well plate for 24 hrs, followed by replacing the DMEM/F12 medium with serum-free DMEM/F12 medium (SFM) containing 5 μg/mL transferrin and 5 ng/mL selenium. Twenty-four hours later, the medium was replaced again with SFM alone or SFM containing each CLA isomer or linoleic acid, a positive control agent, at a concentration of 20 μM. The incubation was continued over a period of 6 days. The number of cells was determined every two days by MTT assay (*19*).

Results and Discussion

The purity of *trans*-10,*cis*-12, *cis*-9,*trans*-11, *trans*-10,*trans*-12 and *trans*-9,trans-11 CLA-Me isomers used was 99.0, 90.3, 95.0 and 96.0%, respectively, when analyzed by GC (*20*). The purity of *trans*-10,*cis*-12 and *cis*-9,*trans*-11 CLA-Me fractions separated from the synthetic CLA in acetone at -68 °C and then -71 °C was 92.5 and 87.3%, respectively, but the purity was further increased to 99.0 and 90.3%, respectively, by urea treatment. Impurities, such as saturated fatty acids, oleic acid, oxidation by-products, *trans,trans*-CLA isomers and *cis,cis*-CLA isomers, were easily removed from the *trans*-10,*cis*-12 CLA-Me fraction by urea treatment, but not from the *cis*-9,*trans*-11 CLA-Me fraction. Interestingly, the *trans*-10,*trans*-12 or *trans*-9,*trans*-11 CLA-Me fraction was not a single compound, but contained a mixture of positional isomers of *trans,trans* CLA-Me, when analyzed by Ag^+-HPLC. The *trans*-10,*trans*-12 CLA-Me fraction contained 2.8% *trans*-12,*trans*-14, 14.9% *trans*-11,*trans*-13, 34.3% *trans*-10,*trans*-12, 33.8% *trans*-9,*trans*-11, 11.6% *trans*-8,*trans*-10, and 2.6% *trans*-7,*trans*-9 CLA-Me, whereas the *trans*-9,*trans*-11 CLA-Me contained 1.5% *trans*-12,*trans*-14, 10.2% *trans*-11,*trans*-13, 33.8% *trans*-10, *trans*-12, 38.5% *trans*-9,*trans*-11, 13.8% *trans*-8,*trans*-10, and 2.2% *trans*-7,*trans*-9 CLA-Me.

Linoleic acid (20 μM) treatment enhanced the proliferation of NCI-N87 cells relative to control. This effect was maximized by 4 days of incubation (142% of control).

In contrast, all CLA isomers tested significantly inhibited the proliferation of the cells over a period of 6 days. The efficacy of *trans*-9, *trans*-11 CLA on inhibition was very similar to that of *trans*-10,*trans*-12 CLA, but much higher than that of *trans*-10,*cis*-12 CLA or *cis*-9,*trans*-11 CLA. No significant difference was seen in the efficacy of *trans*-10,*cis*-12 CLA from that of *cis*-9,*trans*-11 CLA. At day 6, the proliferation rate of the cells treated with 20 μM *trans*-10,*trans*-12 CLA or *trans*-9,*trans*-11 CLA isomer was found to be 83% (17% inhibition) and 62% (38% inhibition), respectively, relative to control. These results suggest that the CLA isomers showed a divergent cytotoxicity against NCI-N87 cells; *trans/trans* isomers exhibited a stronger effect than their corresponding *cis/trans* isomers. Many studies have shown that a mixture of CLA isomers inhibits the growth of human cancer cells (*5-8*), but they did not clarify the inhibitory activity of individual CLA isomers.

The mechanistic action of anti-proliferative activity of the mixture of CLA isomers is poorly understood. However, it is, in part, attributed to the alterations in eicosanoid metabolism (*21*) and/or peroxidation of CLA (*7*). We believe that eicosanoid metabolism is more strongly altered by *trans/trans* CLA isomers than *cis/trans* CLA isomers. The chemical structure of *trans/trans* CLA isomers closely resembles the straight chain of stearic acid, which is, in turn, preferentially incorporated into the SN-2 position of membrane phospholipids. This might inhibit the process of elongation and desaturation of linoleic acid required for the biosynthesis of arachidonic acid, and thus, alter the eicosanoid metabolisms and/or inhibiting phospholipaseA_2 activity. Further research looking for the mechanistic action of anti-proliferative activity of individual CLA isomers is under way.

Acknowledgements

This study was supported by a grant from KOSEF (2000-1-22000-001-3) .

References

1. Ha, Y.L.; Grimm, N.K.; Pariza, M.W. *Carcinogenesis* **1987**, *8*, 1881-1887.
2. Ha, Y.L.; Strokson, M.; Pariza, M.W. *Cancer Res.* **1990**, *50*, 1097-1101.
3. Ip, C.; Jiang, C.; Thompson, H.J.; Scimeca, J.A. *Carcinogenesis* **1997**, *18*, 755-759.

4. Liew, C.; Schut, H.A.J.; Chin, S.F.; Pariza, M.W.; Dashwood, R.H. *Carcinogenesis* **1995**, *16*, 3037-3043.
5. Cunningham, D.C.; Harrison, L.Y.; Shultz, T.D. *Anticancer Res.* **1997**, *17*, 197-204.
6. Durgam, V.R.; Fernandes, G. *Cancer Letters* **1997**, *116*, 121-130.
7. Schonberg, S.; Krokan, H.E. *Anticancer Res.* **1995**, *15*, 1241-1246.
8. Shultz, T.D; Chew, B.P.; Seaman, W.R. *Anticancer Res.* **1992**, *12*, 2143-2146.
9. Cook, M.E.; Miller, C.C.; Park, Y.; Pariza, M.W. *Poultry Sci.* **1993**, *72*, 1301-1305.
10. Park, Y.; Albright, K.J.; Liu, W.; Storkson, J.M.; Cook, M.E.; Pariza, M.W. *Lipids* **1997**, *32*, 853-858.
11. Thom, E. A *Pilot study with the aim of studying the efficiency and tolerability of Tonalin CLA on the body composition in humans*, Medstat Res. Ltd., Oslo, Norway, **1997**, 1-5.
12. Lee, K.N.; Kritchevsky, D.; Pariza, M.W. *Arteriosclerosis* **1994**, *108*, 19-25.
13. Chin, S.F.; Storkson, J.M.; Albright, K.J.; Cook, M.E.; Pariza, M.W. *J. Nutr.* **1994**, *124*, 2344-2349.
14. Park, Y.; Storkson, J.M.; Albright, K.J.; Liu, W.; Cook, M.E.; Pariza, M.W. *Lipids* **1999**, *34*, 235-241.
15. Park, C.W.; Park, S.J.; Kim, S.J.; Kim, J.K.; Kim, Y.R.; Park, K.A.; Kim, J.O.; Ha, Y.L. *J. Agric. Food Chem.* (accepted).
16. Kim, Y.R.; Lee, Y.H.; Park, K.A.; Kim, J.O.; Ha, Y.L. *Kor. J. Food Sci. Nutri.* **2000**, *5*, 10-14.
17. Park, S.J.; Kim, S.J.; Kim, J.K.; Kim, Y.R.; Park, G.B.; Shim, K.H.; Kim, J.O.; Ha, Y.L. *Lipids* (submitted).
18. Sehat, N.; Rickert, R.; Mossoba, M. M.; Kramer, J. K. G.; Yurawecz, M. P.; Roach, J. A. G.; Adlof, R. O.; Morehouse, K. M.; Fritsche, J.; Eulitz, K. D.; Steinhart, H.; Ku, Y. *Lipids* **1999**, *34*, 407-413.
19. Denizot, F.; Lang, R. *J. Immunological Methods* **1986**, *89*, 271-277.
20. Kim, S.J.; Park, K.A.; Park, J.H.Y.; Kim, J.O.; Ha, Y.L. *J. Food Sci. Nutr.* **2000**, *5*, 86-92.
21. Merrill, A.H. Jr.; Schroeder, J.J. *Annu. Rev. Nutr.* **1993**, *13*, 539-559.

Chapter 11

Green Tea Extracts Prevent the Dioxin Toxicity through the Suppression of Transformation of the Aryl Hydrocarbon Receptor

Itsuko Fukuda[1], Atsushi Kaneko[1], Yoshiyuki Yabushita[1], Iwao Sakane[2], Takami Kakuda[2], Kazuki Kanazawa[1], Gen-ichi Danno[1], and Hitoshi Ashida[1,*]

[1]Department of Biofunctional Chemistry, Faculty of Agriculture, Kobe University, Kobe 657–8501, Japan
[2]Central Research Institute, Ito En, Ltd., Shizuoka 421–0516, Japan

2,3,7,8-Tetrachlorodibenzo-*p*-dioxin (TCDD), the most toxic compound of dioxins expresses toxicities such as teratogenesis, immunosuppression, body weight loss, and cancer promotion through transformation of the aryl hydrocarbon receptor (AhR). To investigate whether tea components suppress transformation of AhR, rat hepatic cytosol fraction was treated with green tea components followed by addition of TCDD. Transformed AhR was detected by an electrophoretic mobility shift assay with a double-strand oligonucleotide probe corresponding to dioxin responsive element. The ethyl acetate- and the hexane-partitioned fractions from green tea extracts blocked AhR transformation dose-dependently. The active components in the ethyl acetate-partitioned fraction were flavonoids. The hexane-partitioned fraction contained sterols, chlorophylls, pheophytins and carotenoids. Chlorophylls and lutein, one of the carotenoids, suppressed transformation of AhR effectively. These results suggest that drinking green tea, which contains various suppressive compounds on transformation of AhR, would reduce the dioxin toxicity.

Introduction

Environmental contaminants, polyhalogenated aryl hydrocarbons (PAHs) such as polychlorinated dibenzo-*p*-dioxins, polychlorinated dibenzofurans and coplanar polychlorinated biphenyls are serious health concern, because of their toxicities and relics in our body. PAHs express toxicities such as teratogenesis, immunosuppression, body weight loss, and cancer promotion through transformation of the aryl hydrocarbon receptor (AhR); PAHs bind to a cytosolic AhR, and after transformed AhR translocates to nucleus with AhR nuclear translocator (Arnt), AhR/Arnt complex binds to the specific enhancer element, called dioxin responsive element (DRE) (*1*, *2*). The binding of transformed AhR to DRE sequences, various genes exist in downstream region, for example, one of the drug metabolizing enzymes, cytochrome P4501A (CYP1A) is accelerated to express. CYP1A protein activates other procarcinogenic compounds as heterocyclic amines and makes them ultimate carcinogens (*3*). The toxicity of dioxins is correlated with their affinities to AhR, and the most toxic compound is 2,3,7,8-tetrachlorodibenzo-*p*-dioxin (TCDD) (*4*). It is difficult to suppress transformation of AhR by certain drugs, because dioxins invade our body mainly with diet unexpectedly. Although their toxicities differ among species and sexes (*5*, *6*), suppression by food components expects the reduction of their toxicities.

It has been reported that some synthetic and natural flavonoids act as antagonists for AhR, and suppress its transformation (*7-11*). Here, we focused on green tea, because it contains abundant flavonoids and they have a habit of drinking green tea through or after meal in Japan. Green tea possesses many beneficial effects, i.e., anti-tumor effects, anti-oxidative effects, among others. Recently report (*12*) showed that green tea extracts suppressed CYP1A gene expression, and this means catechins act as antagonists for AhR. However, our previous study (*7*) demonstrated suppressive effects of catechins on transformation of AhR were weak. In this study, we, therefore, investigated that which components in green tea can suppress transformation of AhR under the *in vitro* system using rat hepatic cytosol.

Materials and Methods

Extraction and Fractionation of Green Tea Leaves

Green tea leaves (*camellia sinensis*) were obtained from Shizuoka prefecture in Japan, and tea leaves (*Sen-cha*, 500 g) were extracted with 3 L of 75% ethanol two times, and the extracts were lyophilized and used as the ethanol extracts. The ethanol extracts were suspended in 1 L of distilled water and partitioned stepwise with *n*-hexane, chloroform, ethyl acetate, and *n*-butanol, 2 L each 3 times and each fraction was collected and lyophilized (Figure 1). The *n*-hexane-partitioned fraction was subjected to a centrifugal liquid-liquid partition chromatography (Sanki LLB-M, Tokyo, Japan) in *n*-hexane-90% ethanol (1:1, v/v), and separated to 13 fractions. Partition was performed under the following conditions: mobile phase, 120 mL of 90% ethanol following 240 mL of *n*-hexane; centrifugation at 1,200 rpm; and flow rate of 3 mL/min. A portion of the same volume of each fraction was applied on a thin-layer chromatography (TLC) plate (silica gel, 0.25 mm thick, 60 F_{254}; Merck, Germany), and separated with chloroform-methanol (50:1, v/v). Separated bands were scraped off and extracted with suitable solvent. Compounds in each band were identified using NMR.

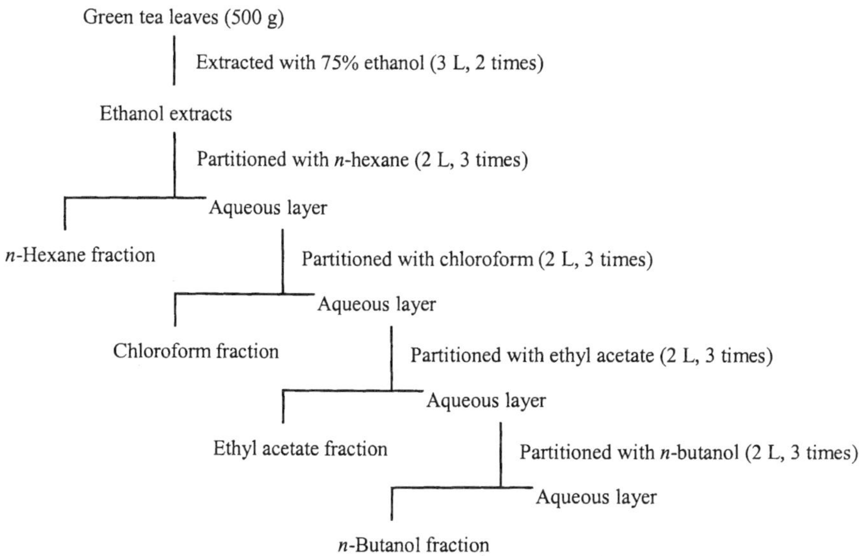

Figure 1. Extraction and fractionation of green tea leaves.

Assessment of Suppressive Effects of Green Tea Extracts

The rat hepatic cytosol fraction was prepared as described previously (*7*). The cytosol fraction (4.0 mg/ml protein) was incubated with various concentrations of green tea extracts 10 min prior to addition of 1 nM TCDD (AccuStandard, New Heaven, CT, USA) at 20°C for 2 h to lead transformation of AhR. Transformed AhR was detected by electrophoretic mobility shift assay (EMSA) using a ^{32}P-labeled dioxin responsive element (DRE) oligonucleotide probe as described previously (*7*).

Results

To investigate the effects of green tea components on transformation of AhR by TCDD, green tea leaves were extracted with 75% ethanol as shown in Figure 1. The suppressive effects of the ethanol extracts on transformation of AhR were first examined. The ethanol extracts completely suppressed TCDD-induced transformation at 400 μg/ml, and did not cause the transformation of AhR themselves (Figure 2).

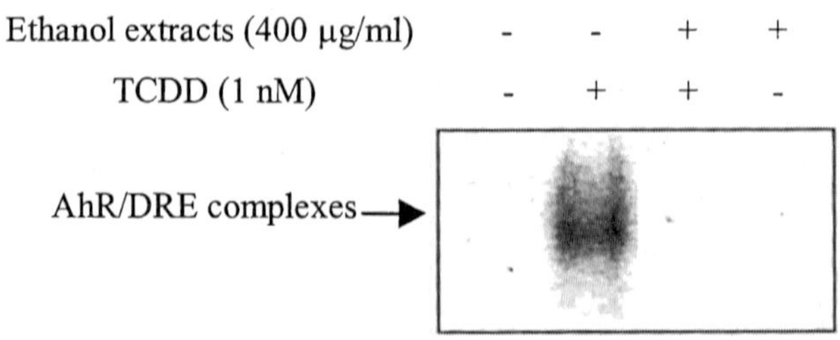

Figure 2. The ethanol extracts from green tea suppressed transformation of AhR. The rat hepatic cytosol fraction was incubated with ethanol extracts (400 μg/ml) and TCDD (1 nM) at 20°C for 2 h. Transformed AhR was detected by EMSA using ^{32}P-labeled DRE. Arrow indicates the specific bands of AhR/DRE complexes.

The ethanol extracts were separated to 5 fractions by partition with various solvents as described in Materials and Methods. Obtained fractions were subjected to EMSA to survey the most suppressive fraction. All of the fractions decreased transformation of AhR by TCDD (Figure 3). Particularly, the *n*-hexane- and the ethyl acetate-partitioned fractions effectively suppressed it to the control levels.

The main components in the ethyl acetate-partitioned fraction are flavonoids. The suppressive effects of flavonoids on transformation of AhR were already demonstrated using authentic compounds, and catechins showed weaker effects than flavones and flavonols (*7*). Thus, it is suggested that the suppressive compounds in the ethyl acetate-partitioned fraction are flavones and flavonols. The *n*-hexane-partitioned fraction contained a lot of pigments such as chlorophylls, pheophytins, carotenoids and so on. Which components in the *n*-hexane fraction could suppress transformation of AhR was further investigated. A portion of the same volume of the *n*-hexane-partitioned fractions was separated with TLC as described in Materials, and detected visible compounds (Figure 4A). The suppressive effects of obtained 13 fractions on the transformation were examined (Figure 4B). Fraction-7, -8 and -9 contained rich pigments and completely suppressed transformation of AhR at 5 μg/ml.

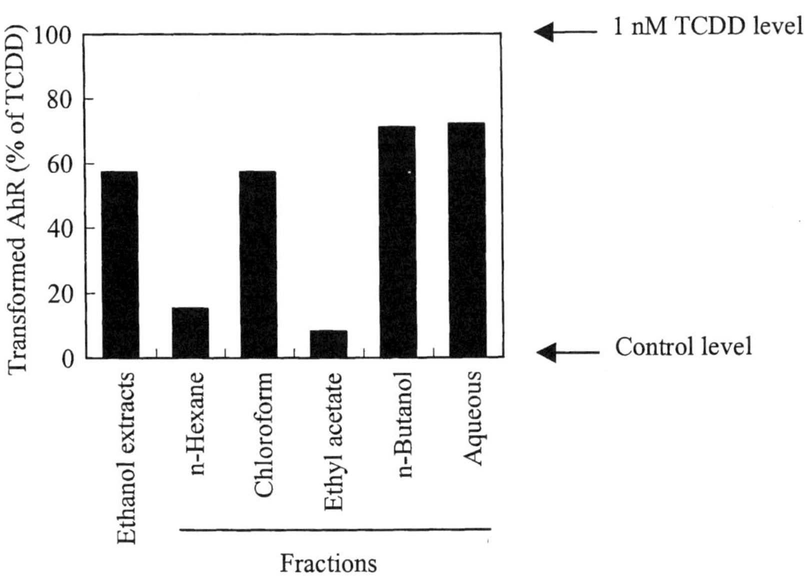

Figure 3. Suppressive effects of green tea extracts and partitioned fractions on transformation of AhR. The rat cytosol fraction was incubated with partitioned fractions (100 μg/ml each) and TCDD (1 nM). Transformed AhR was detected by EMSA. Density of the specific bands were analyzed and calculated as % of TCDD-treated ones.

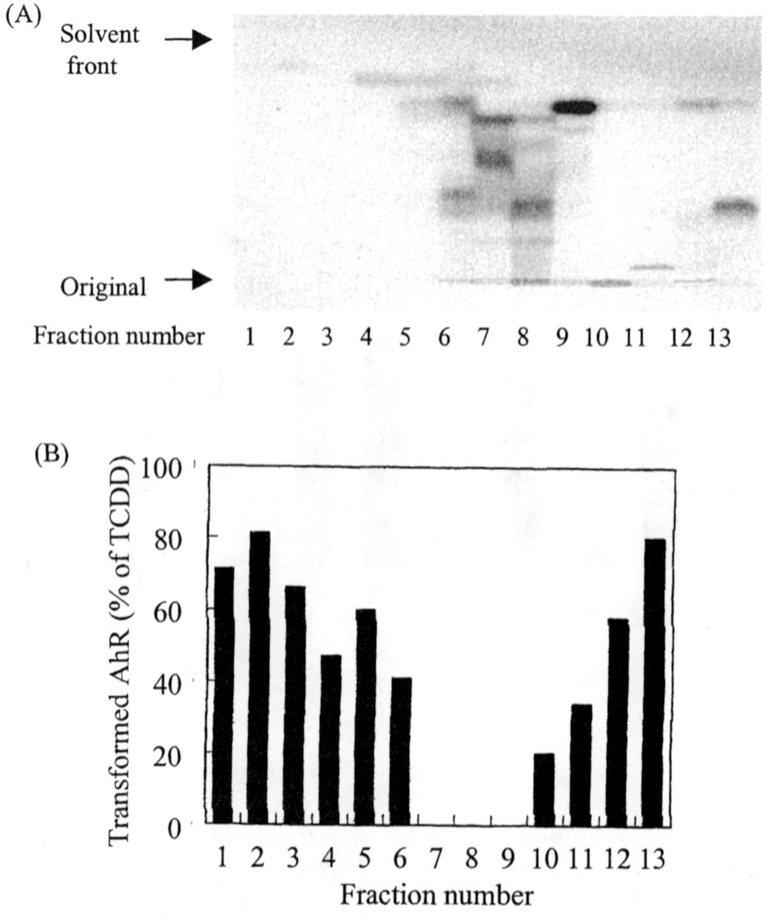

Figure 4. Suppressive effects of the n-hexane fractions on transformation of AhR. The n-hexane fraction was separated by centrifugal partition chromatography as shown in Materials and Methods and obtained 13 fractions. (A) Obtained fractions were separated by TLC as described in Materials. (B) The cytosol was incubated with these fractions (5 μg/ml) and TCDD (1 nM). Transformed AhR was detected by EMSA. Density of the specific bands were analyzed and calculated as % of TCDD-treated ones.

From these fractions, chlorophylls, pheophytins, sterols and carotenoids were identified (data not shown), and the suppressive effects of identified compounds on transformation of AhR by TCDD were examined by EMSA as shown in Table. Chlorophylls showed a strong suppressive effect, though pheophytins showed weak effects. Since both chlorophylls and pheophytins have porphyrin rings, the structure of the rings may not be associated with their suppressive effects. Regarding carotenoids contained in fraction-7, -8 and -9, lutein suppressed effectively, while sterols and carotenes did not affect.

Table I. The Compounds in the *n*-Hexane Fraction and their Effects on Transformation of AhR

Compounds	*Suppressive effect*
Chlorophylls	strong
Pheophytins	weak
Sterols	negative
Carotenes	negative
Lutein	strong

The compounds identified from the *n*-hexane fraction-7, -8 and -9, and their suppressive effects were examined at various concentrations against 1 nM TCDD. Transformed AhR was detected by EMSA, and the 50% inhibitory concentration (IC_{50} value) of compounds against TCDD-induced transformation was determined. Strong, IC_{50} value 5 μM; weak, 5 < IC_{50} value 50 μM; negative, 50 μM < IC_{50} value

Discussion

Green tea extracts, especially, the *n*-hexane- and the ethyl acetate-partitioned fractions suppressed transformation of AhR effectively (Figure 3). The ethyl acetate-partitioned fraction contains mainly polyphenols such as catechins, flavonols and flavones. Our previous report (*7*) demonstrated that flavones and flavonols suppress transformation of AhR at their dietary levels, but catechins did not. These results suggest that effective compounds in the ethyl acetate-partitioned fraction on the suppression of the transformation are flavones and flavonols. On the other hand, effective compounds in the *n*-hexane-partitioned fraction have been unknown yet. In the present study, certain pigments also suppressed transformation of AhR.

We identified several compounds from the *n*-hexane fraction (Table). Especially, chlorophylls and lutein showed suppressive effects. These pigments are widely distributed among vegetables and fruits, and can be obtained easily from plant-based diet. Chlorophylls have been considered not to be absorbed in our body and excreted as pheophytins. However recently, it was reported that chlorophyll derivatives incorporates into Caco-2 cells (*13*). Moreover, bilirubin can directly induce CYP1A1 gene expression through transformation of AhR (*14*). These reports indicate the possibility that chlorophylls and their metabolites may at least in part, incorporate into the body and act as the antagonists for AhR. Regarding lutein, this compound is absorbed in our bodies (*13*, *15*, *16*), and some carotenoids induce CYP1A gene expression (*17*, *18*). Therefore, chlorophylls and lutein are effective compounds in green tea to suppress transformation of AhR.

Green tea leaves contain effective compounds such as flavones, flavonols, chlorophylls, and lutein on the suppression of transformation of AhR induced by TCDD. Drinking green tea or eating tea leaves positively may increase the physiological concentration of these compounds in our body and prevent the toxicity of dioxins, which invade our body unexpectedly.

References

1. Rowlands J. C.; Gustafsson J. A. *Crit. Rev. Toxicol.*, **1997**, 27, 109-134
2. Safe S. H. *Crit. Rev. Toxicol.*, **1994**, 24, 87-149
3. Code E. L.; Crespi C. L.; Penman B. W.; Gonzalez F. J.; Chang T. K.; Waxman D. J. *Drug. Metab. Dispos.*, **1997**, 25, 985-993
4. Heid S. E.; Walker M. K.; Swanson H. I. *Toxicol. Sci.*, **2001**, 61, 187-196
5. Vanden Heuvel J. P.; Lucier G. *Environ. Health Perspect.*, **1993**, 100, 189-200
6. Enan E.; Overstreet J. W.; Matsumura F.; VandeVoort C. A.; Lasley B. L. *Reprod. Toxicol.*, **1996**, 10, 401-411
7. Ashida H.; Fukuda I.; Yamashita T.; Kanazawa K. *FEBS Lett.*, **2000**, 476, 213-217
8. Dertinger S. D.; Nazarenko D. A.; Silverstone A. E.; Gasiewicz T. A. *Carcinogenesis*, **2001**, 22, 171-177
9. Guo M.; Joiakim A.; Reiners J. J. Jr. *Biochem. Pharmacol.*, **2000**, 60, 635-642
10. Reiners J. J. Jr.; Lee J. Y.; Clift R. E.; Dudley D. T.; Myrand S. P. *Mol. Pharmaxol.*, **1998**, 53, 438-445
11. Ciolino H. P.; Yeh G. C. *Br. J. Cancer*, **1999**, 79, 1340-1346
12. Williams S. N.; Shih H.; Guenette D. K.; Brackney W.; Denison M. S.; Pickwell G. V.; Quattrochi L. C. *Chem.-Biol. Interact.*, **2000**, 128, 211-229
13. Ferruzzi M. G.; Failla M. L.; Schwartz S. J. *J. Agric. Food Chem.*, **2001**, 49, 2082-2089
14. Sinal C. J.; Bend J. R. *Mol. Pharmacol.*, **1997**, 52, 590-599

15. O'Neill M. E.; Thurnham D. I. *Br. J. Nutr.*, **1998**, 79, 149-159
16. Krinsky N. I.; Russett M. D.; Handelman G. J.; Snodderly D. M. *J. Nutr.*, **1990**, 120, 1654-1662
17. Gradelet S.; Astorg P.; Pineau T.; Canivenc M. C.; Siess M. H.; Leclerc J.; Lesca P. *Biochem. Pharmacol.*, **1997**, 54, 307-315
18. Gradelet S.; Leclerc J.; Siess M. H.; Astorg P. O. *Xenobiotica.*, **1996**, 26, 909-919

Chapter 12

Preventive Effects of Food Components on Caspase-8-Mediated Apoptosis Induced by Dietary Carcinogen, Trp-P-1, in Rat Mononuclear Cells

Takashi Hashimoto[1], Wakana Ito[2], Takashi Furuyashiki[2], Takashi Sano[2], Ken-ichiro Minato[3], Masashi Mizuno[1], Kazuki Kanazawa[1], Gen-ichi Danno[1,2], and Hitoshi Ashida[1,2,*]

[1]Division of Life Science, Graduate School of Science and Technology and [2]Department of Biofunctional Chemistry, Faculty of Agriculture, Kobe University, Nada-ku, Kobe 657–8501, Japan
[3]Miyagi Agricultural College, Sendai 982–1125, Japan

3-Amino-1,4-dimethyl-5*H*-pyrido[4,3-*b*]indole (Trp-P-1), a contaminant in diet, induces apoptosis in immunocytes such as splenocytes and thymocytes. In rat mononuclear cells (MNCs), Trp-P-1 also induces apoptosis, in which caspase-8 dominated the caspase cascade. Since Trp-P-1-induced apoptosis in immunocytes may be led to immunodeficiency, it is important for a living body to prevent the apoptosis. Although Trp-P-1 increased the generation of reactive oxygen species, both ascorbic acid and α-tocophrol did not inhibite the apoptosis. This indicates that the induction of apoptosis was not mediated through reactive oxygen species. On the other hand, certain food components such as dopamine, myricetin, robinetin, delphinidin, pyrogallol, and gallic acid inhibited Trp-P-1-induced apoptosis. Thus, these food components in our dairy diet may prevent chemical-induced cytotoxicity in immunocytes.

Introduction

3-Amino-1,4-dimethyl-5*H*-pyrido[4,3-*b*]indole (Trp-P-1) is a tryptophan pyrolysate and formed in cooked meat and fish. For example, the broiled beef contains 0.21 ng/g in Trp-P-1, and sardine 13 ng/g (*1, 2*). This compound is known as a potent carcinogen in the liver of rodents (*3*). According to the *in vivo* study, administrated Trp-P-1 was detectable in plasma for longer than 3 weeks (*4*) and detected in various kinds of tissues including the liver, spleen and thymus (*5*). Thus, Trp-P-1 is considered to be absorbed in and transported to various tissues through blood and lymph. We have demonstrated that Trp-P-1 induces apoptosis in rat hepatocytes (*6-8*), splenocytes and thymocytes (*9*). Our recent study showed Trp-P-1 also induced apoptosis in mononuclear cells (MNCs; including lymphocytes and monocytes) from rats and human peripheral blood (*10*).

Apoptosis is characterized by morphological and biochemical changes (*11*), and mediated through caspase cascade, in which either caspse-8 or -9 is initially activated by death receptor- and mitochondria-mediated pathway, respectively. Apoptosis plays an important role in maintaining homeostasis, and it is achieved through cytokines and cell communications, and changes in intracellular conditions during embryogenesis, metamorphosis, normal tissue turnover, thymic selection, and cell-mediated cytotoxicity (*12-14*). In such cases, apoptosis is works as a programmed cell death. On the other hand, apoptosis as the cytotoxicity, which is not programmed, is induced by many chemicals. For example, etoposide, an anticancer drug induces cytotoxic apoptosis in normal thymocytes as the side effect of the pharmaceutical action against cancer (*15*). Trp-P-1-induced apoptosis is also considered to be a cytotoxic action to immunocytes, and the excess apoptosis may cause diseases including immunodeficiency.

Certain natural compounds possess anti-apoptotic effects. For example, ascorbic acid and α-tocopherol prevent apoptosis caused by serum withdrawal in HL-60 cells with the antioxidative effects (*16*). Caffeic acid inhibits ceramide-induced apoptosis in U937 cells through the inhibition of protein tyrosine kinase activity (*17*). Quercetin inhibits hydrogen peroxide-induced apoptosis via intervention in the activator protein 1 (AP-1) -mediated apoptotic pathway (*18*). Epigallocatechin-3-gallate and theaflavins inhibits arsenite-induced apoptosis through the decrease in phosphorylation of Erks and JNKs (*19*). Therefore, it is important to know whether these natural compounds show inhibitory effects on Trp-P-1-induced apoptosis. In this study, we demonstrated that Trp-P-1 induced caspase-8-initiated apoptosis in rat MNCs, and that certain food components inhibited Trp-P-1-induced apoptosis.

Materials and Methods

Materials

Trp-P-1 acetate form was purchased from Wako Pure Chemical Industries (Osaka, Japan) and dissolved in 20 mM in dimethyl sulfoxide (DMSO). Peptide inhibitors of caspases, acetyl (Ac)-IETD-aldehyde (CHO) and Ac-LEHD-CHO against caspase-8 and caspase-9, respectively, were purchased from Peptide Institute (Osaka, Japan), ascorbic acid and α-tocopherol were from Nacalai Tesque (Kyoto, Japan), and trolox were from Sigma Chemicals (St. Louis, MO). For the screening anti-apoptotic food factors, the following compounds were used; catechins from Kurita Kogyo (Tokyo, Japan), dopamine from Nacalai Tesque, myricetin, robinetin and delphinidin from Extrasynthese (Genay, France), and pyrogallol and gallic acid from Wako Pure Chemical Industries. All other chemicals were of the highest quality commercially available.

Preparation and Culture of Rat Mononuclear Cells

All animal treatment in this study conformed to the "Guidelines for the care and use of experimental animals, in Rokkodai Campus, Kobe University". Mononuclear cells were prepared from male Wistar rats (7 to 8 weeks old; Japan SLC, Shizuoka, Japan) and cultured at 1×10^6 cells/ml in RPMI 1640 medium (Nissui Pharmaceutical, Tokyo, Japan) containing 5% fetal bovine serum (Dainippon Pharmaceutical, Tokyo, Japan), 1 mM glutamine, and 1mg/ml kanamycin.

Assay for DNA Fragmentation

DNA fragmentation was measured according to the previous report (*9*).

Assay for Caspase Activity

Caspase activity was measured using fluorogenic tetrapeptide substrates as described previously (*9*). The substrates (Peptide Institute, Osaka, Japan) used were Ac-YVAD-methycoumarylamide (MCA) for caspase-1-like proteases, Ac-DEVD-MCA for caspase-3-like proteases, Ac-DMQD-MCA for caspase-3, Ac-

VEID-MCA for caspase-6, Ac-DQTD-MCA for caspase-7, Ac-IETD-MCA for caspase-8, and Ac-LEHD-MCA for caspse-9.

Measurement of ROS

Intracellular ROS was measured using 2',7'-dichlorofluorescein diacetate (DCFH-DA) as described previously (*20*). MNCs were pretreated with 100 μM DCFH-DA for 1 h, and treated with Trp-P-1 for another 1 h. The cells were twice washed with PBS, and formed 2',7'-dichlorofluorescein was spectrofluorometrically measured at excitation and emission wavelengths of 495 and 530 nm, respectively.

Screening of Anti-Apoptotic Food Components

In this study, 30 kinds of food components were subjected on the screening for the inhibition of Trp-P-1-induced apoptosis. MNCs were incubated with each food component in the medium for 1 h, followed by addition of 10 μM Trp-P-1. Anti-apoptotic action was evaluated as a suppressive effect of food components on DNA fragmentation.

Results and Discussion

Dietary Carcinogen, Trp-P-1 Induces Apoptosis in Mononuclear Cells

Dietary carcinogen, Trp-P-1, is considered to affect blood components, because orally administered Trp-P-1 was detected in plasma for, at least, 3 weeks (*4*). To investigate the effects of this compound on the cytotoxicity in immunocytes of blood, rat MNCs from blood, which mainly consist of lymphocytes and monocytes, were treated with 10 μM Trp-P-1 for 4 h. Trp-P-1 markedly increased DNA fragmentation characterizing apoptosis (Figure 1). In addition, this compound reduced cell viability time- and dose-dependently and caused apoptotic morphological changes such as cell shrinkage and nuclear fragmentation (data not shown). It is, therefore, suggested that intake of Trp-P-1 as a contaminant in diet may induce apoptosis in immunocytes of blood.

Trp-P-1 Activates Caspase-8 as An Apical Caspase

Cysteine proteases, caspases family, form an apoptotic signaling cascade, and play an important role in execution of apoptosis. However, caspase-1 and -4 in the family are not involved in the cascade directly and rather associated with inflammatory responses. Trp-P-1-induced apoptosis is mediated through the activation of caspase-3-like proteases (caspase-3 and -6) but not that of caspase-1-like proteases (caspase-1 and -4) in rat splenocytes and thymocytes (*9*) and in hepatocytes (*21*). In MNCs also, Trp-P-1 activated caspase-3-like proteases but not caspase-1-like proteases (Figure 2). Caspase cascade takes two pathways, i.e. death receptor- and mitochondria-dependent pathways: the former is dominated by caspase-8, and the latter is by caspase-9 (*22*). After either initiator caspase is activated, apoptotic executioners, caspase-3, -6, and -7 are activated, and these caspases activate or inactivate the intracellular substrates specifically (*23*). Caspase-3, -6, -7, -8, and -9 (Figure 3) were markedly activated in 10 μM Trp-P-1-treated MNCs (white bars) in comparison with the control cells (black bars) 3 h after treatment. Thus, Trp-P-1 activates most of caspases related with apoptosis. To investigate which initiator caspase-8 or -9 dominates Trp-P-1-induced apoptosis, cells were pretreated with 50 μM specific peptide inhibitor for caspase-8 (Ac-IETD-CHO) or caspase-9 (Ac-LEHD-CHO) for 1 h followed by treatment with 10 μM Trp-P-1 for another 3 h. Ac-IETD-CHO completely inhibited the activation of caspase-3, -6, -7, and -9 to the control level (dotted bars), although Ac-LEHD-CHO slightly suppressed caspase-3, -6, -7, and -8 (slashed bars). According to the time course experiments, the activities of caspase-3, -6, and -8 were induced time-dependently and reached to the maximum level at 3 h (Figure 4). Caspase-8 was significantly activated 1 h after treatment and followed by the activation of caspase-3 and -6. These results indicate that caspase-8 dominates other caspases in Trp-P-1-induced apoptosis.

ROS Is Not Involved in The Induction of Apoptosis, Though Trp-P-1 Increased Intracellular ROS

ROS mediates apoptosis induced by certain inducers such as cytokines, drugs and toxins, and so on; for example, tumor necrosis factor in human breast cancer MCF-7 cells (*24*), gallic acid in promyelocytic leukemia HL-60RG cells (*25*), endosulfan in human T-cell leukemia Jurkat T cells (*26*), dopamine and cyanide in PC12 cells (*27*), and 1-methyl-4-phenylpyridium ion in PC12 cells (*28*). Moreover, we reported that the intraperitoneally administration of Trp-P-1 into rats increased the level of thiobarbituric acid reactive substances, a common marker of lipid peroxidation, in the liver (*29*). The increase in ROS was investigated in MNCs using DCFH-DA 1 h after treatment when caspase-8 already activated. Trp-P-1 increases intracellular ROS in a dose-dependent manner (Figure 5). At 10 μM, an increase in ROS was not significant, though it

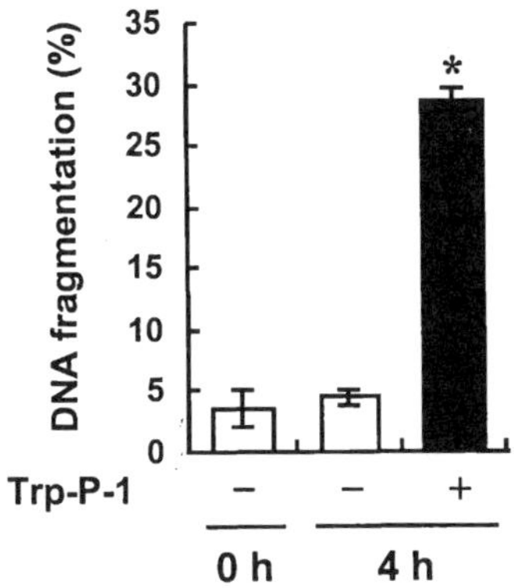

Figure 1. Trp-P-1 induces DNA fragmentation in rat MNCs. Rat MNCs were cultured with or without 15 μM Trp-P-1 for 4 h. DNA fragmentation was measured as described in Materials and Methods. Data represent the means ± S.D. of triplicate experiments. Asterisks indicate significant differences from 0 h-cells (Student's t-test, $P < 0.05$).

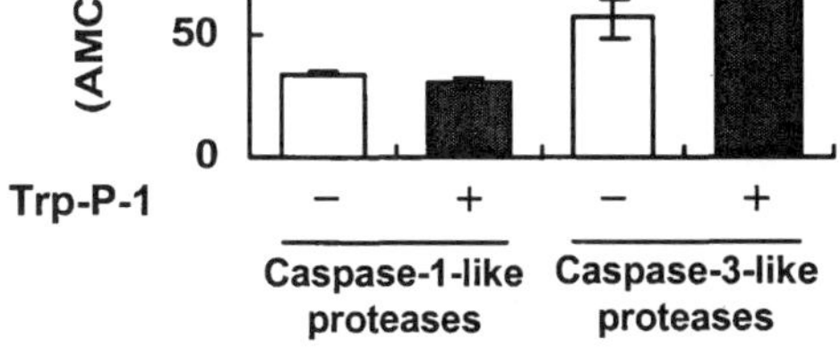

Figure 2. Trp-P-1 activated caspase-3-like proteases. MNCs were cultured with or without 10 μM Trp-P-1 for 3 h. Whole cell lysate was prepared and subjected to the assay for caspase-1- and -3-like protease activities using their peptide substrates, Ac-YVAD-MCA and Ac-DEVD-MCA, respectively, as described in Materials and Methods. Caspase activity was calculated as the amounts of AMC released from substrates per min. Data represent the means ± S.D. of triplicate experiments. Asterisks indicated significant difference from corresponding control (Student's t-test, $P < 0.05$).

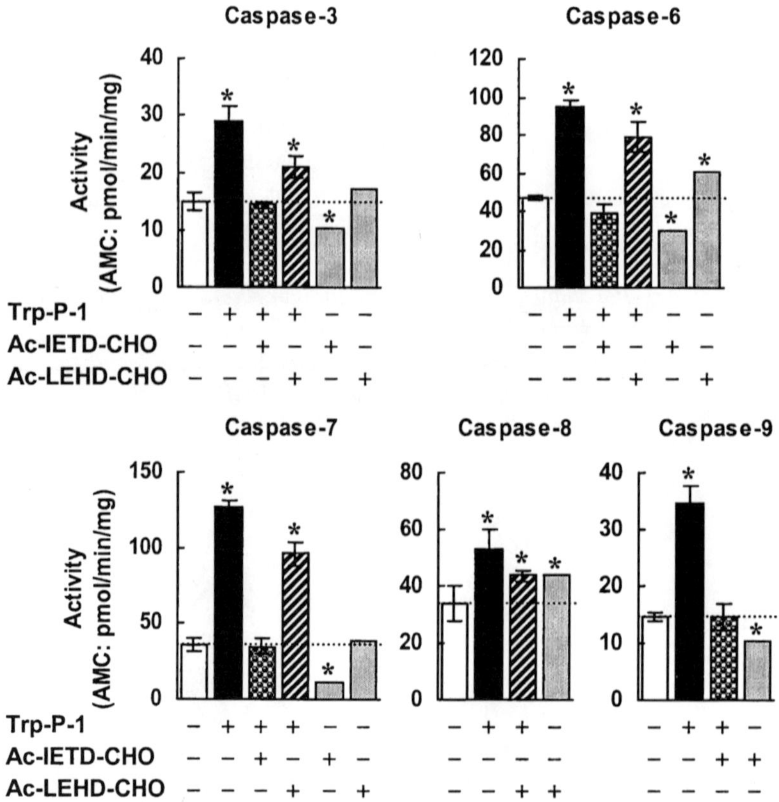

Figure 3. Caspase-8 dominates Trp-P-1-induces apoptosis. MNCs were pretreated with 50 μM peptide inhibitors of caspase-8 (Ac-IETD-CHO) or caspase-9 (Ac-LETD-CHO) for 1 h, and treated with 10 μM Trp-P-1 for 3 h. Whole cell lysate was prepared and measured caspase activity as described in Materials and Methods. Data represent the means ± S.D. of triplicate experiments. Asterisks indicated significant difference from corresponding control (Student's t-test, $P < 0.05$).

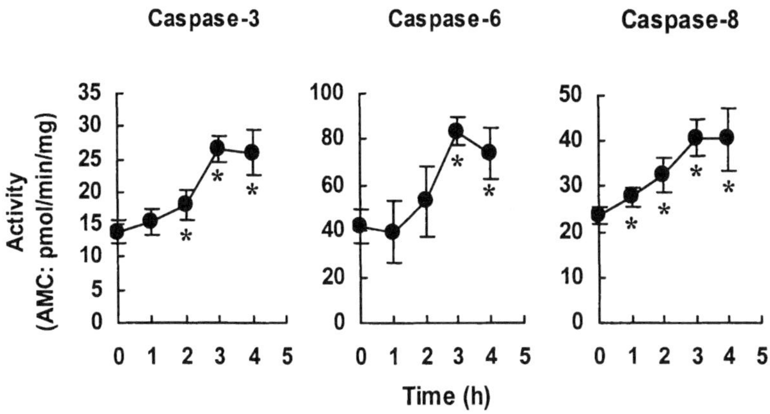

Figure 4. Caspase-8 was activated 1h after treatment. MNCs were treated with 10 μM Trp-P-1 for the indicating time, and caspase-3, -6 and -8 were measured as described in Materials and Methods. Data represent the means ± S.D. of triplicate experiments. Asterisks indicate significant differences from 0 h-cells (Student's t-test, P < 0.05).

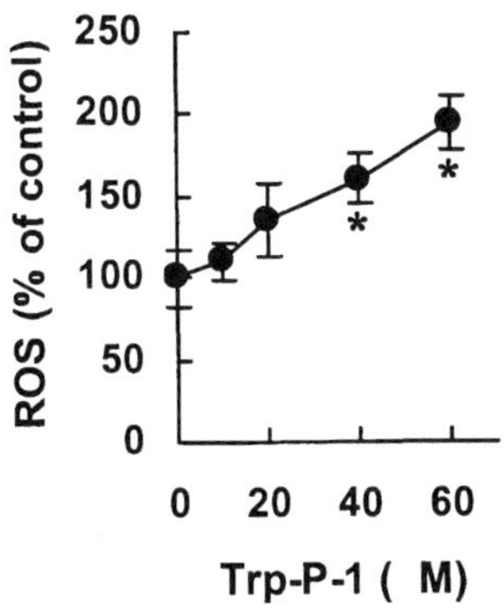

Figure 5 Trp-P-1 produced ROS in MNCs. MNCs were pretreated with 100 μM DCFH-DA for 1h, and treated with the indicated concentrations of Trp-P-1 for further 1 h. The intracellular ROS was quantified spectrofluorometrically as the formed 2',7'-dichlorofluorescein and expressed as % of control. Data represent the means ± S.D. of triplicate experiments. Asterisks indicated significant difference from corresponding control (Student's t-test, P < 0.05).

was reported that the generation of a small amounts of ROS involved in apoptosis, and the marked increase in ROS caused necrosis (ROS). To investigate the effects of antioxidants on Trp-P-1-induced apoptosis, cells were pretreated with 50 and 100 μM ascorbic acid, α-tocopherol, or trolox (water-soluble vitamin E) for 1 h and treated with 10 μM Trp-P-1 for 4 h. These antioxidants did not affect the DNA fragmentation as an apoptotic marker (Figure 6). Although 100 μM trolox showed slight suppression, it seems due to the cytotoxicity because trolox itself increased DNA fragmentation. These results suggest that the generation of ROS is not involved in Trp-P-1-induced apoptosis.

Screening of Anti-Apoptotic Food Components

To investigate whether food components can prevent the cytotoxicity of Trp-P-1, the effects of 30 food components on Trp-P-1-induced DNA fragmentation were measured. The IC_{50} value of each food component was calculated and shown in Table. Myricetin, delphinidin, and robinetin showed anti-apoptotic effects with the IC_{50} value at 18, 10, and 8 μM, respectively. These flavonoids have a triol structure in their B-ring. On the other hands, flavonoids with the diol structure in their B-ring, such as quercetin and rutin, did not affect Trp-P-1-induced DNA fragmentation. Since gardenin A, which has three methoxy groups in the B-ring, did not affect DNA fragmentation, the anti-apoptotic action seems to require the triol structure in the B-ring. Moreover, pyrogallol and gallic acid also showed a potent inhibition with IC_{50} value at 2 and 3 μM, while 1,2,4-benzentriol, α-resocylic acid, β-resocylic acid, and protocatechuic acid did not. Thus, a benzene ring with the triol structure seems to be associated with the anti-apoptotic activity. Since ROS is not involved in the apoptosis (Figure 6), the inhibitory mechanism of the triol structure against apoptotic action is considered to be independent of the antioxidative actions of the triol. Gallocatechins, such as, GC, EGC, GCg and EGCg, showed the same IC_{50} value at 20μM, though these gallocatechins caused cytotoxicity at 10 μM (data not shown), indicating that their inhibitory mechanism was due to the cytotoxicity but not to anti-apoptotic effects.

Dopamine showed a potent inhibition (IC_{50} value; 15 μM). It was reported that Trp-P-1 is taken up into PC 12 cells through dopamine uptake system (*30*), and the uptake of Trp-P-1 into immunocytes was also inhibited by dopamine (data not shown). Therefore, the inhibitory mechanism of dopamine is considered to be due to the competitive effects on the uptake of Trp-P-1.

It is reported that caffeic acid inhibits ceramide-induced apoptosis in U937 cells by the inhibition of protein tyrosine kinase activity (*17*). Quercetin inhibits hydrogen peroxide-induced apoptosis via intervention in the AP-1-mediated apoptotic pathway (*18*). Caffeic acid and quercetin did not inhibit the DNA fragmentation in this study. Therefore, Trp-P-1-induced apoptosis is unlikely to depend on the activations of protein tyrosine kinase and AP-1.

Table. Effects of food factors on DNA fragmentation.

Food components	*IC_{50} (μM) on DNA fragmentation*
Capsaicine	No effect up to 10 μM
Sesamin	No effect up to 10 μM
Sesamol	No effect up to 10 μM
Curcumin	No effect up to 10 μM
Lycopene	No effect up to 10 μM
Dopamine	15 μM
Myricetin	18 μM
Quercetin	No effect up to 50 μM
Rutin	No effect up to 10 μM
Daizein	No effect up to 10 μM
Genistein	No effect up to 10 μM
Robinetin	8 μM
Delphinidin	10 μM
Gardenin A	No effect up to 10 μM
Catechin	No effect up to 200 μM
Epicatechin	No effect up to 200 μM
Gallocatechin (GC)	20 μM
Epigallocatechin (EGC)	20 μM
Catechin Gallate	No effect up to 200 μM
Epicatechin Gallate	No effect up to 200 μM
Gallocatechin Gallate (GCg)	20 μM
Epigallocatechin Gallate (EGCg)	20 μM
Teaflavine	12 μM
Pyrogallol	2 μM
Gallic acid	3 μM
Caffeic acid	No effect up to 10 μM
1,2,4-Benzentriol	No effect up to 10 μM
α-resocylic acid	No effect up to 10 μM
β-resocylic acid	No effect up to 10 μM
Protocatechuic acid	No effect up to 10 μM

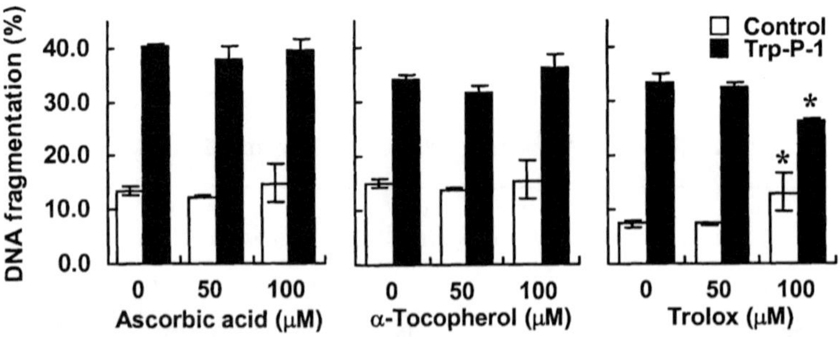

Figure 6. Ascorbic acid and α-tocophorol do not inhibit DNA fragmentaion. MNCs were pretreated with 50 and 100 μM ascorbic acid, α-tochopherol, and trolox for 1 h followed by treatment with 10 μM Trp-P-1 for 4 h. DNA fragmentation was measured as described in Materials and Methods, and expressed as % of control. Data presented is as the means ± S.D. of triplicate experiments. Asterisks indicated significant differences from corresponding control (Student's t-test, $P < 0.05$).

Conclusion

Trp-P-1 induces caspase-8-mediated apoptosis in MNCs derived from blood, and this apoptosis may be concerned with a cause of diseases such as immunodeficiency. The results in the present study suggest that our daily food contains certain components to prevent Trp-P-1-induced apoptosis in immunocytes.

References

1. Wakabayashi, K.; Nagao, M.; Esumi, H.; Sugimura, T. *Cancer Res.* **1992,** *52*, 2092s-2098s.
2. Yamaizumi, Z.; Shiomi, T.; Kasai, H.; Nishimura, S.; Takahashi, Y.; Nagao, M.; Sugimura, T. *Cancer Lett.* **1980,** *9*, 75-83.
3. Matsukura, N.; Kawachi, T.; Morino, K.; Ohgaki, H.; Sugimura, T.; Takayama, S. *Science* **1981,** *213*, 346-347.
4. Manabe, S.; Kanai, Y.; Wada, O. *Environ. Mol. Mutagen.* **1989,** *14*, 34-41.
5. Brandt, I.; Kowalski, B. I.; Gustafsson, J.-Å.; Rafter, J. *Carcinogenesis* **1983,** *4*, 1291-1296.

6. Ashida, H.; Adachi, H.; Kanazawa, K.; Danno, G. In *Functional Foods for Disease Prevention II, Medical Plants and Other Foods;* Osawa, T.; Shibamoto, T.; Terao, J. Eds.; American Chemical Society: Washington, DC, 1998; pp 88-100.
7. Ashida, H.; Shiotani, B.; Adachi, H.; Hashimoto, T.; Kanazawa, K.; Danno, G. *Biosci. Biotechnol. Biochem.* **1998,** *62*, 2283-2287.
8. Ashida, H.; Kihara, K.; Shiotani, B.; Hashimoto, T.; Kanazawa, K.; Danno, G. *Biosci. Biotechnol. Biochem.* **2000,** *64*, 2021-2024.
9. Hashimoto, T.; Ashida, H.; Sano, T.; Furuyashiki, T.; Shiotani, B.; Kanazawa, K.; Danno, G. *Mutat. Res.* **2000,** *457*, 57-67.
10. Hashimoto, T.; Ashida, H.; Sano, T.; Furuyashiki, T.; Hatanaka, Y.; Minato, K.; Mizuno, M.; Nomura, K.; Kumatori, A.; Kanazawa, K.; Danno, G. *Biochem. Biophys. Acta* **2001,** *1539*, 44-57.
11. Wyllie, A., H.; Kerr, J., F., R.; Currie, A., R. *Int. Rev. Cytol.* **1980,** *68*, 251-306.
12. Arends, M. J.; Wyllie, A. H. *Int. Rev. Exp. Pathol.* **1991,** *32*, 223-254.
13. Ellis, R. E.; Yuan, J. Y.; Horvitz, H. R. *Annu. Rev. Cell Biol.* **1991,** *7*, 663-698.
14. Cohen, J. J.; Duke, R. C.; Fadok, V. A.; Sellins, K. S. *Annu. Rev. Immunol.* **1992,** *10*, 267-293.
15. Sun, X.-M.; Carthew, P.; Dinsdale, D.; Snowden, R. T.; Cohen, G. M. *Toxicol. Appl. Pharmacol.* **1994,** *128*, 78-85.
16. Barroso, M. P.; Gomez-Diaz, C.; Lopez-Lluch, G.; Malagon, M. M.; Crane, F. L.; Navas, P. *Arch. Biochem. Biophys.* **1997,** *343*, 243-248.
17. Nardini, M.; Leonardi, F.; Scaccini, C.; Virgili, F. *Free Radic. Biol. Med.* **2001,** *30*, 722-733.
18. Ishikawa, Y.; Kitamura, M. *Kidney Int.* **2000,** *58*, 1078-1087.
19. Chen, N. Y.; Ma, W. Y.; Yang, C. S.; Dong, Z. *J. Environ. Pathol. Toxicol. Oncol.* **2000,** *19*, 287-295.
20. Rosenkranz, A. R.; Schmaldienst, S.; Stuhlmeier, K. M.; Chen, W.; Knapp, W.; Zlabinger, G. J. *J. Immunol. Methods* **1992,** *156*, 39-45.
21. Shiotani, B.; Nonaka, Y.; Hashimoto, T.; Kihara, K.; Kanazawa, K.; Danno, G.; Ashida, H. *Carcinogenesis* **2001,** *22*, 693-700.
22. Thornberry, N. A.; Lazebnik, Y. *Science* 1998, *281*, 1312-1316.
23. Cohen, G. M. *Biochem. J.* **1997,** *326*, 1-16.
24. Manna, S. K.; Zhang, H. J.; Yan, T.; Oberley, L. W.; Aggarwal, B. B. *J. Biol. Chem.* **1998,** *273*, 13245-13254.
25. Inoue, M.; Sakaguchi, N.; Isuzugawa, K.; Tani, H.; Ogihara, Y. *Biol. Pharm. Bull.* **2000,** *23*, 1153-1157.

26. Kannan, K.; Holcombe, R. F.; Jain, S. K.; Alvarez-Hernandez, X.; Chervenak, R.; Wolf, R. E.; Glass, *J. Mol. Cell Biochem.* **2000,** *205*, 53-66.
27. Jones, D. C.; Gunasekar, P. G.; Borowitz, J. L.; Isom, G. E. *J. Neurochem.* **2000,** *74*, 2296-2304.
28. Seaton, T. A.; Cooper, J. M.; Schapira, A. H. *Brain Res.* **1997,** *777*, 110-118.
29. Ashida, H.; Kanazawa, K.; Danno, G. *Biosci. Biotechnol. Biochem.* **1994,** *58*, 55-59.
30. Naoi, M.; Takahashi, T.; Ichinose, H.; Wakabayashi, K.; Sugimura, T.; Nagatsu, T. *Neurosci. Lett.* **1989,** *99*, 317-322.

Chapter 13

A Tryptophan Pyrolysis Product, 3-Amino-1,4-dimethyl-5*H*-pyrido[4,3-*b*]indole (Trp-P-1) but Not Its Metabolite Induces Apoptosis in Primary Cultured Rat Hepatocytes

Induction of CYP 1A Interfaces Trp-P-1-Induced Apoptosis

Bunsyo Shiotani[1], Hitoshi Ashida[1,2,*], Yuji Nonaka[1], Takashi Hashimoto[1], Kazuki Kanazawa[1], and Gen-ichi Danno[1,2]

[1]Division of Life Science, Graduate School of Science and Technology and [2]Department of Biofunctional Chemistry, Faculty of Agriculture, Kobe University, Nada-ku, Kobe 657–8501, Japan

Heterocyclic amines, which are formed during the daily cooking process, are the typical carcinogen and considered to be one of the major causes of human cancer. Their carcinogenic or mutagenic activity has been well studied, but the cytotoxicity to normal cells is little known. Previously, we demonstrated that Trp-P-1 also induces apoptosis to primary cultured rat hepatocytes. However, it is not clear which form, intact Trp-P-1 or its metabolite, induces apoptosis. In the carcinogenic process, the *N*-hydroxylation of Trp-P-1 catalyzed by cytochrome P450 (CYP) 1A subfamily is necessary to show its carcinogenic effects. In the present study, whether the induction of CYP 1A affects cytotoxic and apoptotic effects of Trp-P-1 was investigated using β-naphthoflavone (β-NF) pretreated rats hepatocytes. Pretreatment with β-NF of rats suppressed Trp-P-1-induced apoptosis in primary cultured hepatocytes. In the same cultures, metabolites of Trp-P-1 were increased. These results suggest that intact Trp-P-1 but not its metabolites induce apoptosis in hepatocytes.

The presence of heterocyclic amines (HCAs) in cooked foods is well documented. The HCAs are potent mutagens in the Ames test and have been found to be carcinogenic in rodents and non-human primates (*1*). Human exposure to HCAs is substantiated by the presence of HCAs and their metabolites in the urine, and the detection of HCA-DNA adducts in different tissue samples of healthy people consuming a normal diet (*2*). One of HCAs, 3-amino-1,4-dimethyl-5*H*-pyrido[4,3-*b*]indole (Trp-P-1) is formed by tryptophan pyrolysis. HCAs including Trp-P-1 require metabolic activation by cytochrome P450 (CYP) 1A subfamily in the first step and subsequently by *N*-*O*-acetyl transferase to form DNA adducts (*3-7*). Formation of DNA adducts is generally regarded as contributing to genetic mutations.

Another heterocyclic amine, 2-amino-1methyl-6-imidazo[4,5-*b*]pyridine (PhIP) shows a mutagenic activity with a similar mechanism to Trp-P-1. PhIP induced apoptosis in the colon with typical morphology of apoptosis, and PhIP-induced apoptosis was accelerated by administration of β-naphthoflavone (β-NF), which is a well known inducer of CYP 1A1 and 1A2 (*8*). Since PhIP requires metabolic activation by CYP 1A2 to exert genotoxic activities, the modulating effect of β-NF on PhIP-induced apoptosis is through a CYP 1A2-dependent mechanism. It was previously reported that Trp-P-1 showed the strongest cytotoxicity to primary cultured rat hepatocytes among the eleven heterocyclic amines examined (*9*) and exposure of hepatocytes to Trp-P-1 resulted in DNA fragmentation and nucleosomal ladder formation characteristic of apoptotic cells (*9, 10*). Moreover, intact Trp-P-1 without activation interacted with DNA (*11*) and induced chromosomal aberrations in CHO cells (*12*), suggesting that Trp-P-1 causes DNA damage in mammalian cells without metabolic activation to the *N*-hydroxyl form. It is, therefore, important to know which form, intact Trp-P-1 or a metabolite, induces apoptosis to hepatocytes. In this study, Trp-P-1-induced apoptosis in hepatocytes from rats treated with β-NF to induce CYP 1A (*13*) was examined and the possibility that the Trp-P-1 induced apoptosis without being metabolized by CYP 1A was demonstrated.

Materials and Methods

Materials

Trp-P-1 acetate form and phenobarbital sodium salt were purchased from Wako Pure Chemical Industries, Ltd. (Osaka, Japan). Corn oil, and β-naphthoflavone were purchased from Nacalai Tesque, Inc. (Kyoto, Japan). Anti-rat CYP1A1 antiserum was purchased from Daiichi Pure Chemicals Co., Ltd. (Tokyo, Japan). An antibody to caspase-3 was purchased from Santa Cruz Biotechnology, Inc. (Santa Curz, CA). Secondary antibody to goat IgG was purchased from Wako Pure Chemical Industries, Ltd. (Osaka, Japan). All other chemicals were of the highest quality commercially available.

Animal Treatment

All animal experiments in this study were performed in accordance with the "Guidelines for the care and use of experimental animals, of Rokkodai Campus, Kobe University". Male Wistar rats, obtained from Japan SLC, Inc. (Shizuoka, Japan), weighing 200-250 g, were housed in suspended steel cages, provided with commercial chow and water *ad libitum*, and maintained under a controlled environment (temperature 25°C, humidity 60%, and 12-h light / 12-h dark cycle) and used for the preparation of hepatocytes. Rats were treated with β-NF (80 mg/kg body weight/day) in corn oil for 3 consecutive days by i.p. injection. Control rats were administered an equal amount of corn oil vehicle alone.

Hepatocyte Isolation And Culture Conditions

Hepatocytes were isolated from rats by *in situ* perfusion of the liver with collagenase solution by the method of Tanaka *et al.* (*14*). Isolated hepatocytes were suspended at a concentration of 5×10^5 cells/ml in William's medium E with 1 nM insulin, 1 nM dexamethasone, 100 mg/l kanamycin, 10 kIU/ml aprotinin and 5% fetal bovine serum. The cells were seeded on plastic multi-well plates or dishes (Becton Dickinson Co., Ltd., Franklin Lakes, NJ) pre-coated with collagen type I, then cultured under an atmosphere of 95% air-5% CO_2 at 37°C for 2 h or 20h. Hepatocytes were treated with various concentrations of Trp-P-1 in dimethyl sulfoxide (DMSO) for various times as indicated in each figure. Parallel dishes were treated with vehicle alone to obtain control samples (maximum concentration of DMSO in the medium was 0.1%, v/v).

Western Blotting Analysis

Hepatocytes isolated from treated rats were cultured for 2 or 20 h and rinsed twice with 1.15% KCl. They were homogenized with 7 strokes of a Teflon homogenizer in 1.15% KCl, and the homogenate was centrifuged at 10,000 *g* for 20 min at 4°C. The supernatant was centrifuged at 100,000 *g* for 1 h at 4°C, and the resultant pellet was resuspended in a solution (0.1 M Tris, pH 7.4, 20% glycerol and 1 mM phenylmethylsulfonylfluoride (PMSF)) and used as the microsomal fraction. For detection of CYP 1A, aliquots of 10 μg of microsomal protein were separated on 10% gels. The nuclear protein extraction was performed as described previously (*10*). For determination of cleavage of caspase-3, aliquots of 30 μg of nuclear protein were separated on 15% gels. After SDS-PAGE, proteins were transferred onto the PVDF membranes followed by blocking of the nonspecific binding sites with 10% FBS in TBST buffer (10 mM Tris-HCl, pH 8.0, 150 mM NaCl, and 0.06% Tween 20) at 4°C overnight. The membranes were washed with TBST buffer four times for 5 min each time and incubated with respective primary antibodies for 1 h. After washing with TBST buffer under the same conditions, the membranes were incubated with the secondary antibody conjugated with horseradish peroxidase for 30 min. Specific immune complexes were visualized with the ECL detection system (Amersham Pharmacia Biotech).

CYP Enzyme Activity

Hepatic microsomal 7-ethoxyresorufin *O*-dealkylase (EROD) activity was determined according to the method of Burke *et al.* (*15*) using fluorescence spectrophotometer with excitation and emission wavelengths of 530 and 585 nm, respectively.

Cell Viability Measurement

Cell viability test was performed by using MTT (3-[4,5-dimethylthiazol-2-yl]-2,5-diphenyltetrazolium bromide) test according to the method of Mosmann *et al.* (*16*).

Analysis of DNA Fragmentation

Hepatocytes were treated with Trp-P-1 and then lysed with 200 μl of TE buffer (10 mM Tris-HCl, pH 7.4, and 10 mM EDTA) containing 0.5% SDS. The resultant lysate was incubated with 500 μg/ml RNase A at 50°C for 30 min and then with 500 μg/ml proteinase K at 50°C for 60 min. After addition of 0.5 M NaCl and 1 mM EDTA (final concentrations), DNA was precipitated in 50% isopropanol at -20°C overnight. DNA precipitate was obtained by centrifugation at 17,000 *g* for 20 min, washed with 70% ethanol, and resuspended in TE buffer. DNA was resolved by 2% agarose gel electrophoresis in TBE buffer (89 mM Tris-HCl, 89 mM borate, and 2 mM EDTA). After electrophoresis, the gel was stained with ethidium bromide and visualized on a UV transilluminator.

Detection of Trp-P-1 And Its Metabolite on HPLC

Detection of metabolites derived from Trp-P-1 during primary culture was performed by the method described by Minamoto and Kanazawa (*17*) with some modifications. Briefly, intracellular metabolites and Trp-P-1 were extracted with ethyl acetate from these cells. The metabolites were detected using a HPLC (Hitachi L-7100) equipped with a UV detector (Hitachi L-7420) and electrochemical detector (ECD; IRICA Σ 875) connected in series. An Inertsil column, ODS (i.d. 4.6 × 150 mm), was maintained at 35 °C. The mobile phase consisted of 40 mM potassium phosphate monobasic (pH 4.6)-acetonitrile (80/20, v/v) containing 0.1 mM EDTA and 0.05% acetic acid and the flow rate was 1.0 ml/min. The UV detector was set at 267 nm, λ_{max} of Trp-P-1. ECD with a glassy carbon electrode was set at +600 mV versus Ag/AgCl, the optimal voltage for detecting metabolites under conditions in which various interfering substances were present.

Results

Induction of CYP 1A in Hepatocytes from β-NF-Treated Rats

The level and activity of CYP 1A in the hepatocytes from β-NF-treated rats were examined. In hepatocytes from control rats, CYP 1A was detected very slightly. β-NF markedly increased the level of CYP 1A in hepatocytes cultured for 2 h, but the level of CYP 1A decreased during 20 h in culture (Figure. 1A). The same tendency was observed in the EROD activity, which is generally regarded as CYP 1A activity: β-NF increased the activity, and this increase was diminished during culture (Figure 1B).

Trp-P-1-Induced Apoptosis Was Interfered in Hepatocytes from β-NF-Treated Rats

Trp-P-1 decreased the cell viability in cultures from control rats in a time-dependent manner in both 2 h- and 20 h-cultures. After 2 h-culture, hepatocytes from β-NF-treated rats showed a significant tolerance to the cytotoxicity of Trp-P-1 (Figure 2). However, in 20 h-cultured hepatocytes from β-NF-treated rats, the cell viability decreased compared with cells cultured for 2 h. The difference of susceptibility between 2 h- and 20 h-cultured hepatocytes from β-NF-treated rats correlated with the decrease in the level/activity of CYP 1A (Figure 1). During apoptotic process, it was recognized that the most likely candidate in the caspase cascade is caspase-3 (*18*). Trp-P-1 caused cleavage of inactive procaspase-3 to the p20-subunit in control rats, and this cleavage was suppressed in 2 h-cultured hepatocytes from β-NF-treated rats after treatment with Trp-P-1 (Figure 3). After 20 h-culture, this suppression was weaken. Treatment with Trp-P-1 resulted in nucleosomal ladder formation as a characteristic of apoptotic cells in 20 h-cultured hepatocytes from control rats (Figure 4). In hepatocytes from β-NF-treated rats, the ladder formation by Trp-P-1 was suppressed. Thus, Trp-P-1-induced apoptosis was suppressed in hepatocytes isolated from β-NF-treated.

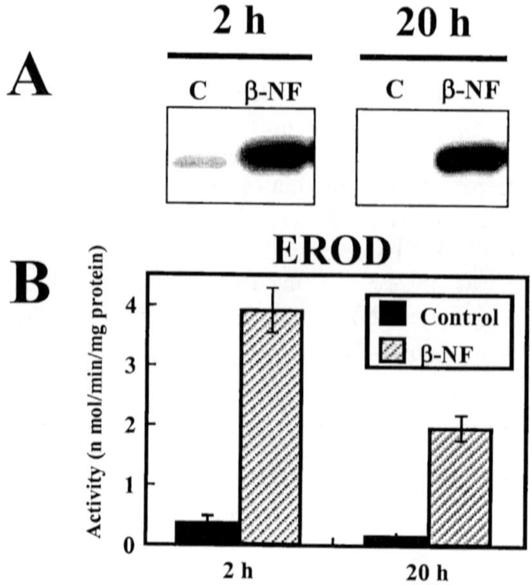

Figure 1. Expression of CYP 1A1 in β-NF-treated rat hepatocytes. Hepatocytes were isolated from β-naphthoflavone (β-NF) and corn oil (Control)-treated rats. After culture for 2 or 20 h, microsomal proteins were prepared from hepatocytes and loaded onto a 10% SDS-polyacrylamide gel (10 μg protein, each). (A) CYP 1A level by Western blotting (B) EROD activity were measured as described in Materials and methods. Values are presented as means ±S.D. (n=3).

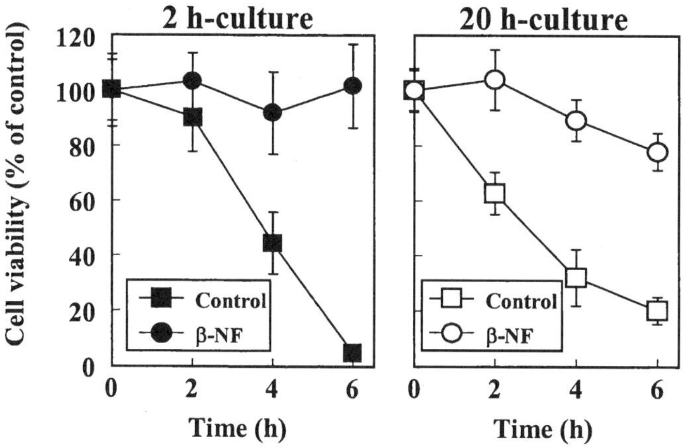

Figure 2. Suppression of the cytotoxicity induced by Trp-P-1 in β-NF-treated rat hepatocytes. Hepatocytes were isolated from β-naphthoflavone (β-NF) and corn oil (Control)-treated rats and cultured for 2 or 20 h. The cells were treated with Trp-P-1 (30 μM) for 2, 4, and 6 h and cell viability was determined by MTT test. Data are presented as means ±S.D. (n=10).

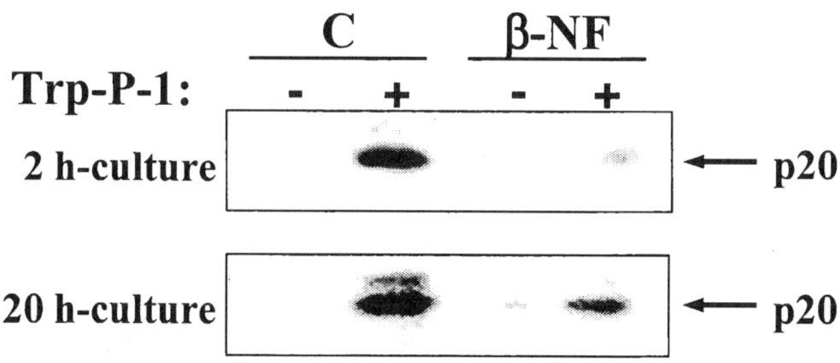

Figure 3. Suppression of caspase-3 activation by Trp-P-1 in β-NF-treated rat hepatocytes. Hepatocytes were isolated from β-naphthoflavone (β-NF) and corn oil (C)-treated rats and cultured for 2 (upper panel) or 20 h (lower panel). Cleavage of caspase-3 was analyzed in nuclear protein extracts from the cultured cells after treatment with Trp-P-1 (30 μM) for 4 h by Western blotting as described in the Materials and Methods.

Changes in The Levels of Metabolites of Trp-P-1 and Intact Trp-P-1 in Hepatocytes Isolated from β-NF-Treated Rats

Trp-P-1 was incorporated into hepatocytes from control rats in a time-dependent manner by 1 h, and the uptake increased linearly without detection of the metabolites, when the cells were treated with various concentrations of Trp-P-1 (data not shown). When the production of metabolites was measured after various treatment periods of Trp-P-1 in 2 h-cultured hepatocytes from β-NF treated rats, the ECD positive metabolites increased within the 30 min treatment period (Figure 5). In 20 h-cultured hepatocytes, the levels of metabolites were also increased but levels were less than those of 2 h-cultures. These results suggested that Trp-P-1 was metabolized to other forms in hepatocytes conserving with the high CYP 1A activity.

Discussion

In the present study, we investigated whether the intracellular level/activity of CYP 1A affected the cytotoxic and apoptotic effects of Trp-P-1 on rat hepatocytes. The results demonstrated that Trp-P-1-induced apoptosis was diminished in hepatocytes expressing CYP 1A at a high level by *in vivo* treatment with β-NF to rats. A decrease in the level/activity of CYP 1A during culture altered the cytotoxicity of Trp-P-1 to hepatocytes from β-NF-treated rats.

Similar to other HCAs, Trp-P-1 requires metabolic activation to cause mutagenicity. The major pathway for the activation involves *N*-hydroxylation, which is catalyzed by CYP 1A subfamily. Upon activation, Trp-P-1 has been found to react with DNA and forms DNA adducts. In the present study, the CYP 1A level/activity in hepatocytes from β-NF-treated rats was markedly higher than control hepatocytes. Although Trp-P-1 induced apoptosis to hepatocytes from control rats, it did not induce to hepatocytes from β-NF-treated rats. The difference of the sensitivity to Trp-P-1 in both hepatocytes might be due to the level/activity of CYP 1A, since 2 h-cultured hepatocytes from β-NF-treated rats with high level/activity of CYP 1A showed tolerance to Trp-P-1-induced apoptosis and this tolerance was weakened in 20 h-cultured hepatocytes with lower CYP 1A. Moreover, the results showed that induction of CYP 1A by β-NF in hepatocytes increased the ECD-positive metabolites, mainly *N*-hydroxy-Trp-P-1. Thus, these observations suggest that intact Trp-P-1, but not its metabolites, induced apoptosis in hepatocytes. It remains, however, a possibility that other factors, which are altered by β-NF-treatment, may cause the tolerance to the apoptogenic activity of intact Trp-P-1 instead of CYP 1A.

It is now assumed that some of the damaged cells are successfully recovered by an intrinsic repair system, however, if those are defective in repair, the cells will not undergo apoptosis. One of the HCAs, PhIP has been reported to induce apoptotic response in colonic epithelium accelerated by β-NF administration (*8*).

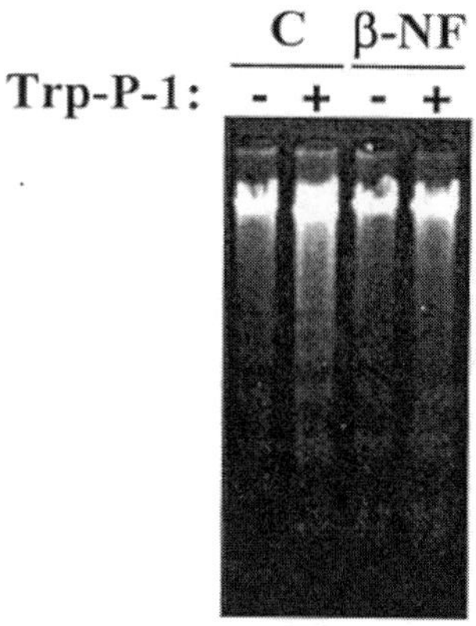

Figure 4. Suppression of DNA fragmentation caused by Trp-P-1 in β-NF-treated rat hepatocytes. Hepatocytes were isolated from β-naphthoflavone (β-NF) and corn oil (C)-treated rats and cultured for 20 h. These hepatocytes were treated with Trp-P-1 for 6 h, and DNA fragmentation was analyzed by 2% agarose gel electrophoresis.

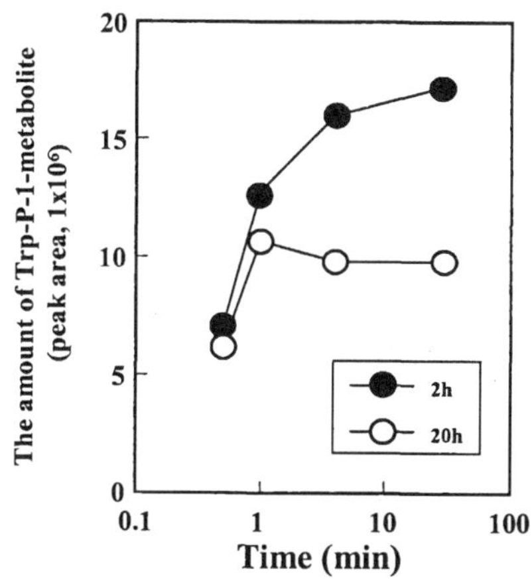

Figure 5. The levels of metabolites derived from Trp-P-1 in hepatocytes from β-NF-treated rats during culture. Hepatocytes were isolated from β-naphthoflavone (β-NF) and cultured for 2 or 20 h. The cells were treated with Trp-P-1 (30 μM) for 0.5, 1, 4 or 30 min. The amounts of metabolites derived from Trp-P-1 were determined by HPLC with ECD as described in the Materials and Methods.

It is also reported that PhIP-induced apoptosis is through a mismatch repair dependent pathway (*19*). In our previous study, intact PhIP did not induce apoptosis to primary cultured hepatocytes from normal rats. Taken together, PhIP-induced apoptosis may be due to the formation of DNA adducts after metabolic activation by CYPs. However, Trp-P-1 induced apoptosis without being metabolized by CYP 1A suggests that this apoptosis might not be dependent on the DNA adducts formation. It has been reported that intact Trp-P-1 inhibits topoisomerases, which affect DNA excision repair, by intercalation into DNA (*20*) resulting in DNA double-strand break. Chemotherapeutic agents that inhibit topoisomerases induce apoptosis (*21*). Therefore, it is possible that intact Trp-P-1 inhibits topoisomerases causing to severe DNA damage and induces apoptosis in normal hepatocytes with low levels of CYP 1A.

References

1. *Food Borne Carcinogens: Heterocyclic Amines;* Nagao, M.; Sugimura, T., Eds.; John Wiley and Sons: Hoboken, NJ, 2000; p 390.
2. Schut, H.A.; Snyderwine, E.G. *Carcinogenesis* **1999,** *20*, 353-368.
3. Mita, S.; Yamazoe, Y.; Kamataki, T.; Kato, R. *Biochem. Pharmacol.* **1983,** *32*, 1179-1182.
4. Ishida, Y.; Negishi, C.; Umemoto, A.; Fujita, Y.; Sato, S.; Sugimura, T.; Thorgeirsson, S. S.; Adamson, R. H. *Toxicol. In Vitro*, **1987,** *1*, 45-48.
5. Ishii, K.; Ando, M.; Kamataki, M.; Kato, R.; Nagao, M. *Cancer Lett.***1980,** *9*, 271-276.
6. Mita, S.; Ishii, K.; Yamazoe, Y.; Kamatati, T.; Kato, R.; Sugimura, T. *Cancer Res*. **1981,** *41*, 3610-3614.
7. Hashimoto, Y.; Shudo, K.; Okamoto, T. *Biochem. Biophys. Res. Commun.* **1980,** *96*, 355-362.
8. Hirose, Y.; Sugie, S.; Yoshimi, N.; Matsunaga, K.; Hara, A.; Mori, H *Cancer lett.* **1998,** *123*, 167-172.
9. Ashida, H.; Shiotani, B.; Adachi, H.; Hashimoto, T.; Kanazawa, K.; Danno, G. *Biosci. Biotechnol. Biochem.***1998,** *62*, 2283-2287.
10. Asida, H.; Adachi, H.; Kanazawa, K.; Danno, G. In *Functional Foods For Disease: Prevention II-Medical Plants and Other Food;* Ogawa, T.; Shibamoto, T.; Terao, J. Eds.; American Chemical Society: Washington, DC, 1998, pp 88-100.
11. Mihara, Y.; Doi, M.; Inohara, T.; Kawamura, M.; Hamanaka, N.; Ishida, T. *Biochem. Biophys. Res. Commun.***1997,** *240*, 803-806.
12. Sasaki, Y. F.; Yamada, H.; Shimoi, K., Kinae, N.; Tomita, I.; Matsumura, H.; Ohta, T.; Shirasu, Y. *Mutat. Res*. **1992,** *269*, 79-95.
13. Guengerich, F. P.; Dannan, G. A.; Wright, S. T.; Martin, M. V.; Kaminsky, L. S. *Biochemistry* **1982**, *21*, 6019-6030.

14. Tanaka, K.; Sato, M.; Tomita, Y.; Ichihara, A. *J. Biochem. Tokyo* **1978,** *84*, 937-946.
15. Burke, M. D.; Mayer, R. T.; *Chem. Biol. Interact.* **1983,** *45*, 243-258.
16. Mosmann, T. *J Immunol. Methods* **1983,** *65*, 55-63.
17. Minamoto, S.; Kanazawa, K. *Analytical Biochemistry* **1995,** *225*, 143-148.
18. Leist, M.; Jaattela, M. *Nat. Rev. Mol. Cell Biol.* **2001,** *2*, 589-598.
19. Duc, R.; Leong-Morgenthaler, P. M. *Mutat. Res.* **2001**, *486*, 155-164.
20. Funayama, Y.; Nishio, K.; Wakabayashi, K.; Nagao, M.; Shimoi, K.; Ohira, T.; Hasegawa, S.; Saijo, N. *Mutat. Res.* **1996,** *349,* 183-191.
21. Scott, H. K. *Biochim. Biophys. Acta* **1998,** *1400*, 195-211.

Chapter 14

Simulation of TNF-α and NO Production from Murine Macrophage by Water-Soluble Polysaccharides from *Isaria japonica*

Sachiko Kawakami[1,2], Ken-ichiro Minato[3], Toshikatsu Imamura[4], Yasuo Aizono[5], and Masashi Mizuno[1,*]

[1]Graduate School of Science and Technology, Kobe University, Kobe 657–8501, Japan
[2]The Tottori Mycological Institute, Tottori 689–1125, Japan
[3]Miyagi Agricultural College, Sendai 982–0215, Japan
[4]Aseptic Sericulture System Laboratory, Kyoto 601–8203, Japan
[5]Faculty of Agriculture, Kobe University, Kobe 657–8501, Japan

Antitumor polysaccharide from *Isaria japonica* was chromatographically isolated and purified from the hot-water soluble fractions as an index of TNF-α and NO production from murine peritoneal macrophages. Molecular weight of the purified polysaccharide was approximately 8,200 by high performance size exclusion Chromatography. TNF-α and NO production with 500 μg/ml of the purified polysaccharide were significantly enhanced to 365.9 pg/ml and 37.3 μM, respectively, as compared with those of saline, being 2.2 pg/ml and 13.8 μM, respectively. The purified polysaccharide did not cross-react with anti-β-1,3- and anti-β-1,6-glucan antibodies, suggesting that it might have a different structure with novel antitumor polysaccharides such as lentinan, gliforan and schizophyllan.

Polysaccharides from mushrooms are known to exhibit anti-tumor activity (*1-8*). These polysaccharides do not show any direct cytotoxicity against tumor cells (*9-12*) as their activities are caused by potentiation of the immune response. Recently, it has been reported that the anti-tumor polysaccharides stimulate the secretion of tumor necrosis factor (TNF)-α from macrophages (*13*) . TNF-α, an endogenous factor with tumor-selective cytotoxicity, is recognized as an important host defense molecule that affects tumor cells. It has been reported that lentinan stimulates NK cell activity (*14*) and several macrophage functions, e.g. the release of TNF-α (*15*). Nitric oxide (NO), a free-radical gas, is synthesized by nitric oxide synthase (NOS) (*16*) and mediates diverse functions, including vasodilation, neurotransmission, inhibition of platelet aggregation, immunoresponse, and inflammation (*17*). Furthermore, recent studies have demonstrated that murine macrophages stimulated with TNF-α (*18*) produce NO via expression of the inducible NOS gene (*16*), and that reactive nitrogen intermediates play a significant role in tumoricidal and microbicidal activities (*17,18*). Thus, it seems that TNF-α and NO serve as factors that exhibit anti-tumor cell activity and a wide variety of physiological activities in the immune system.

Isaria japonica belongs to Clavicipitaceae in CLAVICIPITALES in ASCOMYCOTINA and has been researched traditionally for its medicinal and physiological function. Indeed, the fruiting bodies have been used in Korea to treat cancer. Takano et al. (*19*) have reported that *Isaria japonica* significantly enhanced the production of anti-sheep red blood cell plaque forming cells by oral ingestion. Recently, an apoptosis-inducing compound, 4-acetyl-12,13-epoxyl-9-trichothecene-3,15-diol, was isolated from the methanol extract of *Isaria japonica*, and the apoptosis-inducing activity at 10 nmol/l concentration was further confirmed by a nuclear morphological change, a ladder pattern of internucleosomal DNA fragmentation, and activation of caspase-3 (*20*). However, the anti-tumor polysaccharide in *Isaria japonica* has not been known. In this study, the immunomodulating polysaccharides was justified as an index of TNF-α and NO production from murine peritoneal macrophages.

Materials and Methods

Materials

Isaria japonica was a gift from Aseptic Sericulture System Laboratory (Kyoto, Japan). Mouse rTNF-α and lipopolysaccharide were purchased from Wako Pure Chemicals Industries (Osaka, Japan) and Difco Laboratories (Detroit,

MI), respectively. All other chemicals were of the highest quality commercially available.

Extraction of hot water-soluble fractions

The fresh fruit body of *Isaria japonica* was homogenized with liquid nitrogen using a Waring blender and lyophilized. The lyophilized mushroom (60 g) was extracted three times with 85% ethanol (600 ml) at 80°C for 3 h and filtrated. The combined extracts were evaporated and defatted by extraction for 12h with 1.5 times volume of chloroform. The aqueous layer was lyophilized as the MI fraction. The residues after extractions with ethanol were extracted three times with hot-water (600 ml) for 6 h and filtrated. Ethanol (2400 ml) was added to the filtrate four times and centrifuged at 8,000 g for 30 min. The pellet was dissolved in water and dialyzed against distilled water through a cellulose tube. The residual solution was concentrated to a small volume by evaporation and then lyophilized (MII fraction). The supernatant, after centrifugation, was evaporated and dialyzed against distilled water. The residual solution was concentrated to a small volume by evaporation and then lyophilized (MIII fraction).

Isolation of an active polysaccharide from hot water- soluble fraction

The MII fraction (100 mg) in distilled water was separated by a DEAE-Sepharose CL-6B column (2.6 x 30 cm). The column was eluted with 500 ml of 1/15 M phosphate buffer (pH 7.2) and then eluted with a stepwise elution of 300 ml each using same buffer containing 0.2 and 0.6 M NaCl. The active fraction (15 mg) was further subjected to gel filtration on a Toyopearl HW-55S (1.6 x 94 cm) equilibrated with 1/9 M phosphate buffer (pH 7.2). Each collected fraction was dialyzed and lyophilized. The active fraction (20mg) was redissolved in 800 μl of 1/15 M phosphate buffer (pH 7.2) and the second anion exchange chromatography was performed on a Mono Q HR5/5 (0.5 x 5cm) with a FPLC system (LCC-551, Amersham Pharmacia Biotech) using a linear gradient elution from 0 M to 1 M NaCl in 1/15 M phosphate buffer (pH 7.2). To confirm the molecular weight, the active fraction (1mg) was subjected to high performance size exclusion chromatography (HP-SEC). The column was joined SB-G guard column (6.0 x 50 mm; Shodex denko), SB-805 HQ (6.0 x 50 mm, Showa denko), and SB-803 HQ (8.0 x 300 mm, Showa denko) in tandem. The peak was detected by UV detector (2487 Dual λ Absorbance Detector ,Waters) and RI detector (2410 Referactive index Detector, Waters). The sample (40μl, 2mg/ml) was eluted with 1/15 M phosphate buffer (pH 7.2) at a flow rate of 0.8 ml/min for 45min and the column temperature was maintained at 40°C.

Pullulan kit (Shodex STANDARD P-82) was used as a standard. The data was analyzed by HP-SEC analysis soft (Millemmium 32-J, Waters).

Preparation of peritoneal macrophages

All animal treatments in this study conformed to the "Guidelines for the care and use of experimental animals, in Rokkodai Campus, Kobe University". Peritoneal macrophages were isolated from mice (BALB/c, Japan SLC Co, Japan) that had been injected intraperitoneally with 2 ml of 4.05% (w/v) fluid thioglycollate medium 3 day prior to peritoneal lavage with 10 ml serum-free RPMI 1640 medium. The collected cells were washed with RPMI 1640 and cultured in RPMI 1640 containing 5% fetal calf serum at a density of $0.5x10^6$ cells / well. The cells were plated on a 24 flat-bottom well microculture plate and then incubated for 2 h at 37°C and 5% CO_2. After removing the nonadherent cells, the monolayered macrophages were stimulated with sample solution for 24 h at 37°C and 5% CO_2. At the end of the incubation, culture supernatant was collected by centrifugation at 300 x *g* for 5 min.

Measurement of TNF-α activity

TNF-α activity was measured by closely following the procedure given by Kerékgyártó *et al.* (*15*). TNF-α in culture supernatants obtained from untreated or activated macrophages was measured by a biological assay using actinomycin D-treated L-929 mouse fibroblast cells. Recombinant murine TNF-α (Wako Pure Chemcal, Co) was used as a standard. Briefly, L929 cells were plated on a 96-well flat-bottom microculture plate at a density of $2x10^4$ cells/ml in a complete medium containing 1 μg/ml actinomycin D. Culture supernatant of peritoneal mecrophages was added to the plates. After 20 h incubation at 37°C, the remaining viable cells were fixed and stained with 0.1% crystal violet, and absorbance was measured at 570 nm.

Nitrite assay

The macrophages prepared above were plated at a density of $1x10^6$ cells/well in 24-well plates. After 24 h incubation, synthesis of NO was determined by an assay of culture supernatants for nitrite (NO_2^-), the stable reaction product of NO with molecular oxygen, as described by Stuehr and Nathan (*21*). Briefly, 100 μl of Griess reagent was added to 100 μl of each supernatant in 96-well plates, and the absorbance was measured at 570 nm.

Molecular weight determination

The molecular weight of the purified polysaccharide was determine using the following standard pullulans (Showa Denko, Japan): P-400 (Molecular weight: 380,000), P-200 (186,000), P-100 (100,000), P-50 (48,000), P-20 (23,700) and P-10 (12,200) by HP-SEC.

Results and Discussion

Isolation of polysaccharides from *Isaria japonica*

The fractionation of polysaccharides in *Isaria japonica* is shown schematically in Figure 1. Fractions of MI, MII, and MIII from fruiting bodies were separated by extraction with 85% ethanol solution and hot-water. Each fraction (100 μg/ml) was measured for production of TNF-α and NO. The production of TNF-α from macrophage stimulated with MI, II, and III was 0.10 ± 0.04, 1459.96 ± 188.63, and 1348.34 ± 428.92 pg/ml, respectively. The production of NO from macrophage stimulated with MI, II, and III was 4.53 ± 0.88, 20.50 ± 2.80, and 14.61 ± 1.73 μM, respectively (Figure 2). The hot-water fraction (MII) which showed the highest activity was separated into 5 fractions using a DEAE-Sepharose CL-6B column (Figure 3). The production of TNF-α from macrophage stimulated with MII-1, 2, 3, 4 and 5 was 301.7 ± 8.6, 391.1 ± 6.6, 359.5 ± 5.4, 603.8 ± 11.6, and 597.8 ± 5.0 pg/ml, respectively. The production of NO from macrophage stimulated with MII-1, 2, 3, 4 and 5 was 7.70 ± 1.01, 17.79 ± 0.15, 14.72 ± 0.69, 16.56 ± 1.61 and 18.14 ± 0.09 μM, respectively (Figure 4). Thus, MII-4 and fraction 5 (10 μg/ml) showed a higher specific activity in both assays. As the yield of MII-5 fraction was higher than that of MII-4 (Figure 3), MII-5 fraction was further fractionated by Mono Q column. As shown in Figure 5, three fractions were detected. The production of TNF-α from macrophage stimulated with MII-5-a-1, MII-5-a-2, and MII-5-a-3 was 349.0 ± 38.4, 400.0 ± 53.4, and 389.3 ± 15.1 pg/ml, respectively. The production of NO from macrophage stimulated with MII-5-a-1, MII-5-a-2, and MII-5-a-3 was 22.26 ± 0.46, 37.26 ± 5.86 and 30.51 ± 2.72 μM, respectively (Figure 6). Though MII-5-a-2 and 3 fractions showed the highest activity in the production of TNF-α and NO from murine macrophages, MII-5-a-3 fraction was recovered more than MII-5-a-2 fraction. MII-5-a-3 fraction was collected and supplied to the instrumental analyses.

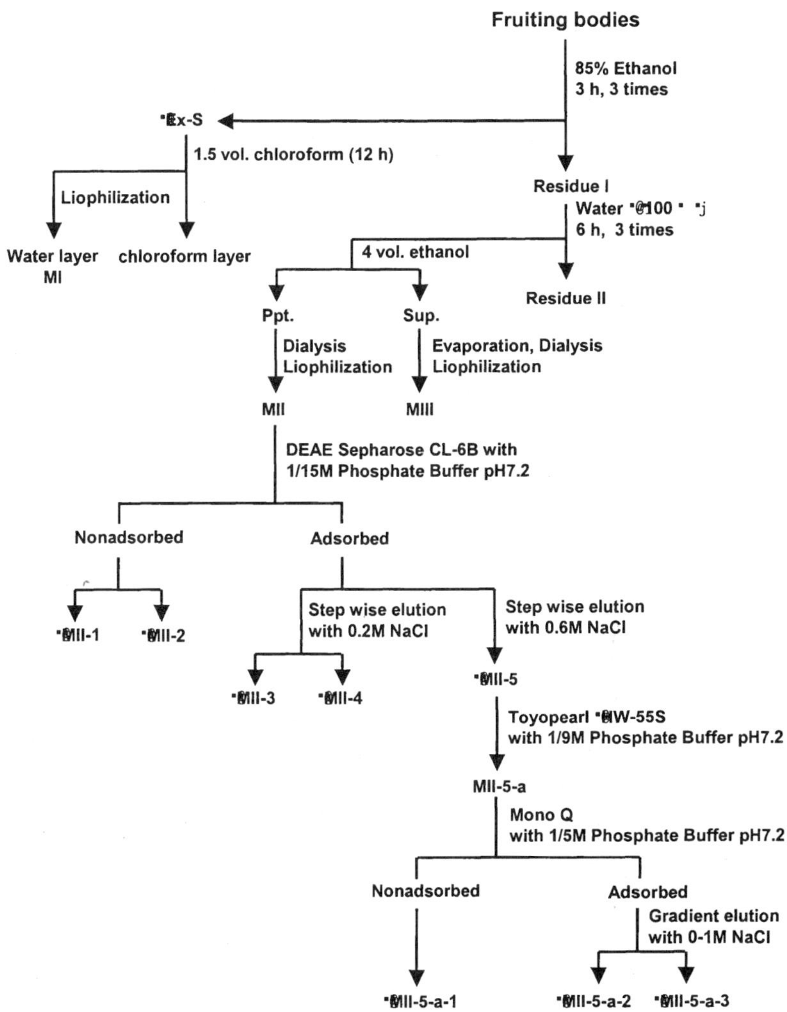

Figure 1. Extraction of polysaccharides from Isaria japonica and fractionation of hot-water-soluble fraction into MII-5-a-3.

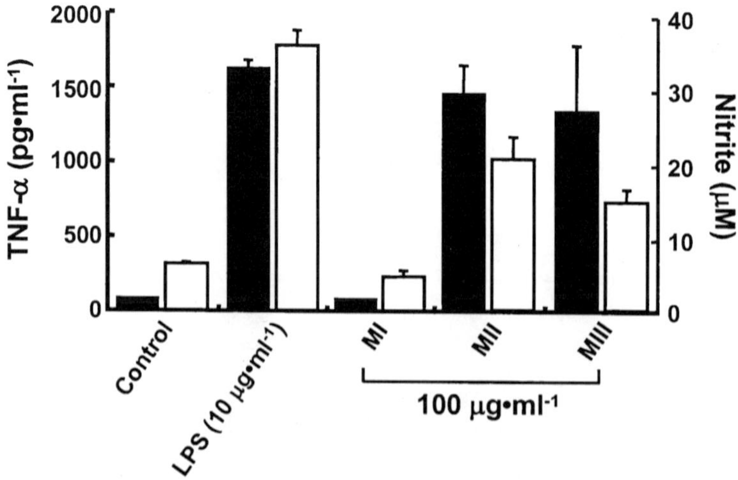

Figure 2. Effects of MI, MII, and MIII fraction on production of TNF-α (black bars)and NO (white bars) from murine peritoneal macrophages of BALB/c. All values are means ± SE of triplicate measurements. LPS (10 μg/ml) was used as positive control.

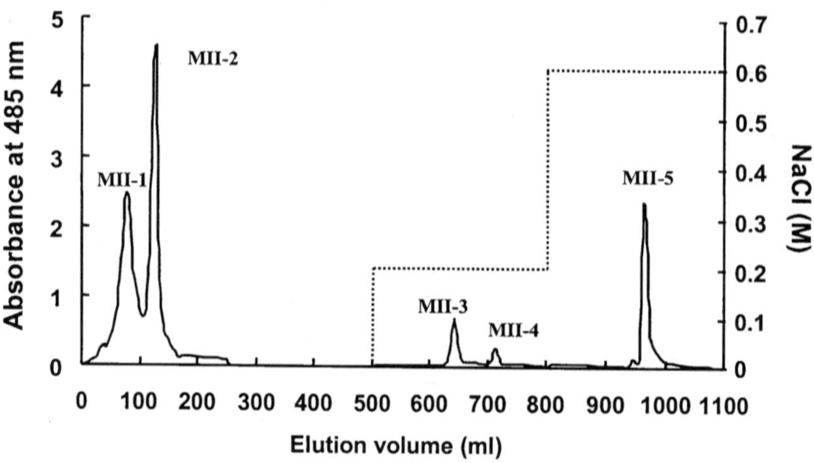

Figure 3. Elution profile of MII fraction from hot-water extraction in Isaria japonica on a column of DEAE-Sepharose CL-6B column. MII (100 mg) was eluted with 1/15 M phosphate buffer (pH 7.2) and the same buffer containing 0.2 or 0.6M NaCl in step wise elution. The sugar content of each fraction was measured at 485.0 nm by the phenol-sufluric acid method.

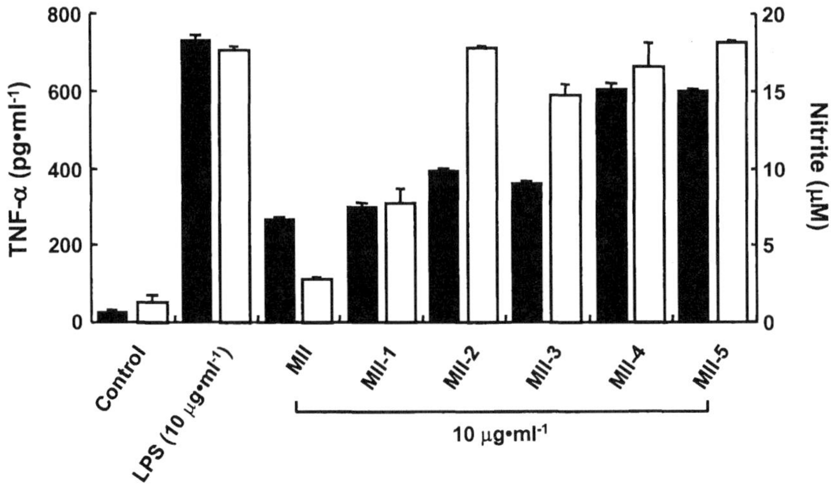

Figure 4. Effects of MII and MII-1, 2, 3, 4, and 5 fraction on production TNF-α (black bars)and NO (white bars) from murine peritoneal macrophages of BALB/c. All values are means ± SE of triplicate measurements. LPS (10 μg/ml) was used as positive control.

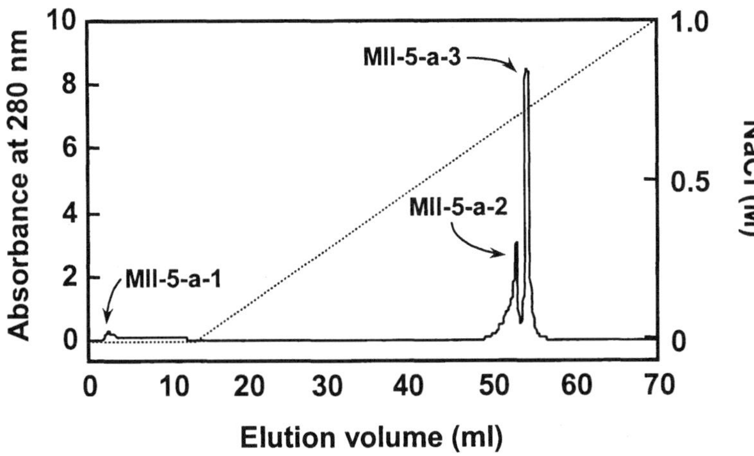

Figure 5. Elution profile of MII-5-a fraction on a column of Mono Q column in FPLC. MII-5 (20 mg) was eluted with 1/15 M phosphate buffer (pH 7.2) and then with a gradient elution between 0 and 1 M NaCl in the same buffer. The sugar content of each fraction was measured as described in Figure 1.

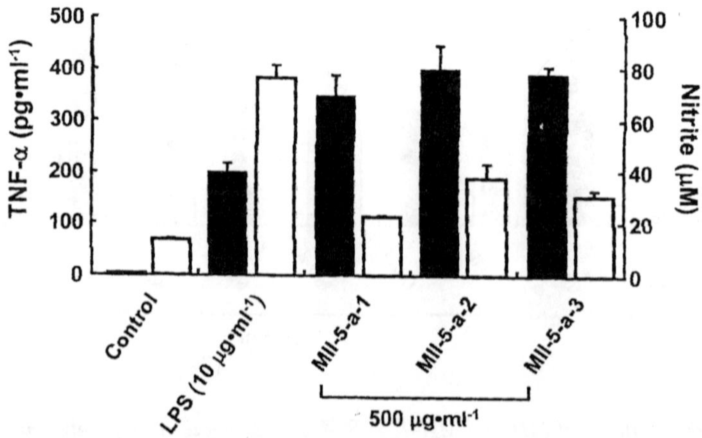

Figure 6. Effects of MII-5-a-1, 2, and 3 fraction on production TNF-α (black bars)and NO (white bars) from murine peritoneal macrophages of BALB/c. All values are means ± S.E. of triplicate measurements. . LPS (10 μg/ml) was used as positive control.

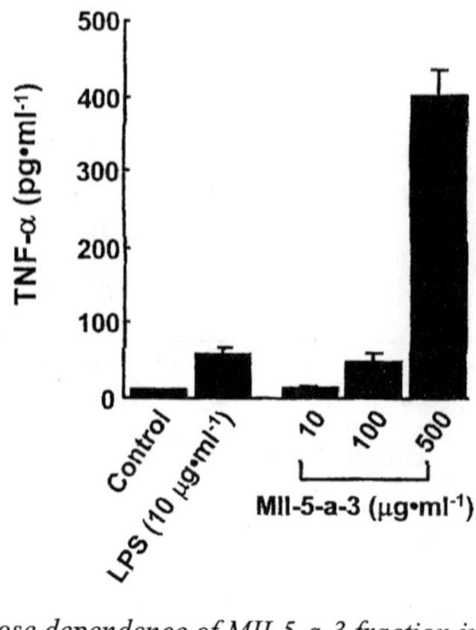

Figure 7. Dose dependence of MII-5-a-3 fraction in terms of TNF-α production from murine peritoneal macrophages of BALB/c at several concentrations. The results are expressed as means ± S.E. for three wells.

Characterization of MII-5-a-3 fraction

The molecular weight was determined chromatographically to be approximately 8,200. As molecular weight of anti-tumor polysaccharides has been reported to be at least 400,000 (*22*), MII-5-a-3 might be a new anti-tumor polysaccharide. The purified fraction MII-5-a-3 showed TNF-α production in a dose-dependent manner at concentrations ranging from 10 to 500 μg/ml (Figure 7). TNF-α production with 500 μg/ml MII-5-a-3 was enhanced to more than 400 pg/ml as compared to that of saline, and was significantly higher than that of 10 μg/ml lipopolysaccharide (LPS). Moreover, TNF-α production with 100 μg/ml was almost at the same level as that of LPS (10 μg/ml). To obtain information about its structure, the TMS analysis of MII-5-a-3 was carried out. The components of this fraction were arabinose and xylose whose mole ratio was 2:1 (data not shown). Other sugars were not detected. These results suggest that MII-5-a-3 is composed of arabinane as its main chain. Furthermore, MII-5-a-3 did not cross-react with the specific antibodies against β-1,3-glucan possessed β-1,6-glucose side chain and β-1,6-glucan possessed β-1,3-glucose side chain (data not shown), suggesting that the structure of this polysaccharide was completely different from other novel anti-tumor polysaccharides such as lentinan (*22*), schizophyllan (*2*) and gliforan (*23*). As the anti-tumor polysaccharides were generally composed mainly of β-1,3-glucan or β-1,6-glucan, MII-5-a-3 might be a new polysaccharide. Further studies are needed to confirm the structure of this compound.

References

1. Chihara, G.; Maeda, Y.; Hamuro, J.; Sasaki, T.; Fukuoka, F. *Nature*, **1969,** *222,* 687.
2. Komatsu, N.; Okubo, S.; Kikumoto, S.; Kimura, K.; Saito, G. *Gann*, **1969,** *60,* 137-144.
3. Nanba, H.; Hamaguchi, A.; Kuroda, H. *Chem. Pharm. Bull.*, **1987,** *35,* 1162.
4. Mizuno, T.; Inagaki, R.; Kanao, T.; Hagiwara, T.; Nakamura, T.; Ito, H.; Shimura, K.; Sumiya, T.; Asakura, A. *Agric. Biol. Chem.* **1990**, *54,* 2897.
5. Mizuno, M.; Shiomi, Y.; Minato, K.; Kawakami, S.; Ashida, H.; Tsuchida, H. *Immunopharmacology*, **2000**, *46,* 113.
6. Mizuno, M.; Morimoto, M.; Minato, K.; Tsuchida, H. *Biosci. Biotech. Biochem.*, **1998**, *62,* 434.
7. Mizuno, M.; Minato, K.; Ito, H.; Kawade, M.; Terai, H.; Tsuchida, H. *Biochem. Mol. Biol. Int.*, **1999**, *47,* 707.
8. Kawagishi, H.; Nomura, A.; Mizuno, T.; Kimura, A.; Chiba, S. *Biochim. Biophys. Acta.*, **1990**, *1034,* 247.

9. Maeda Y.Y.; Chihara, G. *Int. J. Cancer*, **1973,** *11,* 153-161.
10. Kobeyashi, H.; Matsunaga K.; Fujii, M. *Cancer Epidemiol. Biomarkers Prev.,* **1993**, *2,* 271-276.
11. Ladanyi, A.; Timar, J.; Lapis, K. *Cancer Immunol Immun.,* **1993,** *36,* 123-126.
12. Mizutani, Y.; Yoshida, O. *J. Urology*, **1991,** *145,* 1082-1087.
13. Okazaki, M.; Adachi, Y.; Ohno, N.; Yadomae, T. *Biol. Pharm. Bull.,* **1995,** *18,* 1320-1327.
14. Nanba, H.; Kuroda, H. *Chem. Pharm. Bull.,* **1987,** *35,* 2459-2464.
15. Kerékgyártó, C.; Virág, L.; Tankó, L.; Chihara, G.; Fachet, J.; *Int. J. Immunopharmacol.,* **1996**, *18,* 347-353.
16. Xie, O.-W.; Cho, H.J.; Calaycay, J.; Mumford, R.A.; Swiderek, K.M.; Lee, T.D.; Ding, A.; Troso, T.; Nathan, C. *Science,* **1992**, *256,* 225-228.
17. Lowenstein, C.J.; Snyder, S.H.; *Cell*, **1992,** *70,* 705-707.
18. Lorsbach, R.B.; Murphy, W.J.; Lowenstein, C.J.; Snyder, S.H.; Russell, S.W. J. *Biol. Chem.,* **1993,** *268,* 1908-1913.
19. Takano, F.; Kikuchi, Y.; Fushiya, S.; Hojo, H.; Nozoe, S.; Yahagi, N.; Yahagi, R.; Kondo, Y. *Biol. Pharm. Bull.,* **1996,** *19,* 641-643.
20. Oh, G.S.; Hong, K.H.; Oh, H.; Pae, H.O.; Kim, I.K.; Kim, N.Y.; Kwon, T.O.; Shin. M.K.; Chung, H.T. *Biol. Pharm. Bull.,* **2001,** *24,* 785-789.
21. Stuehr, D.J.; Nathan, C.F.; *J. Exp. Med.,* **1989,** *169,* 1543-1555.
22. Chihara, G.; Hamuro, J.; Maeda, Y.Y.; Arai, Y.; Fukuoka, F.; *Cancer Res.,* **1970,** *30,* 2776-2781.
23. Adachi, Y.; Ohno, N.; Osawa, M.; Sato, K.; Oikawa, S.; Yadomae, T. *Chem. Pharm. Bull.,* **1989,** *37,* 1838-1843.

Chapter 15

Role of Histone Acetyltransferase and Deacetylase in the Retinoic Acid-Induced Differentiation of F9 Cells

Chunyuan Jin[1,2], Hongie Li[1,2], Masami Horikoshi[3], Kailai Sun[2], and Kazunari K. Yokoyama[1,*]

[1]Gene Engineering Division, RIKEN (The Institute of Physical and Chemical Research), Bioresource Center, 3–1–1 Koyadai, Tsukuba, Ibaraki 305–0074, Japan
[2]Department of Medical Genetics, China Medical University, Shenyang 110001, Peoples Republic of China
[3]The University of Tokyo, 1–1–1 Yayoi, Bunkyo-ku 113–0032, Japan

Up-regulation of the *c-jun* gene is a critical event in the retinoic acid (RA)-mediated differentiation of embryonal carcinoma F9 cells. Activation transcription factor-2 (ATF-2), adenovirus E1A associated p300 protein (p300) and Jun dimerization protein (JDP2) cooperate in the regulation of transcription of the *c-jun* gene. ATF-2 was found to be a novel histone acetyltransferase (HAT) and it acetylated specifically both histone H2B and histone H4. Motif A, of the HAT domain, was responsible for stimulation of the transcription of *c-jun* gene, in conjunction with HAT of p300. By contrast, JDP2 served as a repressor of AP-1 and inhibited the transactivation of the *c-jun* gene by p300/ATF-2, by recruitment of histone deacetylase complex (HDAC3), thereby repressing the RA-induced transcription of the *c-jun* gene and then inhibiting the RA-mediated differentiation of F9 cells. These results suggest that HDAC3/JDP2 and p300/ATF-2 complex play a critical role in controlling the differentiation of F9 cells, in response to RA.

Murine F9 cells, a line of embryonal carcinoma (EC) cells derived from a teratocarcinoma (*1*), can be induced to differentiate to distinct types of endoderm-like cells by exposure to retinoic acid (RA) (2). The RA-mediated differentiation is associated with dramatic changes in gene expression, including a rapid increase in the rate of transcription of the *c-jun* gene (*3,4*). Moreover, constitutive expression of the *c-jun* gene results in differentiation of various lines of EC cells, such as F9 and P19 cells (*4-6*), suggesting that the induction of the transcription of *c-jun* by RA plays an important role in such differentiation. It has been demonstrated that both RA and adenovirus E1A can stimulate the activity of the *c-jun* promoter and increase the level of endogenous c-jun mRNA (*4,7-11*). The *c-jun* gene encodes a major component of the AP-1 transcription factor that is expressed in many organs during murine development as well as in the adult mouse (*12*). Murine embryos with null mutations in the *c-jun* gene die at midgestation, a phenomenon that suggests an essential function for the product of this gene in murine development (*13,14*). A sequence element in the *c-jun* promoter, designated DRE (differentiation response element), is necessary and sufficient for the RA-induced expression of the *c-jun* gene (*11*). This element binds the differentiation regulatory factor (DRF) complex, of which one component is the adenovirus E1A-associated protein p300 (*16*), which has histone acetyltransferase activity (HAT) (*17-19*), and another component is activating transcription factor-2 (ATF-2), which is a DNA-binding subunit of the DRF complex (*20,21*).

Activation transcription factor-2 (ATF-2; also known as [cAMP-response element (CRE) BP-1] is a member of the ATF/CRE-binding (CREB) family of transcription factors and has a basic region leucine zipper motif (bZip domain) (*22,23*). This motif is necessary for the formation of heterodimers with other members of the ATF family, as well as with members of the Jun/Fos family of factors. The motif is also required for the binding of homodimers of ATF-2 to DRE. ATF-2 and p300 interact with each other in the DRF complex and cooperate in the control of transcription in response to differentiation-inducing signals, such as RA or E1A.

ATF-2 has an intrinsic HAT activity

Various coactivators of transcription, such as GCN/5 (*24*), p300/CBP (*18,25*), PCAF (*19*), ACTR (*25*), SRC-1 (*26*), TAFII250 (*27*) and p/CIP (*28*), have recently been identified as histone acetyltransferases (HATs), an observation that suggests that the ability to catalyze acetylation might be linked to the ability to serve as a transcriptional activator and that such an activity might be involved in the regulation of expression of many genes, as well as in the remodeling of nucleosomes (*29*). We have previously demonstrated that ATF-2 interacts with the region that includes the active site of the HAT domain of the coactivator p300 to control transcription of the *c-jun* gene upon treatment of F9 cells with retinoic acid (RA) or adenovirus E1A (*30*). Therefore, we postulated that ATF-2 might affect the intrinsic HAT activity of p300 (*18,25*). To examine this possibility, the HAT activity of p300 *in vitro* in the presence and in the absence of ATF-2 was monitored. Both a recombinant glutathione S-transferase-p300 (GST-p300) fusion protein that contained a HAT domain [amino acids (a.a.) 1195-1810] and GST-ATF-2 were generated in *Escherichia coli* and their relative HAT activities determined. As reported previously (*17,18*), the HAT domain of p300 was responsible for the HAT activity of p300 *in vitro*, while GST itself had no HAT activity. The HAT activity of p300 was enhanced after incubation with ATF-2. To our surprise, significant HAT activity was still observed when ATF-2 was incubated with p300 that lacked the HAT domain and that had no detectable HAT activity per se, suggesting that the residual HAT activity might have been due to ATF-2.

Possible enhancement of HAT activity by ATF-2 that might be detectable *in vivo* was then examined. The HAT activity of immunoprecipitates obtained with p300-specific or ATF-2-specific antibodies was assayed. Incubation of proteins in extracts of Hela cells with antibodies against p300 or against ATF-2 immunoprecipitated the respective factors that specifically acetylated histones was carried out. The immunoprecipitates obtained with antibodies against c-Jun or p21 had no HAT activity *in vitro*. Therefore, it appeared that ATF-2 might have HAT activity. Assuming that nucleosomes would be the targets for HAT activity *in vivo*, we examined the purified ATF-2 protein for its ability to acetylate free histones and histones in mononucleosomes. ATF-2 preferentially acetylated human histones H2B and H4, both as free histones and as histones bound within mononucleosomes (Fig. 1A) but it did not acetylate histones H3 and H2A (Figs. 1A and 1B).

This finding was further confirmed in experiments that involved *in vitro* phosphorylation by JNK and "in gel HAT assay" using phosphorylated ATF-2 proteins. The phosphorylation of ATF-2 appears to play a key role in stimulating the HAT activity of ATF-2 and in promoting DRE-dependent transcription (*31*). Moreover, the HAT domain of ATF-2 exhibited significant homology to motif A of HATs in the PCAF family and the conserved amino acids at 296, 297 and 299 in motif A were critical for the intrinsic HAT activity of ATF-2 [Fig. 1C]. Our findings provide evidence of a novel phenomenon with respect to the functions of sequence-specific transcription factors. It appears that sequence-specific transcription factors target specific promoters and then recruit various HATs to these specific promoters to enhance transcription. Moreover, it was demonstrated here that a sequence-specific factor, ATF-2, itself has intrinsic HAT activity; ATF-2 might also recruit other HATs that are required for transcriptional activation. Nucleosomal histone acetylation is believed to be a critical step in the modulation of chromatin structures associated with transcriptional activation (*32,33*). Here, it is demonstrated that RA induces dramatic hyperacetylation at endogenous target genes through the HAT activity

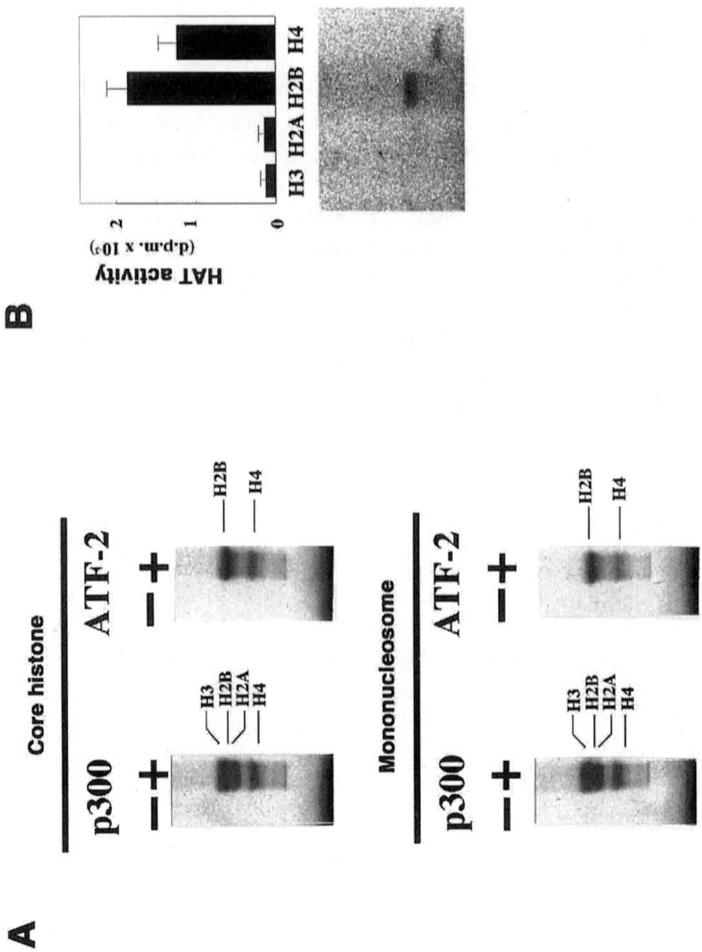
A
Core histone
p300
ATF-2
− +
− +
H3
H2B
H2A
H4
H2B
H4
Mononucleosome
p300
ATF-2
− +
− +
H3
H2B
H2A
H4
H2B
H4
B
HAT activity
(d.p.m. x 10-3)
0
1
2
H3 H2A H2B H4

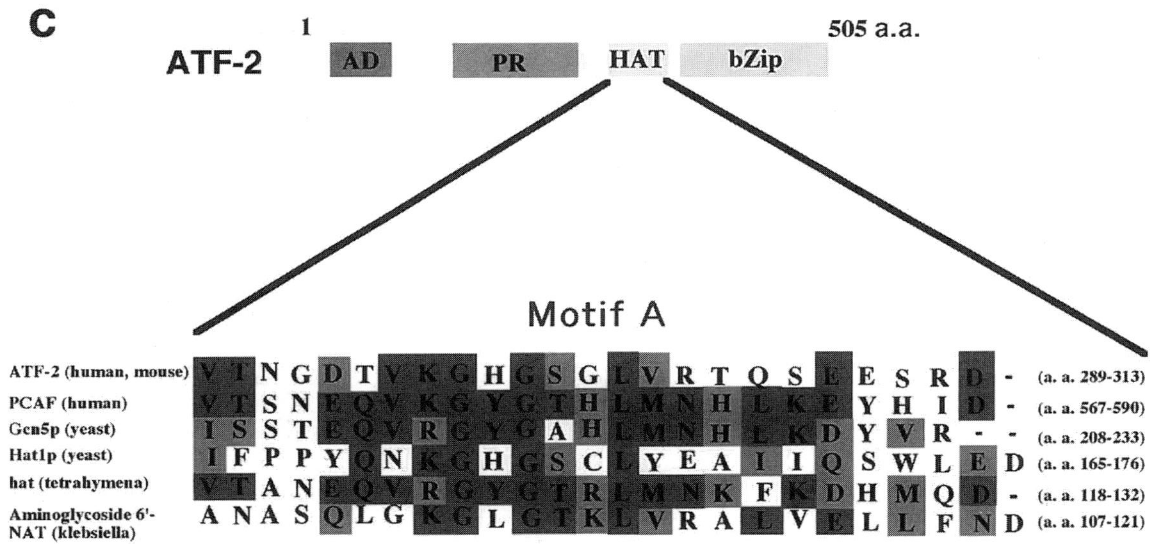

Figure 1. ATF-2 selectively acetylated histones H2B and H4 in vitro. *A, Core histone (33μg, upper panel) or mononucleosome (3μg, lower panel) were incubated with no enzyme (-), with GST-p300 (+) or with GST-ATF-2 (+) as indicated.* ***B****, Purified human histones (H3, H2B, H2A or H4, 0.1 μg of each) was used in a filter binding assay (upper panel) and in an assay with analysis by PAGE (lower panel).* ***C****, Sequence alignment of ATF-2 and members of the PCAF family [45]. Red and pink boxes indicated the same and related amino-acids, respectively. (Reproduced with permission from reference 31. Copyright 2000 McMillan.)*

of ATF-2. To assess directly whether RA-dependent induction of gene expression was correlated with changes in states of histone acetylation, levels of histone acetylation at target genes of ATF-2 was analyzed using a chromatin immunoprecipitation (ChIP) assay (*34*). Thus, an *in vivo* assay of chromatin acetylation demonstrated that RA enhanced the hyperacetylation of H4 by p300/ATF-2 at the ATF-2 target DRE in the *c-jun* promoter. The p300- and CBP-specific ribozyme expressing F9 clones, on the other hand, were not associated with such enhancement of acetylation of all four histones species in the p300 specific-immunoprecipitates. Thus, the possibility that the acetylation of H2B and H4 is caused by other HAT proteins other than ATF-2 and p300/CBP cannot be ruled out. However, these results suggest that treatment of F9 cells with RA enhances the histone acetyltranferase activity of ATF-2. This HAT activity promotes the acetylation of chromatin of ATF-2's target genes, such as *c-jun*, particularly at the chromatin in the DRE region of the *c-jun* promoter, *in vivo*.

Role of histone acetyltransferase activity of ATF-2

The specificity of the histone acetylation catalyzed by ATF-2 is intriguing. Individual heterodimers are quite stable during the assembly of a stable nucleosome core (*35*). Thus, the H2B:H4 interface is a likely site for initial disruption of histone-histone interactions upon unfolding of the nucleosome *in vitro* and *in vivo*. It is possible that ATF-2, a specific DNA-binding factor, might play a key role in the control of the stability of the H2B:H4 interaction by acetylation and/or by direct binding to a specific site on DNA. However, the possibility that nonhistone proteins, such as p53 (*36*), EKLF (*37*), GATA-1 (*38*), TFIIE (*27*) and TFIIF (*27*), might be targets of the HAT activity of ATF-2 cannot be ruled out. Acetylation of the regulatory domains, of these factors by ATF-2 might lead to a dramatic increase in DNA-binding activity and stimulate transcription, as in the case of p53 (*36*).

The possibility exists that ATF-2 has two distinct HAT activities, namely, the intrinsic activity of ATF-2 itself and the HAT activity associated with the p300 coactivator. ATF-2 and p300 might have overlapping actions in terms of substrate specificity, with each protein being required for optimal acetylation for the activation of transcription. It is now important to determine the way in which ATF-2 and p300 function cooperatively and regulate each others activities. In conclusion, as shown here, ATF-2 has intrinsic HAT activity and that the HAT activity of ATF-2 and subsequent DRE-mediated transcription of *c-jun* gene are modulated by phosphorylation.

JDP2 is an inhibitory subunit of the DRF

In a yeast-two hybrid screening with ATF-2 as the bait to identify additional proteins in DRF complex, JDP2, a repressor of AP-1, was isolated as a candidate protein of other members of DRF (*39*). Further studies confirmed that JDP2 is an inhibitory DNA-binding subunit of DRF on the basis of the following observations. First, JDP2 bound directly to the DRE as homodimers or as heterodimers with ATF-2; second, in the electrophoresis migration shift assay (EMSA), bands that corresponded to DRF were shifted still further upon addition of antibodies against JDP2 (Fig. 2A); third, JDP2 interacted directly with ATF-2 *in vivo* and *in vitro* , as well as in a yeast two hybrid system (*39*); and, finally, overexpresson of JDP2 repressed DRE-mediated transactivation by ATF-2 and p300.

Repression of the RA-mediated transcription of the *c-jun* gene by JDP2

Since DRE is both necessary and sufficient for the RA-induced expression of the *c-jun* gene (*11*), repression by JDP2 of the DRE-dependent transcription induced by ATF-2 and p300 implies a role for JDP2 in regulation of the RA-mediated transcription of the *c-jun* gene. In a CAT assay using F9 cells, which had been stably transfected with the -730/+874 c-jun-CAT reporter, both transiently and stably expressed JDP2 repressed the CAT activity that was mediated by the *c-jun* promoter in response to RA. Furthermore, when the cells, which had been stably transfected with JDP2 expressing vector, were treated with RA for different times and then monitored the level of the transcription of the *c-jun* gene by Northern blotting analysis, overexpression of JDP2 delayed and decreased the extent of RA-induced transcription of the *c-jun* gene, as compared to that in cells transfected with the empty vector alone (Fig. 2B). These results suggested that JDP2 inhibits the RA-induced expression of the *c-jun* gene mediated through DRE within *c-jun* promoter.

Block of the RA-induced differentiation of F9 cells by JDP2

Inhibition of transcription of the *c-jun* gene by JDP2 led us to investigate the role of JDP2 in the RA-induced differentiation of F9 cells. As expected, overexpression of JDP2 repressed RA-mediated differentiation, with a delay in and a decrease in the extent of morphological changes associated with differentiation (Fig. 3A), as well as repression of the transcription of RA-inducible genes and genes for markers of differentiation, such as collagen 4α1, laminin B1 and Hoxa-1. The inhibitory effect of JDP2 on differentiation might involve regulation of the transcription of *c-jun*, in view of the key role of *c-jun* in differentiation and of the activity of JDP2 as a negative regulator of the expression of this gene. It is also possible that JDP2 inhibits differentiation, not only via suppression of transcription of *c-jun* but also, by direct repression of expression of other RA-inducible genes and/or genes for markers of differentiation.

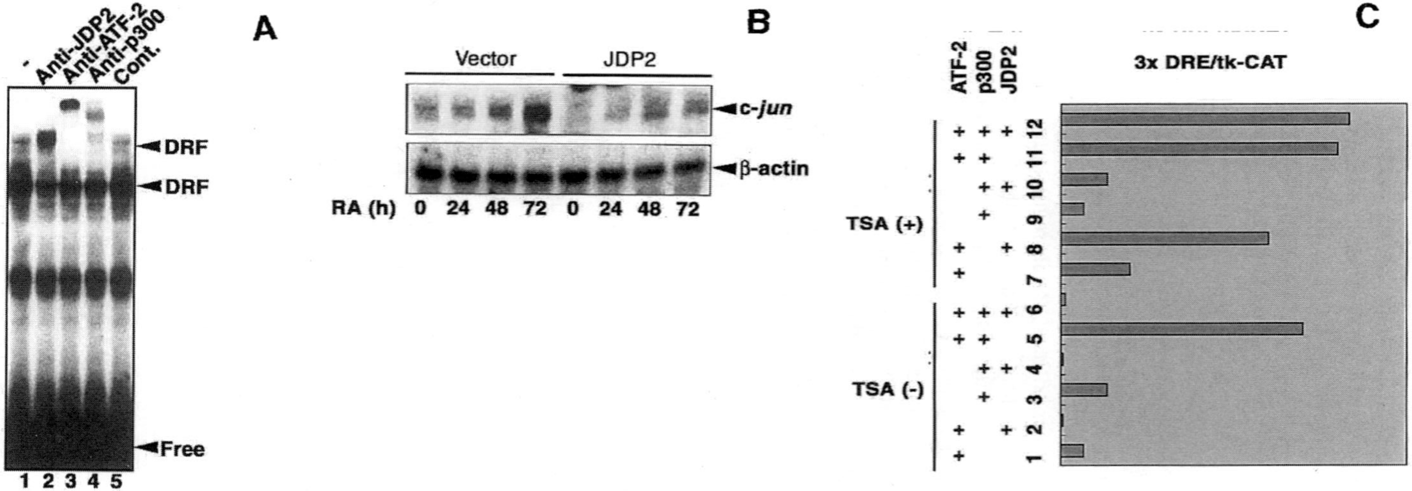

Figure 2. ***JDP2 is a component of the DRF complex.*** *A, EMSA assay with DRE as a probe. Nuclear extracts from F9 cells were incubated without (lane 1) or with antibodies against (Anti-) JDP-2, ATF-2, p300 and control antibody (lanes 2-5, respectively) and mixtures were analyzed by EMSA with DRE as the DNA probe. The position of DRF is indicated.* ***B****, JDP2 represses RA-induced transcription of the c-jun gene. F9 cells that had been stably transfected with empty vector (Vector) or JDP2 expressing vector (JDP2) were incubated with 1 μM RA for the indicated times and levels of c-jun and β-actin transcripts were determined by Northern blotting.* ***C****, Treatment with TSA reverses repression by JDP2. F9 cells were transfected with 3x DRE/tk-CAT in presence or absence of pECE-ATF-2, pACT-p300 and pcDNA-JDP2. Then, 8 h after transfection, the cells were incubated with or without TSA (100 ng/ml) for 16 h and assayed for CAT activity. The results are shown of one of three experiments that gave similar results.*

Mechanism of function of JDP2

JDP2 was initially isolated based on its ability to interact specifically with the AP-1 transcription factor c-Jun (*39*). JDP2 is a relatively small (163 amino acids), ubiquitously expressed bZIP protein that can form stable heterodimers with c-Jun, JunB or JunD, and acts as repressor of c-Jun and c-Jun/c-Fos heterodimer (*39*). JDP2 also interacts with ATF-2 both *in vitro* and *in vivo* via its bZIP domain and binds to the cAMP-response element (CRE) to repress the CRE-dependent transcription that is mediated by ATF-2 (*39*). Thus, it is likely that JDP2, as an AP-1 repressor, might be involved in a variety of transcriptional responses that are associated with progression of the cell cycle, cell differentiation, apoptosis and tumorigenesis (*40-45*). In fact, an inhibitory role of JDP2 in regulating UV-induced apoptosis through suppression of the expression of p53 was reported recently (*46*). However, details of the physiological role of JDP2 remain unknown and the mechanisms by which JDP2 acts also remain to be clarified. Aronheim *et al.* (*47*) proposed that JDP2 might repress the transcriptional activity of *c-jun* by forming a stable c-Jun/JDP2 heterodimer and competes with activators for binding to c-Jun. Alternatively, JDP2 might enhance the binding of c-Jun to the promoter, thereby providing further inhibition via competition with active heterodimers for binding to the same elements. However, in the case of the repression by JDP2 of ATF-2-mediated transactivation, the repression of transcription of the *c-jun* gene by JDP2 depended on an HDAC with, most probably, recruitment of HDAC3 to the DRE of the *c-jun* promoter. This conclusion is confirmed by the observation that the suppression by JDP2 of DRE-mediated transactivation by ATF-2 and p300 was reversed when cells were treated with TSA, an HDAC-specific inhibitor (Fig. 2C) and by the observation that the immunoprecipitates obtained with antibodies specific for JDP2 had HDAC activity. Moreover, association of JDP2 with HDAC3 was confirmed by a demonstration of their interaction *in vivo* and by their co-existance in a DRF complex, as determined by EMSA and the ChIP assay (Fig. 3B). Furthermore, augmentation of the repressive activity of JDP2 by enhanced expression of HDAC3 also suggested a functional relationship between JDP2 and HDAC3.

Role of JDP2 in the commitment of F9 cells to RA-induced differentiation

A very low level of c-Jun, a major component of the AP-1 transcription factor, is expressed in undifferentiated F9 cells. Levels of endogenous *c-jun* mRNA begin to rise dramatically within 18-24 h of the start of exposure to RA and reach a steady state after 60-72 h (*44*). The mechanisms of transactivation of the *c-jun* gene in stimulated F9 cells are relatively well understood but it is unclear how the expression of the gene is maintained in an inhibited state in non stimulated F9 cells but can respond rapidly to RA. It is possible that JDP2, acting as a repressive component of DRF, might have properties consistent with a role in inhibiting the expression of *c-jun* in non stimulated F9 cells and in the

A

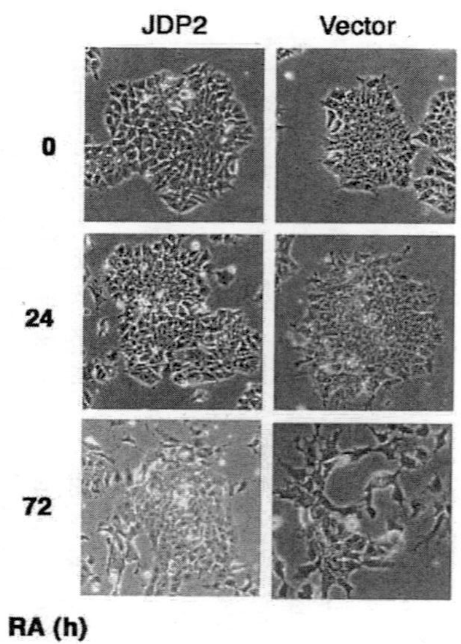
JDP2
Vector
0
24
72
RA (h)

C

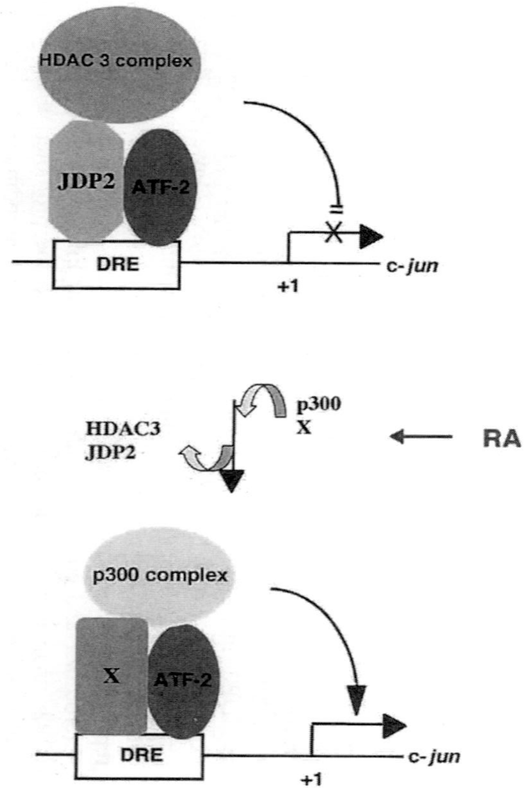
HDAC 3 complex
JDP2
ATF-2
DRE
+1
c-jun
HDAC3
JDP2
p300
X
RA
p300 complex
X
ATF-2
DRE
+1
c-jun

B

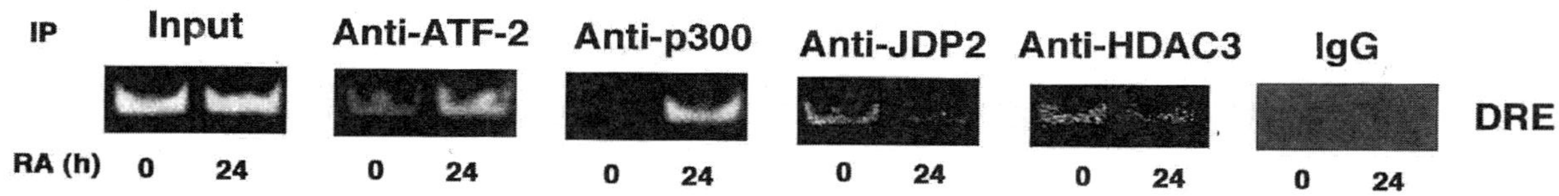

Figure 3. JDP2 blocks RA-mediated differentiation of F9 cells. *A, F9 cells that had been stably transfected with empty vector (Vector) of JDP2 expressing vector (JDP2) were incubated without or with 1 μM RA. The cells were then photographed at the indicated times after exposure to RA under a phase-contrast microscope (magnification, 125x).* ***B****, Alterations in binding to DRE of components of DRF. Soluble chromatin was prepared from F9 cells that had been incubated with (24 h) or without RA (0 h) and it was immunoprecipitated (IP) with various antibodies (Anti-) as indicated. The same extracts were incubated with mouse IgG for the nonspecific precipitation of chromatin. Precipitated genomic DNA was analyzed by PCR using primers that corresponded to the sequence that spanned the DRE. The left panel shows the level of DRE that was amplified prior to immunoprecipitation, confirming that equivalent amounts of DNA were present in each sample.* ***C****, Hypothetical model of the role of JDP2 in the commitment of F9 cells to differentiation in response to RA. In undifferentiatied F9 cells, the association of HDAC3 with JDP2, which has interacted with ATF-2, results in deacetylated histones on the DRE, with repression of expression of c-jun. When the cells are exposed to RA, JDP2 and HDAC3 are replaced by p300 and, perhaps, by an unknown factor (X), resulting in hyperacetylation of histones associated with DRE, initiation of transcription of the c-jun gene and, finally, initiation of the differentiation of F9 cells.*

rapid response to stimulation by RA during the commitment of F9 cells to differentiation. This hypothesis is further supported by the observation that, although the level of expression of JDP2 was apparently unchanged, binding of JDP2 to DRE and the association of JDP2 with HDAC3 and with ATF-2 decreased markedly at 24 h after the start of treatment of F9 cells with RA (Fig. 3B). By contrast, binding to DRE of p300 and ATF-2 was significantly enhanced after treatment of cells with RA for 24 h (Fig. 3B). Furthermore, the replacement of the JDP2/HDAC3 combination by the ATF-2/p300 combination in the DRF complex was accompanied by a change in the acetylation status of histones associated with the DRE, from hypo- to hyperacetylation, during the commitment of F9 cells to differentiation in response to RA.

A simple model for the role of JDP2 in regulation of transcription of the *c-jun* gene in F9 cells is presented (Fig. 3C). In this model, JDP2, which has interacted with ATF-2 and bound to DRE, recruits HDAC3 to the DRE in undifferentiated F9 cells, thereby, maintaining the deacetylated status of histones and repressing the expression of the *c-jun* gene. When the cells are exposed to RA, JDP2 and HDAC3 are replaced by p300/ATF-2 and, perhaps, by another unknown factor (X), with resultant hyperacetylation of histones associated with the DRE and initiation of activation of the *c-jun* gene. The levels of recruitment of the HDAC3/JDP2 complex and the p300/X complex might be critical for determination of the choice between the undifferentiated state and the commitment of cells to differentiation in response to RA.

Taken together, it is likely that the relative extent of histone acetylation by p300/ATF-2 and deacetylation by HDAC3/JDP2, respectively, play a critical role in determining the stage of undifferentiation or of differentiation of F9 cells, in response to RA.

References

1. Bersteine, E. G.; Hooper, M. L.; Grandchamp, S.; Ephrussi, B. (1973). *Proc. Natl. Acad. Sci.* **1973**, *70,* 3899-3903.
2. Strickland, S.; Mahdavi, V. *Cell* **1978**, *15*, 393-403.
3. de Groot, R.P.; Schoorlemmer, J.; van Genesen, S. T.; Kruijer, W. *Nucleic Acids Res.* **1990**, *18*, 3195-3202.
4. Yang-Yen, H. F.; Chiu, R.; Karin, M. *Nature New Biol.* **1990**, *2*, 351-361.
5. de Groot, R.P.; Kruyt, F.A.E.; van Genesen, S.T.; Kruijer, W. *EMBO J.* **1990**, *9*, 1831-1837.
6. Yamaguchi-Iwai, Y.; Satake, M.; Murakami, Y.; Sakai, M.; Muramatsu, M.; Ito, Y. *Proc. Natl. Acad. Sci.* **1990**, *87*, 8670-8674.
7. van Dan, H.; Offringa, R.; Moijer, I.; Stein, B.; Smits, A. M.; Herrich, P.; Bos, J.L.; van der Eb, A. *J. Mol. Cell. Biol.* **1990**, *10*, 5857-5864.
8. de Groot, R.P.; Foulkes, N.; Mulder, M.; Krujer, W.; Sassow-Corci, P. *Mol. Cell. Biol.* **1991**, *4*, 192-206.

9. de Groot, R. P.; Rales, D.; Kruijer, W. *Nucleic Acids Res.* **1991**, *19*, 1585-1591.
10. Kitabayashi, I.; Chiu, R.; Gachelin, G.; Yokoyama, K. *Nucleic Acids Res.* **1991**, *19*, 644-655.
11. Kitabayashi, I.; Kawakami, Z.; Chiu, R.; Ozawa, K.; Matsuoka, T.; Toyoshima, S.; Umesono, K.; Evans, R. M.; Gachelin, G.; Yokoyama, K. *EMBO J.* **1992**, *11*, 167-175.
12. Angel, P.; Karin, M. *Biochim. Biophys. Acta.* **1991**, *1072*, 129-157.
13. Hilberg, F.; Aguzzi, A.; Howells, N.; Wagner, E. F. *Nature* **1997**, *365*, 179-181.
14. Johnson, R.S.; van Liger, B.; Papaioannou, V.E.; Spiegelman, B. M. *Genes & Dev.* **1993**, *7*, 1309-1317.
15. Eckner, R.; Yao, T.-S.; Oldread, E.; Livingston, D.M. *Genes & Dev.* **1994**, *8*, 869-884.
16. Kitabayashi, I.; Eckner, R.; Arany, Z.; Chiu, R.; Gachelin, G.; Livingston, D.M.; Yokoyama, K. *EMBO J.* **1995**, *14*, 3496-3509.
17. Bannister, A.J.; Kouzarides, T. *Nature* **1996**, *384*, 641-643.
18. Ogryzko, V.W.; Schiltz, R.L.; Russanova, V.; Howard, R.H.; Nakatani, Y. *Cell* **1996**, *87*, 953-959.
19. Yang, X.J.; Ogryzko, V.V.; Nishikawa, J.; Howard, B.H.; Nakatani, Y. *Nature* **1996**, *382*, 319-324.
20. Kawasaki, H.; Song, J.; Eckner, R.; Ugai, H.; Chiu, R.; Taira, K.; Shi, Y.; Jones, N.; Yokoyama, K.K. *Genes & Dev.* **1998**, *12*, 233-245.
21. Kawasaki, H.; Eckner, R.; Yao, T-P.; Taira, K.; Chiu, R.; Livingston, D.M.; Yokoyama, K. *Nature* **1998**, *393*, 284-289.
22. Hai, T.; Fiu, F.; Coukos, W.J.; Green, M.R. *Genes & Dev.* **1989**, *3*, 2083-2090.
23. Maekawa, T.; Skura, H.; Ishi-Kanei, C.; Sudo, T.; Yoshimura, T.; Fujisawa, J.; Yoshida, M.; Ishii, S. *EMBO. J.* **1989**, *8*, 2023-2028.
24. Brownell, J.E.; Zhou, J.; Ranalli, T.; Kabayashi, R.; Edmondson, D.G.; Roth, S.Y.; Allis, C.D. *Cell* **1996**, *84*, 843- 851.
25. Chen, H.; Lin, R.J.; Schiltz, R.l.; Chakravarti, D.; Nash, A.; Nagy, L.; Privalsky, M.L.; Nakatani, Y.; Evans, R.M. *Cell* **1997**, *90*, 569-580.
26. Spencer, T.E.; Jenster, G.; Burcin, M.M.; Allis, C.D.; Zhou, J.; Mizzen, C.A.; McKenna, N.J.; Onate, S.A.; Tsai, S.Y.; Tsai, M-J.; O'Malley, B.W. *Nature* **1997**, *389*, 194-198.
27. Imhof, A.; Yang, X.J.; Ogryzko,V.V.; Nakatani, Y.; Wolff, A.P.; Ge, H. *Curr. Biol.* **1997**, *7*, 689-692.
28. Torchia, J.; Rose, D.W.; Inostroza, J.; Kamei, Y.; Westin, S.; Glass, C.W.; Rosenfeld, M.G. *Nature* **1997**, *387*, 677-684.
29. Struhl, K. *Genes & Dev.* **1998**, *12*, 599-606.
30. Brown, C.E.; Lechner, T.; Howe, L.; Workman, J.L. *TIBS* **2000**, *25*, 15-19.

31. Kawasaki, H.; Schiltz, L.; Chiu, R.; Itakura, K.; Taira, K.; Nakatani, Y.; Yokoyama, K. *Nature* **2000**, *405*, 195-200.
32. Luger, K.; Mäder, A.M.; Richmond, R.K.; Sargent, D.F.; Richmond, T.J. *Nature* **1997**, *389*, 251-259.
33. Gu, W.; Roeder, R.G. *Cell* **1997**, *90*, 595-606.
34. Zhang, W.; Bieker, J.J. *Proc. Natl. Acad. Sci. USA* **1998**, *95*, 9855-9860.
35. Boyes, J.; Byfield, P.; Nakatani, Y.; Ogryzko, V. *Nature* **1998**, *396*: 594-598.
36. Jin, C.; Ugai, H.; Song, J.; Murata, T.; Nili, F.; Sun, K.; Horikoshi, M.; Yokoyama, K.K. *FEBS Lett.* **2001**, *489,* 34-41.
37. Karin, M.; Liu, Z.; G.; Zandi, E. *Curr. Opin. Cell Biol.* **1997**, *9,* 240-246.
38. Vogt, P.; Bos, T.J. *Adv. Cancer Res.* **1990**, *55,* 1-35.
39. Bossy-Wetzel, E.; Yaniv, M. *EMBO J.* **1997**, *16*: 1695-1709.
40. Schreiber, M.; Kolbus, A.; Piu, F.; Szabowski, A.; Muhle-Steinlein, U.; Tian, J.; Karin, M.; Angel, P.; Wagner, E.F. *Genes & Dev.* **1999**, *13*, 607-619.
41. Yong, M.R.; Li, J.-J.; Rincon, M.; Flavell, R.A.; Sashyanarayana, B. K.; Hunziker, R.; Colburn, N. *Proc. Natl. Acad. Sci.* **1999**, *96*, 9827-9832.
42. Piu, F.; Aronheim, A.; Katz, S.; Karin, M. *Mol. Cell. Biol.* **2001**, *21,* 3012-3024.
43. Aronheim, A.; Zandi, E.; Hennemann, H.; Elledge, S.J.; Karin, M. *Mol. Cell. Biol.* **1997**, *17*: 3094-3102.
44. Kitabayashi, I.; Chiu, R.; Evans, R.M.; Gachelin, G.; Yokoyama, K. *Cell Dev. Biol.* **1994**, *30A*, 761-768.
45. Dutnall, R.N.; Tafrov. S.T.; Stermgalanz, R.; Ramakrishnam, V. *Cell* **1998**, *94*, 427-438.

Biomarker and Animal Models

Chapter 16

In Vivo Inhibition of Mammary Carcinogenesis, Formation of DNA–Carcinogen Adducts, and Mammary Proliferation by Dietary Dibenzoylmethane

Chuan-Chuan Lin[1,2], Yao-Ping Lu[1], You-Rong Lou[1], Chi-Tang Ho[2], Harold H. Newmark[1], Christopher MacDonald[3], Keith W. Singletary[3], and Mou-Tuan Huang[1]

[1]Laboratory for Cancer Research, College of Pharmacy, Rutgers, The State University of New Jersey, Piscataway, NJ 08854–8020
[2]Department of Food Science, Cook College, Rutgers, The State University of New Jersey, New Brunswick, NJ 08901–8520
[3]Department of Food Science and Human Nutrition, University of Illinois, Urbana, IL 61801

Dibenzoylmethane (DBM) is a minor constituent in licorice and has anti-inflammatory activity. Feeding 1% DBM in the diet to Sencar mice during both the initiation and post-initiation stages strongly inhibited 7,12-dimethylbenz[a]-anthracene (DMBA)-induced mammary tumorigenesis in both tumor incidence and tumor multiplicity. Feeding 1% DBM in the diet to immature mice for 4-5 weeks decreased uterine wet weight, inhibited proliferation of uterus and mammary gland, and lowered serum estradiol levels. In addition, feeding 1% DBM in the diet to mice increased liver weight and levels of hepatic cytochrome P-450 as well as increased hepatic hydroxylation and glucuronidation of estradiol. In further studies, feeding 1% DBM in the diet to mice at 2 weeks before, during and for a week after DMBA treatment (intubation of 1 mg DMBA in corn oil per mouse once a week for 2 or 5 weeks) markedly inhibited formation of mammary gland DMBA-DNA adducts by a [^{32}P]post-labeling assay. Adding various doses of DBM to an incubation of DMBA with mouse liver microsomes in vitro inhibited DMBA metabolism and formation of DMBA-DNA adducts in a dose-dependent manner. In an assay of competitive binding to estrogen receptors with [^{3}H]estradiol in vitro, DBM showed only weak binding affinity.

Cancer has been a major killer throughout human history. As countries become more industrialized, long term risk factors such as cigarette smoking, unhealthful dietary habits and exposure to dangerous chemicals in the environment seem to be more common (*1*). It is estimated that concers of the lung, colon, breast, and prostate, , account for more than half of all deaths from cancer in the United States. Among these, breast cancer is the most common cancer in women, only second to lung cancer. It is now estimated that 1 in 9 women will expect to develop breast cancer in her lifetime (*2*). Epidemiological data and some laboratory animal studies indicated that certain naturally occurring and synthetic components are able to block the carcinogenic process and inhibit development of some cancers including breast (*3*). Based on the multistage model of chemical carcinogenesis, which consists of initiation, promotion and progression (*4*), chemoprevention may be achieved by interfering with one or several steps in this process.

Dibenzoylmethane (DBM) is a minor constituent of licorice (*5*). DBM somewhat shares chemical and biological properties with curcumin (Figure 1). Both are metal-chelating agents, have anti-inflammatory and anti-tumor promoting activities (*6*). Chemically, curcumin has a β-diketone group with conjugated double bonds, while DBM has a relatively smaller molecular size and lacks phenolic hydroxyl groups and conjugated double bonds, and does not have appreciable antioxidant activity *in vitro* (6). In addition, Dr. Talalay et al. has reported that DBM is a phase-2 enzyme inducer (*7*). Our laboratory and others have shown that dietary DBM strongly inhibited 7,12-dimethylbenz-[a]anthracene (DMBA)-induced mammary carcinogenesis in mice and rats (*8,9*). DBM inhibited benzo[a]pyrene and 1,6-dinitropyrene-DNA adduct formation in human epithelial cells (*10*), protected against free radical DNA damages (*11*), and was used as a sun screening agent (*12*). DBM and certain of its derivatives have anti-mutagenic activity (*13*).

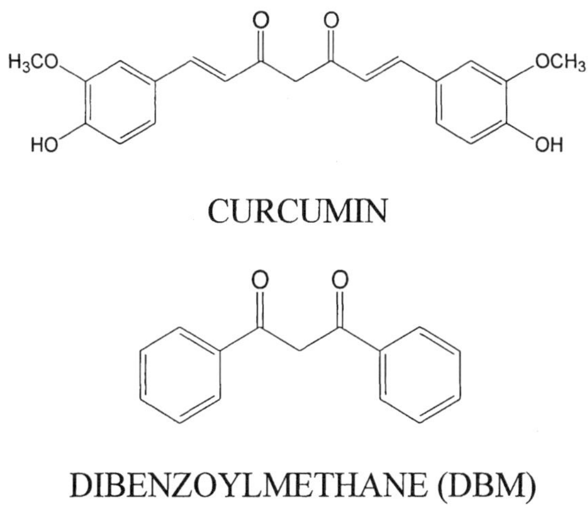

Figure 1. Chemical structures of curcumin and dibenzoylmethane.

Preliminary *in vivo* studies suggested that DBM may have multiple actions toward carcinogenic processes. Based on these results from animal studies, we further investigated the underlying mechanisms of the multiple actions of DBM in the prevention of mammary tumorigenesis through understanding the effects of DBM in the two-stage carcinogenic process (see Figure 2). In this report, we intend to focus on the effect of DBM on the estrogen-dependent promotion considered essential from several lines of evidence (*8-10*).

The studies presented here indicate that dietary DBM decreased uterine wet weight, inhibited proliferation of mammary glands and uterus, decreased formation of mammary gland-DNA adducts and lowered serum estradiol, and triglyceride levels. These biomarker changes suggested that DBM plays an important role in the modulation of endogenous estradiol. Further studies showed that dietary DBM increased liver weight and levels of total hepatic cytochrome P-450 as well as increased hepatic hydroxylation and glucuronidation of estradiol. In addition, in *in vitro* studies, DBM was shown to be able to weakly compete with [^{3}H]-estradiol for estrogen receptor sites (*6,18*). Taken together, these studies could provide insights into understanding the mechanisms involved in the inhibitory action of DBM on mammary tumorigenesis. Therefore, we hope to determine if DBM or a related β-diketone could be considered for extended studies as a potential chemopreventive agent, especially for breast cancer prevention.

Materials and Methods

Dibenzoylmethane, dimethylbenz[a]anthracene, glucose-6-phosphate, glucose-6-phosphate dehydrogenase, nicotinamide adenine dinucleotide phosphate (NADPH), activated charcoal, sodium dodecyl sulfate, estradiol, diethylstilbestrol, hydroxylapatite were purchased from Sigma Chemical Co. (St. Louis, MO). [G-^{3}H] 7,12-dimethylbenz[a]anthracene (specific activity 70 Ci/mmol, 5 Ci/mL)) and [6,7-^{3}H(N)]-estradiol in ethanol (specific activity 40 Ci/mmol, 1 Ci/mL) were purchased from Dupont New England Nuclear Research Products (Boston, MA). Calf thymus DNA was obtained from Miles Laboratory LTD. ScintiVerse and all solvents (HPLC grade) were purchased from Fisher Scientific Co. (Springfield, NJ). AIN-76A diet and 1% DBM in AIN-76A diet were purchased from Research Diets, Inc. (New Brunswick, NJ). BrdU staining kit was purchased from Oncogene Science (Cambridge, MA).

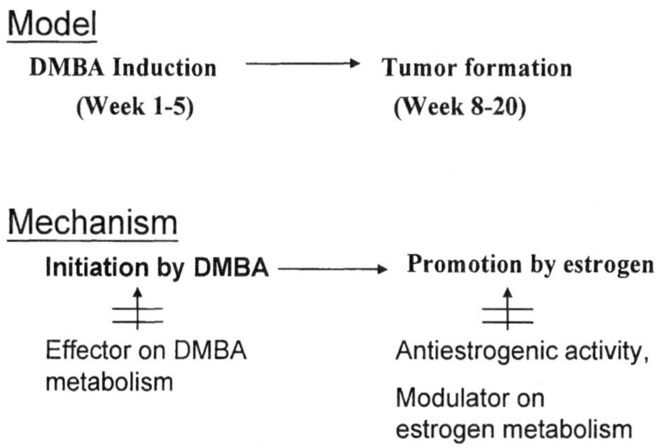

Figure 2. Typical mouse model for DMBA-induced mammary tumorigenesis and possible ways of inhibition.

Animals

Female Sencar mice (3-4 weeks old) were purchased from Charles River Breeding Laboratories (Kingston, NY). The animals were kept in our animal facility for at least one week before use. The mice were given Purina Laboratory Chow 5001 diet and water *ad libitum* and they were kept at a 12 h light/12 h dark cycle during this adaptation period.

Mammary Carcinogenesis Induction in Sencar Mice

DMBA-induced mammary gland tumorigenesis in Sencar mice was produced according to a slight modification of the procedure as described by Fischer (*14*). The mice were intubated with 1 mg DMBA (in 0.1 mL corn oil) once a week for 5 weeks and AIN-76A diet or 1% DBM in AIN-76A diet were given *ad libitum* to mice starting at 2 weeks before the first dose of DMBA, and continuing until the end of the experiment. The sizes of the palpable mammary tumors were measured. Mice with mammary tumor diameters greater than 15 mm were killed. All mice were killed at 20 weeks after the first dose of DMBA. All tumors were examined histopathologically.

Incorporation of Bromodeoxyuridine (BrdU) into DNA of Mammary Gland

Incorporation of BrdU into DNA was performed as described previously (*15*). BrdU, a thymidine analogue that is incorporated into proliferating cells during the S-phase, is detected by a biotinylated monoclonal anti-BrdU antibody and visualized using streptavidin peroxidase and 3,3'-diaminobenzidine, which stains BrdU-containing nuclei a dark brown using a staining kit from Oncogene Science (Cambridge, MA). Briefly, all the animals were injected i.p. with BrdU (50 mg/Kg) and killed 1 hour later. Mammary glands and uterus were removed and stored in a -80^0C freezer for the BrdU labeling index assay.

Determination of Estrous Cycle

For determination of the estrous cycle, vaginal smears were collected 54-60 days postpartum. Smears were fixed in acetone for 10 min at room temperature and then subjected to H & E staining. The estrous cycle averages 4 to 5 days. The estrus phase may last from 9 to 15 hours. The exfoliated cytology is characterized by marked squamification and cornification of the cells and the disappearance of leukocytes. During the latter part of estrus, these cells appear to degenerate and in many cases are recovered in aggregate-like masses of cellular material. All the mice were killed during the estrus phase of the estrous cycle.

Formation of DMBA-DNA Adducts in Mammary Glands

Female Sencar mice (5 weeks old) were randomly divided into 8 groups (9 mice/group) and fed various percentages of DBM in AIN-76A diet as follows: groups 1,5: control AIN-76A; groups 2,6: 0.2% DBM in AIN-76A diet; groups 3,7: 0.5% DBM in AIN-76A diet; groups 4,8: 1% DBM in AIN-76A diet. Two weeks after starting on these diets, the mice were administered 1 mg DMBA in 0.1 ml corn oil once a week for 2 weeks (groups 1-4) or for 5 weeks (groups 5-8). The mice were killed at 24 hours after the last dose of DMBA.

Isolation of Mammary Epithelial Cell Aggregates and DNA

The mice were sacrificed by decapitation and mammary tissues were removed (approx. 12-16 whole mammary fat pads from 3 mice). The mammary tissues were finely minced, transferred to a 20 mL of M199 medium with 40 mg of type II collagenase in a spinner flask. The mixture was gently stirred for 2 hour at 37^{0}C. When the digestion appeared complete, the solution was filtered through a coarse (500 micron) nylon mesh filter. Cells and aggregates were collected by centrifugation at 600 x g for 8 minutes at 4^{0}C and washed by re-suspension in M199 medium. After twice washing and centrifugation, epithelial cell aggregate pellets were subjected to DNA isolation. The genomic DNA from mouse mammary gland was isolated with Easy-DNA kit (Invitrogen, Los Angeles, CA) and pure DNA was quantitated by measuring at A_{260} nm by UV spectrophotometry. The ratio value of absorbance of A_{260}/A_{230} and A_{260}/A_{280} was > 2.4 and 1.8. DNA was quantitated by UV absorption at 260 nm based on the relationship that 1 mg DNA=10 A_{260} units using calf thymus DNA as the standard.

^{32}P-Post-labeling Procedures

The methods for the ^{32}P-post-labeling of mammary DNA as well as identification and quantification of DMBA-DNA adducts on TLC are described in a previous publication (*16*). The adduct numbers designated in Table 3 corresponded to individual DMBA-DNA adducts identified by HPLC (high performance liquid chromatography) cross referencing procedure adapted from Schmeiser *et al* (*17*).

Preparation of Crude Uterine Cytosol from Rat Uteri

Female Sprague-Dawley ovariectomized rats (6 weeks old) were used in this experiment. Estradiol (2 μg in a 100 µL solution containing 10% ethanol in saline) was injected s.c. into the rats once a day for 10 days. Rats were given Lab AIN-76A diet or 0.5% DBM in AIN-76A diet and water *ad libitum*. Rats were sacrificed and the uteri were trimmed, weighed and placed into ice-cold saline.

Rat uteri were collected, weighed and homogenized (100 mg fresh tissue/ml) in tris-EDTA buffer (TE) (10 mM Tris, 1.5 mM EDTA, pH 7.4) in a Kontes glass homogenizer (0-4^{0}C) with a motor driven pestle. The homogenates were centrifuged at 3,000xg for 10 min at 4^{0}C. The supernatant was recentrifuged at 105,000xg for 1 hr at 4^{0}C. The resulting cytosol was diluted to 75 mg tissue/mL TE buffer (5 mg/mL of protein concentration) and stored in a – 20^{0}C freezer for use within 1 month.

Assay for Competitive Inhibition of [^{3}H]-Estradiol Binding to Cytosol

The assay mix contained a 250 μL aliquot of diluted cytosol, 50 μL of 40 nM [^{3}H]-estradiol (specific activity 40 Ci/mmol, 1 Ci/mL) and 50 μL various concentrations of competitor in 20% ethanol-TE buffer. The final concentrations of competitors were 40-40,000 nM of unlabeled estradiol, diethylstilbestrol (DES) or DBM. The mixture was incubated at 30^{0}C for 1 hour and then cooled to 4^{0}C. The bound ligand was separated from free ligand by the addition of 250 μL suspended hydroxylapatite (HAP) in TE buffer (60% v/v).The HAP-cytosol suspension was votexed and centrifuged at 1,000 x g for 10 minutes. The resulting HAP-pellet was washed two times by re-suspension in 1 mL ice-cold TE and centrifuged to remove free [^{3}H]-estradiol. The final washed pellet was extracted with 1 mL 100% ethanol and the bound count was determined by a scintillation counter. Specific binding was determined by subtraction of nonspecific binding (not competed by 300 fold of DES) from the total quantity of bound [^{3}H]-estradiol. Results were expressed as percentage of specific binding versus log concentration of competitor. The data represent an average from triplicate determinations of each sample.

Determination of Several Biomarkers and Intermediate Metabolites in the Serum of 1%DBM-treated Sencar Mice

Female Sencar mice were given AIN-76A diet (n = 15 mice/group) or 1% DBM in the AIN-76A diet (n = 17 mice/group) for 4-5 weeks. During the experiment, water and food consumption and body weights were recorded weekly. At the end of experiment, all mice were killed and parametrial fat pad, uterus, mammary gland and liver weights were measured. The blood samples were collected. The serum was prepared by centrifugation of the collected blood and stored at -80^0C. Determination of the serum estradiol and progesterone concentrations was done by enzyme-linked immunosorbent assay (ELISA) from Oxford Biomedical Research, Inc. (Oxford, MI). The serum was extracted with ethyl ether (or petroleum ether for progesterone assay) and the concentrated residue was dissolved in extraction buffer provided by commercial kit (Oxford Biomedical Research, Inc., Oxford, MI). In a microplate with the corresponding antibody precoated on each well, the samples and enzyme conjugate (estradiol-horseradish peroxidase) were added and the mixture was incubated at room temperature for one hour. During this time, competition for the limited binding sites would take place. After washing 3 times with wash buffer to remove unbound material, the quantity of bound enzyme conjugate was determined by adding substrate (3,3′,5,5′-tetramethylbenzidine and hydrogen peroxide). An optimal color was developed after 30 minutes of incubation and the absorbance reading of each well at 650 nm was measured by a microplate reader. The calculation of hormone concentration in samples was performed according to the manual by using a standard curve.

Concentration of triglyceride was assayed by a commercially available kit (Sigma, St. Louis, MO). Briefly, the triglycerides in the sample were hydrolyzed to glycerol and fatty acids with lipoprotein lipase (Reagent B). After a series of coupled enzymatic reactions catalyzed by glycerol kinase, glycerol phosphate oxidase and peroxidase as well as appropriate substrates (Reagent A), a quinoneimine was produced. The absorbance of both standard and samples at 540 nm was measured and the total glycerol was calculated.

Results

Inhibitory Effect of Dietary DBM on DMBA-induced Mammary Tumorigenesis in Sencar Mice

Mice fed AIN-76A diet in the control group were intubated with 1 mg of DMBA per mouse once a week for 5 weeks. The mice developed DMBA-induced 0.025, 0.50, 0.73 and 1.08 palpable mammary tumors per mouse at 3, 9, 13, or 20 weeks, respectively, after the last dose of DMBA treatment (Table I). Mammary tumors in mice that were killed at 20 weeks after the last dose of DMBA were confirmed histopathologically. The first tumors in control mice appeared at 3 weeks after the last dose of DMBA treatment. In the parallel group of mice fed with 1 % DBM in AIN-76A diet, the first mammary tumor appeared at 18 weeks after the last dose of DMBA treatment, suggesting a mammary tumor latency time of 15 weeks. Tumor incidence in the control mice was 3, 38, 55, or 68% at 3, 9, 13, or 20 weeks after the last of DMBA dosing. Tumor incidence in the 1% DBM treatment mice was 0, 0, 0, or 3% at 3, 9, 13, or 20 weeks after the last DMBA treatment (Table I). The results indicated that 1% DBM dietary dramatically decreased mammary tumor multiplicity and incidence, and increased the time for tumor development.

Table I. Inhibitory effect of feeding 1% dibenzoylmethane in the diet on 7,12-dimethylbenz[a]anthracene-induced mammary carcinogenesis in Sencar mice

	AIN-76A diet		*1% DBM in AIN-76A diet*	
Weeks after last dose of DMBA	*Tumors per mouse*	*Percent of mice with tumors*	*Tumors per mouse*	*Percent of mice with tumors*
3	0.025±0.0	3	0*	0
9	0.50 ±0.05	38	0*	0
13	0.73±0.12	55	0*	0
20	1.08± 0.17	68	0.03*	3

*Statistical difference from the AIN-76A diet group ($P < 0.05$) as determined by the Student's t test. (Data are from Reference *25*)

Inhibitory Effect of Dietary DBM on Proliferation of the Mammary Gland

The inhibitory effect of dietary DBM on proliferation of mammary gland and uterus is shown in Table II. Female Sencar mice were given AIN-76A diet or 1% DBM in AIN-76A diet for 4 to 5 weeks. All mice were killed at an age of 50 - 60 days during the estrus phase of the estrous cycle. 1% DBM in AIN-76A diet for 4-5 weeks inhibited proliferation rate of mammary gland epithelial cells by 53%, uterine epithelium by 23%, and uterine stroma by 77% and uterine wet weight was decreased by 43% (Table II). Under these conditions, total body weight did not significantly change, however, liver weight was increased by 48% (Table II).

Table II. Inhibitory effect of dietary dibenzoylmethane on proliferation of the uterus and mammary gland in Sencar mice

Treatment	*Control Diet*	*1% DBM Diet*	*% Increase (+) or decrease (-)*
Number of mice per group	21	20	-
Body weight (g)	29.3±0.43	28.8±0.61	-
Liver weight (g)	1.63±0.05	2.41±0.07*	+48%
Uterine weight (mg)	225.9±20.4	132.6±14.0*	-43%
BrdU labeling index (BrdU Li)			
Mammary gland (BrdU Li)	7.23±1.91	3.41±0.96*	-53%
Uterine epithelium (BrdU Li)	12.15±2.12	10.57±1.12	-23%
Uterine stroma (BrdU Li)	5.77±1.34	1.32±0.34*	-77%

*Statistical difference from the control diet group ($P < 0.05$) as determined by the Student's t test. (Data are from Reference *25*).

Inhibitory Effect of Dietary DBM on in vivo Formation of DMBA-DNA Adducts in Mammary Gland

An evaluation of the relationship of DBM dose to total and individual ^{32}P-postlabeled adduct formation *in vivo* is presented in Table III. Six spots were detected from the thin layer chromatogram of ^{32}P-postlabeled DMBA-DNA adducts and total binding was calculated as the sum of these six adducts. Four of the six major adducts were previously identified by HPLC cross referencing procedure (*16,17*); Adducts 4 and 8 are derived from the bay region *anti*- and *syn*-dihydrodiolepoxides through reaction with deoxyguanidine (dGuo) and deoxyadenosine (dAdo) respectively, while adducts 6 and 7 are *syn*- and *anti*-dihydrodiolepoxide-derived dGuo adducts, respectively (see Figure 3).

Two types of DMBA treatments were performed in this study. In the two weeks of the DMBA-treated experiment, mice were treated with DMBA once a week for 2 weeks (groups 1-4 in Table III), the total value of adduct quantity in the control group was 244 nmol/mol DNA. In the 5 weeks of DMBA-treated experiment, the mice were treated with DMBA once a week for 5 weeks (groups 5-8 in Table III), the number of total DMBA-DNA adducts in the control group was 125 nmol/mol DNA, which was lower than in the 2 weeks of DMBA treatment. In the 2 weeks of DMBA-treated experiment, the total values of adduct quantity were 244, 71, 78 and 57 for the control, 0.2%, 0.5% and 1% DBM diet, respectively (Table III). A dose-dependent effect was observed where the mice were treated with 1 mg DMBA once a week for 2 weeks during the age of 49 – 56 days (estrus phase). In the groups of mice treated with DMBA once a

Table III. Inhibitory effect of DMBA-DNA adducts in mammary glands

Group	*DMBA treatment*	*DBM dose*	*Adduct quantity (nmol/mol DNA) Adduct number*						
			Total adducts	*1*	*4*	*5*	*6*	*7*	*8*
1	1 mg	0	243.7±25.7	14.2±0.6	91.8±14.1	33.3±3.3	27.8±3.4	12.6±3.6	64.0±10.8
2	once a	0.2%	70.6±4.4*	2.3±0.7	34.0±3.2	4.2±0.8	12.9±0.9	6.1±0.4	11.1±0.8
3	week for	0.5%	78.4±7.3*	4.9±0.2	23.2±3.9	9.8±1.3	11.9±0.4	5.9±1.5	22.9±3.7
4	2 weeks	1.0%	56.6±23.9*	4.8±0.7	16.1±6.9	5.8±2.1	9.4±4.5	4.6±3.4	16.0±6.9
5	1 mg	0	125.3±11.2	4.4±1.12	60.0±2.5	11.3±2.4	18.3±0.9	8.6±0.8	22.7±7.1
6	once a	0.2%	158.0±28.8	11.4±0.1	52.7±19.5	21.0±0.4	21.1±5.2	7.5±0.4	44.4±3.3
7	week for	0.5%	135.1±27.3	9.9±2.3	41.4±10.5	18.5±5.0	19.0±4.4	6.8±4.2	39.4±9.1
8	5 weeks	1.0%	35.1±7.4**	2.0±0.6	10.5±1.7	3. 3±0.5	7.9±1.4	4.8±0.7	6.6±1.0

Adducts 4 and 8 are derived from the bay-region *anti*- and *syn*-dihydrodiolepoxides through reaction with dGuo and dAdo respectively, while adducts 6 & 7 are *syn*- and *anti*-dihydrodiolepoxide-derived dGuo adducts, respectively.

*Statistically different from group 1 ($p<0.05$) as determined by the Student's t test.

**Statistically different from group 5 ($P<0.05$) as determined by the Student's t test.

(Data are from reference *25*)

week for 5 weeks during the age of 49 - 76 days, no effect was observed in lower dosage DBM-diet groups. The lower doses of DBM diet slightly increased certain individual adduct levels resulting in no apparent change in total adducts. Nevertheless, a significant decrease in total binding adducts was observed in the 1% DBM diet (35 nmol/mol), compared to the control AIN-76A diet (125 nmol/mol) (Table III). This treatment was under the same condition as the tumorigenesis experiment (Table I).

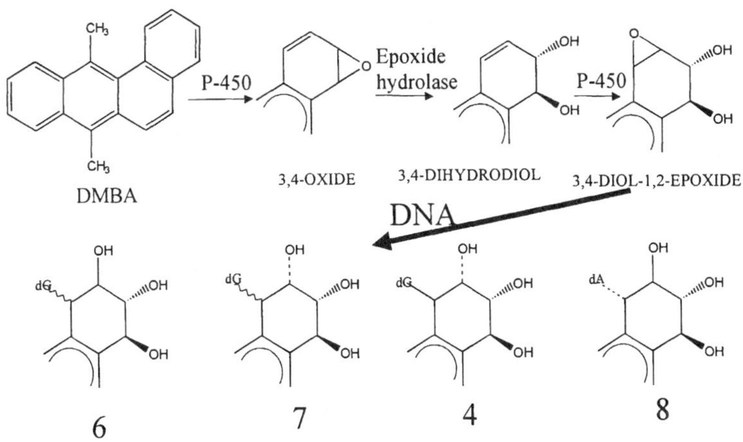

Figure 3. Metabolism of DMBA to bioactivated intermediates and its interaction with DNA to DMBA-deoxyribonucleoside adducts (modified from Reference 16)

The pattern of mouse mammary DMBA-DNA adducts after DMBA dosing reported here is similar to that previously reported in rats (*16,17*). The anti-dGuo adduct 4 was predominant among all the detectable adducts in our mouse model. However, a slight difference in the quantitative proportions of specific adducts was observed. The relative amount of syn-dGuo adduct 8 in the mouse model was considerably more than that in the rat mammary gland. The variation of levels of specific DMBA-DNA adducts between the rat and mouse models may be explained by the difference in DMBA metabolism between species and the condition of DMBA treatment, where DMBA was treated only once in the rat model.

Competitive Estrogen-Receptor Binding Assay Using Rat Uterine Cytosol

In our previous studies, DBM showed inhibitory effect on DMBA-induced covalent binding of [^{3}H]DMBA to mammary gland DNA. Therefore, we subsequently evaluated its influence on hormonal mitogenic action toward tumor promotion. Because of the structural similarity between estradiol (E_2) and DBM, a competitive estrogen-receptor binding assay was used in our studies to examine the inhibitory effects of DBM on estradiol-dependent action.

The competitive binding assay with [^{3}H]-E_2 was used to evaluate the binding affinities of DBM to the rat uterine estrogen receptor (ER). The curves of % [^{3}H]-E2 versus compound concentration is presented in Figure 4. As expected, DES exhibited the most effective affinity at reducing the [^{3}H]-estradiol bound with IC_{50} of 0.4 μM, whereas estradiol showed 10-fold less (IC_{50} = 4 μM). In the case of DBM, weak inhibitory effect was observed, as compared to unlabeled estradiol. Hence, the data showed that DBM was only a weak estrogen-receptor binding ligand.

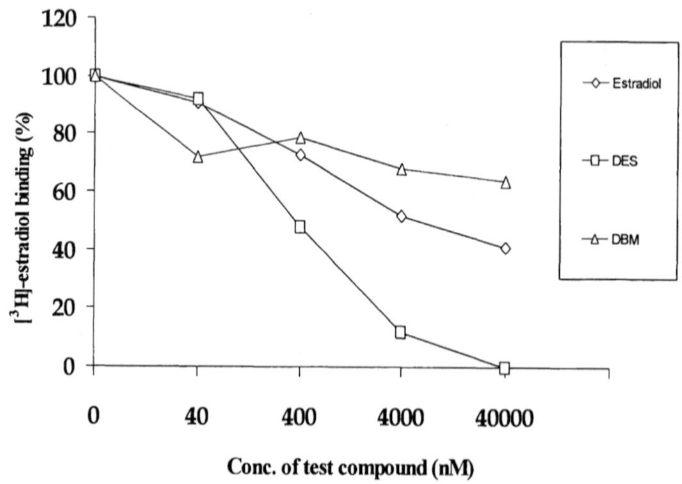

Figure 4. Comparative inhibition of [^{3}H]-17β-estradiol binding to uterine estrogen binding receptors by DMB. (Data are from Reference 18).

Biological Effects of Dietary DBM in Short-term Treatment of Sencar Mice

The results in Table IV indicate that the body weight showed no significant difference between the control diet and 1% DBM diet group after five weeks of administration. The mice fed 1% DBM diet consumed the same amount of food as the control mice, and more water were consumed by 1% DBM diet mice than by control mice. Also, the 1% DBM diet group showed significant reduction (p<0.05) in parametrial fat pad weight, mammary gland weight, but not in uterus weight (p=0.074), while the liver weight was significantly increased (p<0.05) at the end of experiment.

The levels of estradiol and progesterone in serum were measured by ELISA. The results indicated that the concentration of estradiol in 1% DBM group (0.56 ± 0.1 ng/mL) was significantly different (p<0.05) from that in the control diet group (0.21± 0.01 ng/mL). Conversely, no significant difference was observed in the progesterone level (p=0.963). The effect of DBM on fat metabolism was examined by measuring the concentrations of triglyceride. The results indicate that the 1% DBM group showed a marked reduction (approx. 66%) in triglyceride level, compared with the control diet group (Table IV).

Table 4 Biological effects of dietary DBM and measurements of serum concentrations of hormones and lipids in Sencar mice.

Biological effects or substances assayed	*Control diet*	*1% DBM diet*
	n = 15	*n = 17*
Body weight (g)	29.0 ± 1.0	28.3 ± 0.8
Parametrial fat weight (g)	0.58 ± 0.06	0.41 ± 0.05*
Uterus weight (g)	0.20 ± 0.14	0.15 ± 0.02
Mammary gland weight (g)	0.09 ± 0.01	0.07 ± 0.01*
Liver weight (g)	1.64 ± 0.06	2.51 ± 0.09*
Estradiol (pg/mL)	558.1 ± 100.0	211.7 ± 9.6*
Triglyceride (mg/dL)	119.5 ± 3.4	39.5 ± 3.6*
Progesterone (ng/mL)	5.84 ± 1.66	5.75 ± 0.88

*Statistically different from the control AIN-76A diet group (p < 0.05) as determined by the Student's t-test. (Data are from Reference *18*)

Discussion

Estrogen plays an important role in a variety of mammalian physiological processes, especially the development of breast cancer (*19-21*). Epidemiological evidence indicates that the length of exposure of the mammary glands to ovarian-derived estrogenic stimuli is directly proportional to breast cancer risk (*22*). In laboratory studies, estrogen has been reported to increase the proliferation of some human breast cancer cell lines *in vivo* and *in vitro* (*23*).

In this study, we postulated that DBM would influence the mitogenic action of estrogen through interfering either the binding of estrogen to estrogen receptor or its metabolism (see Figure 5). The results of the present study demonstrated an inhibitory effect of dietary DBM on DMBA-induced mammary tumor multiplicity and incidence (Table I). Dietary DBM also reduced the proliferation rate of mammary gland and uterus (Table II), and inhibited formation of DMBA-DNA adducts in mammary glands (Table III). *In vivo* inhibition of the proliferation rate of mammary gland and formation of DMBA-DNA adducts in mammary gland by dietary DBM could explain some of the inhibitory actions of dietary DBM on DMBA-induced mammary carcinogenesis in Sencar mice.

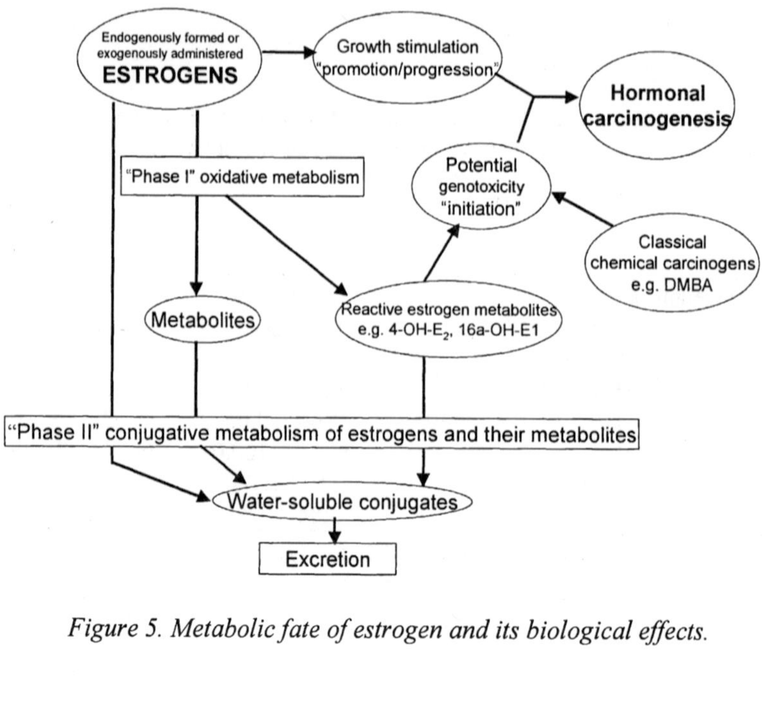

Figure 5. Metabolic fate of estrogen and its biological effects.

The decreased formation of DMBA-DNA adducts by DBM in the mouse model could result from: (a) the influence of DBM on the metabolism of DMBA through phase I and/or phase II enzymatic systems, which would cause the reduction of bioactivated DMBA; (b) the inhibitory effect of DBM on the proliferation rate of mammary gland via the estrogenic hormonal mitogenic pathway. The possibility of the former has been investigated and reported previously (*6,7,10,18*). Singletary's studies also indicated that even though DBM is a potent phase II enzyme inducer, as shown in *in vitro* systems, the inhibitory effect of formation of carcinogen-DNA adducts by DBM in both rat mammary tumorigenesis and human mammary epithelial cell culture system could not be explained by the potent inducing effect of DBM, as indicated by no apparent changes in QR and GST expression (*9,10*). Our studies demonstrate for the first time that DBM lowers the proliferation rate of the mammary gland *in vivo* and produces an inhibitory effect on formation of DMBA-DNA adducts and resulting mammary tumorigenesis.

Feeding 1% DBM in the diet to Sencar mice for 4-5 weeks strongly lowered serum estradiol levels (Table IV). Feeding 1% DBM to Sencar mice increased levels of hepatic cytochrome P450 enzymes as well as increased hepatic hydroxylation and glucuronidation of estradiol (*6*, and Bao *et al.*, private communication) The reduction of serum estradiol could explain the effect of dietary DBM on the decreased proliferation rate of mammary glands and uterus.

In vitro, addition of various doses of DBM to a liver microsomal assay system inhibited hydroxylation of DMBA in a dose-dependent manner (*6,18*). These results might explain how dietary DBM strongly inhibited formation of DMBA-DNA adducts in mammary glands. Further studies in our laboratory indicated that dietary DBM strongly inhibited the accumulation of parametrical fat pads under the abdomen of mice and lowered serum triglyceride levels (Table IV). In addition, the strong reduction of serum triglyceride levels also related to the DBM-induced decrease in serum estrogen level. All these factors could contribute to the observed inhibition of mammary carcinogenesis.

DBM also markedly inhibited skin tumor initiation by DMBA and skin tumor promotion by 12-*O*-tetradecanoylphorbol-acetate (TPA) in CD-1 mice (*24*). Topical application of DBM strongly inhibited ultraviolet B light (UVB)-induced skin tumorigenesis in mice (*24*). Dietary DBM strongly inhibits mammary carcinogenesis, although dietary DBM has some side effects. Consumption of a large amount of DBM in the diet would probably produce a loss of body weight, and increased liver weight and altered lipid and hormone metabolism. However, DBM could be a valuable research tool for studies in lipid, hormone, and drug metabolism related to mammary cancer carcinogenesis and perhaps serve as a model for designing novel chemopreventive agents.

References

1. Greenwald, P. *Sci. Amer.* **1996**, *275*, 96-99.
2. Jordan, V. C. *Br. J. Pharmacol.* **1993**, *111*, 507-517.
3. Wattenberg, L. W. *Cancer Res.* **1993**, *52*, 2085s-2091s.
4. Bertram, J. S.; Kolonel, L. N.; Meyskens, F. L. *Cancer Res.* **1997**, *47*, 3012-3031.
5. Shibata, S. In *Food Phytochemicals for Cancer Prevention II, Teas, Spices, and Herbs*; Ho, C.-T.; Osawa, T.; Huang, M.-T.; Rosen, R. T., Eds.; ACS Symp. Ser. 547, American Chemical Society: Washington DC, 1994; pp 309-321.
6. Lin, C-C. Ph.D. Dissertation, Department of Food Science, Rutgers University, New Brunswick, NJ, 2000.
7. Dinkova-Kostova, A. T.; Talalay, P. *Carcinogenesis* **1999**, *20*, 911 914.
8. Huang, M.-T.; Lou, Y.-R.; Xie, J. G.; Ma, W.; Lu, Y.-P.; Yen, P.; Zhu, B. T.; Newmark, H.; Ho, C.-T. *Carcinogenesis* **1998**, *19*, 1697-1700.
9. Singletary, K.; MacDonald, C.; Iovinelli, M.; Fisher, C.; Wallig, M. *Carcinogenesis* **1998**, *19*, 1039-43.
10. Singletary, K.; MacDonald, C. *Cancer Lett.* **2000**, *155*, 47-54.
11. Damiani, E.; Greci, L.; Parsons, R.; Knowland, J. *Free Rad. Biol. Med.* **1999**, *26*, 809-816.
12. Deleu, H.; Maes, A.; Roelandts, R. *Photodermatol. Photoimmunol. Photomed.* **1992**, *9*, 29-32.
13. Wang, C. Y.; Lee, M. S.; Zukowski, K. *Mutat. Res.* **1991**, *262*, 189-193.
14. Fischer, M. F.; Conti, C. J.; Locniskar, M.; Belury, M. A.; Maldve, R. E.; Lee, M. L.; Leyton, J.; Slaga, T. J.; Bechtel, D. H. *Cancer Res.* **1992**, *52*, 662-666.
15. Lu, Y.-P.; Lou, Y.-R.; Xie, J.-G.; Yen, P.; Huang, M.-T.; Conney, A. H. *Carcinogenesis* **1992**, *18*, 2163-2169.
16. Singletary, K. W.; Parker, H. M.; Milner, J. A. *Carcinogenesis* **1990**, *11*, 1959-1963.
17. Schmeiser, H.; Dipple, A.; Schurdak, M. E.; Randerath, E.; Randerath, K. *Carcinogenesis* **1988**, *9*, 633-638.
18. Lin C.-C.; Ho, C.-T.; Huang, M.-T. *Proc. Natl. Sci. Council, Part B: Life Sci., Taiwan* **2001**, *25*, 158-165.
19. Kumar, V.; Green, S.; Stack, G.; Berry, M.; Jin, J. R.; Chambon, P. *Cell* **1987**, *51*, 941-951.
20. Evans, R. M. *Science* **1988**, *240*, 889-895.
21. Nandi, S.; Guzma, R. C.; Yang, J. *Proc. Natl. Acad. Sci. USA* **1995**, *92*, 3650-3657.

22. Clarke, R.; Hilakivi-Clarke, L.; Cho, E.; James, M. R.; Leonessa, F. In *Dietary Phytochemicals in Cancer Prevention and Treatment.* Plenum Press: New York, 1996; pp. 63-85.
23. Clarke, R.; Brunner, N.; Katzenellenbogen, B. S.; Thompson, E. W.; Norman, M. J.; Koppi, C.; Paik, S.; Lippman, M. E.; Dickson, R. B. *Proc. Natl. Acad. Sci. USA* **1989**, *86*, 3649-3653.
24. Huang, M.-T.; Ma, W.; Xie,. J.-G.; Newmark, H. L. *Proc. Amer. Assoc. Cancer Res.* **1999**, *40*, 260.
25. Lin, C.-C.; Lu, Y.-P.; Lou, Y.-R.; Ho, C.-T.; Newmark, H. H.; MacDonald, C.; Singletary, K. W.; Huang, M.-T. *Cancer Lett.* **2001**, *168*, 125-132.
26. Zhu, B. T.; Conney, A. H. *Carcinogenesis* **1998**, *19*, 1-27.

Chapter 17

Protective Effect of Dibenzoylmethane on Chemically- and UV Light-Induced Skin, Inflammation, Sunburn Lesions, and Skin Carcinogenesis in Mice

Mou-Tuan Huang[1], Yue Liu[1], Jian-Guo Xie[1], Harold H. Newmark[1], and Chi-Tang Ho[2]

[1]Laboratory for Cancer Research, College of Pharmacy, Rutgers, The State University of New Jersey, Piscataway, NJ 08854–8020
[2]Department of Food Science, Cook College, Rutgers, The State University of New Jersey, New Brunswick, NJ 08901–8520

Dibenzoylmethane (DBM) is a minor constituent of licorice and an analogue of curcumin. We previously reported that feeding 1% DBM in the diet strongly inhibited 7,12-dimethylbenzyla[a]anthracene (DMBA)-induced mammary tumorigenesis and formation of leukemias/lymphomas in Sencar mice). In this report, we show that topical application of DBM to the backs of mice inhibited chemical- and ultraviolet light (UV)-induced inflammation, sunburn lesions, and formation of skin tumors in mice. Topical application of DBM inhibited TPA-induced edema of mouse ears and skin tumor promotion in CD-1 mice in a dose-dependent manner. Topical application of 3 – 10 μmol DBM with 5 nmol TPA twice weekly for 16 weeks in CD-1 mice previously treated with DMBA inhibited the number of skin tumors per mouse by 65 – 93%, and percent of mice with tumors was inhibited by 29 – 50%.. Topical application of 10 μmol DBM with mirex (a non-TPA type tumor promoter) 3 times a week for 18 weeks in

DMBA-initiated mice inhibited the mirex-induced number of tumors per mouse by 63%. DBM also strongly inhibited UV-induced skin sunburn lesions and formation of skin tumors in SKH-1 mice. Topical application of 10 μmol DBM to SKH-1 mice previously initiated with DMBA at 10 min prior to each UV (30 mJ/cm^2) irradiation twice a week for 34 weeks inhibited the number of skin tumors per mouse by 91%. Percent of mice with skin tumors was reduced by 44%. In complete UV skin tumorigenic model, topical application of 10 μmol DBM at 10 min before each UV (30 mJ/cm^2) irradiation twice weekly for 34 weeks inhibited the number of skin tumors per mouse by 96%, and percent of mice with tumors was decreased by 48%. Our results indicated that DBM strongly inhibited both chemical- and UV-induced skin inflammation, sunburn lesions and skin tumorigenesis in mice.

Introduction

DBM is a minor constituent of licorice (*1*). The chemical structure of DBM resembles that of curcumin (Figure 1). Both DBM and curcumin contain a central beta-diketone group in conjugation with an unsaturated carbon system which tend to increase enolization of the beta-diketone group. Curcumin has potent antioxidant and anti-inflammatory activities and has been reported to inhibit several types of chemical-induced tumorigenesis in animal models (*2,3*), but curcumin is very poorly absorbed and when administered by injection to rats is rapidly metabolized by reduction of the non-aromatic unsaturated alkyl groups to poorly active metabolites (*4*). DBM is a smaller molecule with anti-inflammatory activity and is a phase-2 enzyme inducer (*5*). DBM appears to be much better absorbed and distributed in tissues *in vivo*. DBM and its derivatives have anti-mutagenic activity (*6*). DBM inhibited benzo[a]pyrene and 1,6-dinitropyrene-DNA adduct formation in human epithelial cells (*7*), and protected against free radical DNA damage (*8*). Recently, our laboratory, and others showed that dietary DBM strongly inhibited 7,12-dimethylbenz[a]anthracene (DMBA)-induced mammary tumorigenesis in mice and rats (*9-11*). In this report, we show that topical application of DBM to the backs of mice strongly protects against chemical-and ultraviolet light-induced skin inflammation, sunburn lesions and tumorigenesis.

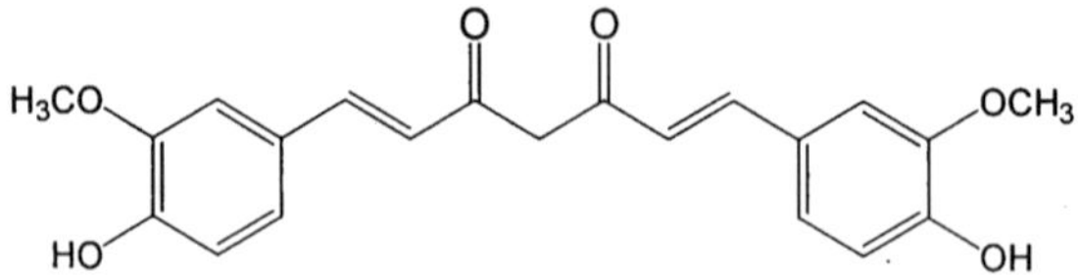

CURCUMIN

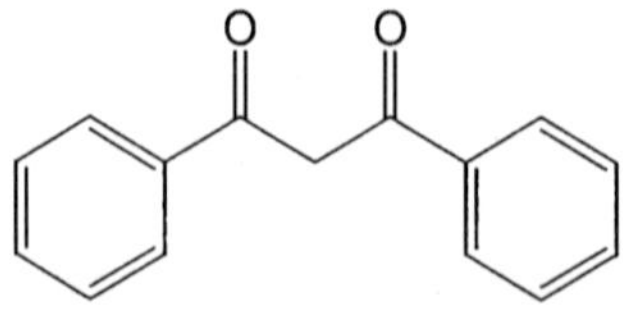

DIBENZOYLMETHANE (DBM)

Figure 1. Chemical structures of curcumin and dibenzoylmethane.

Materials and Methods

DBM and para-aminobenzoic acid (PABA) were purchased from Aldrich Chemical Company, Inc (Milwaukee, WI). DMBA was obtained from Calbiochem-Behringer (San Diago, CA). TPA was purchased from CRC, Inc., (Chanhassen, MN). Mirex was purchased from Fischer Scientific (Springfield, NJ). Female SKH-1 mice (5-6 weeks old) and female CD-1 mice (23 days old or 5-6 weeks old) were purchased from Charles River Laboratories (Kingston, NY) and kept in animal facility at least 1 week before use. Mice were fed a Purina Laboratory Chow 5001 diet and water *ad libitum*.

The UV lamps (FS72T12-UVB-HO; National Biological Corp., Twinsburg, OH) emitted little or no radiation that was < 280 nm and > 375 nm. The UV lamps emitted UVB (280-320 nm; 75-80% of total energy), and UVA (320-375 nm; 20-25% of total energy). The dose of UVB was quantified with a UVB Spectra 305 dosimeter (Daevlin Co., Bryan, OH). The radiation was further calibrated with a Model IL-1700 research radiometer/photometer (International Light, Inc., Newburyport, MA).

For exposure to UV, 10 mice were housed in a 25 cm x 46 cm plastic box. Six boxes (without tops) were placed under 8 UV lamps (51 cm x 183 cm), and the boxes were systemically rotated during the course of the study to compensate for possible small differences in flux at various positions under lamps. The distance between the UV lamps and the backs of mice or the UV detector was 43 cm. The exposure time for a 30 mJ/cm^2 dose of UV was 21-28 seconds.

In Vivo Anti-inflammatory Assay

In vivo ant-inflammatory assay was done according to the following procedure. Both ears of female CD-1 mice (23-25 days old; 5-6 mice per group) were treated topically with 20 µl acetone, TPA (1 nmol) in 20 µL acetone or test compound with TPA (1 nmol) in 20 µL acetone. Five hours later, the mice were killed by cervical dislocation, and 6-mm (diameter) ear punch biopsies were taken and weighed. The increases in weight of ear punches were directly proportional to the degree of inflammation.

DMBA/TPA Two-stage Skin Tumorigenesis

The dorsal region of female CD-1 mice (8-9 weeks old) was shaved with an electric clipper. Two days later, groups of 30 mice were treated topically with 200 nmol DMBA in 200 µL acetone, and control mice received 200 µL acetone alone. After 1 week, mice were treated topically with 200 µL acetone, 5 nmol TPA, or 5 nmol TPA together with test compound in 200 µL acetone twice weekly for 20 weeks. Tumors of at least 1 mm in diameter were counted and recorded every 2 weeks, and the results are expressed as the average number of tumors per mouse and percentage of tumor-bearing mice.

DMBA/UVB Two-stage Skin Carcinogenesis

Female SKH-1 mice (7-8 weeks old) were treated topically with a single dose of DMBA. One week later, the mice were treated topically with 200 µl acetone, DBM (10 µmol), or PABA (10 µmol) in 200 µL acetone prior to each UV (30 mJ/cm^2) twice a week for 34 weeks. Skin tumors greater than 1 mm in diameter were counted and recorded.

Complete UVB Skin Carcinogenesis

Female SKH-1 mice (7-8 weeks old) were treated topical with 200 µl acetone, DBM (10 µmol), or PABA (10 µmol) in 200 µL acetone 10 min prior to each UVB (30 mJ/cm^2) twice weekly for 34 weeks. Skin tumors in diameter greater than 1 mm were counted and recorded.

Results

The Protective Effect of Topical Application of DBM on TPA-induced Skin Inflammation

Anti-inflammatory activity of DBM was evaluated the ability of DBM to inhibit TPA-induced edema of mouse ear (Table I). Topical application of 1 nmol of TPA to mouse ear (24-26 days old) rapidly induced edema of mouse ear. Five hours after TPA application, the average weight of ear punches was increase from an average of 6.8 mg/punch (acetone control group) to 14.2 mg per punch (TPA-treated group). Topical application of DBM at 0.1, 0.3 or 1 µmol of DBM with 1 nmol TPA inhibited TPA-induced ear edema by 39, 45, or 71% respectively. DBM inhibited TPA-induced ear edema in a dose-dependent manner.

The Protective Effect of DBM on TPA-induced Skin Tumor Promotion in CD-1 Mice Previously Initiated with DMBA

Female CD-1 mice initiated with 200 nmol of DMBA and promoted with 5 nmol TPA twice a week for 16 weeks developed an average of 19.5 skin tumors per mouse,. and 93% of mice had skin tumors. Topical application of 3 or 10 µmol of DBM with 5 nmol TPA twice a week for 16 weeks inhibited the number of skin tumors per mouse by 65.1 or 93.3%, and the percentage of mice with skin tumors was decreased by 29 and 49.5%, respectively,(Table II). Additional groups of mice were initiated with DMBA and then treated with acetone or 10 µmol DBM twice weekly for 16 weeks. None of these animals developed tumors, indicating that DBM was not a tumor promoter. DBM inhibited both TPA-induced number of skin tumors per mouse and percent of tumor incidence (Table II).

Table I. Inhibitory Effect of DBM on TPA-induced Edema of Mouse Ear

Treatment	*Number of mice per group*	*Weight of ear punch (mg)*	*Percent inhibition*
Acetone	5	6.80±0.81	-
TPA (1 nmol)	5	14.20±1.25	-
DBM (0.1 μmol) + TPA (1 nmol)	5	11.31±1.41	39
DBM (0.3 μmol) + TPA (1 nmol)	5	10.87±1.35	45
DBM (1.0 μmol) + TPA (1 nmol)	5	8.95±1.01	71*

Female CD-1 mice (24-25 days old; 5 mice per group) were treated topically with 20 μL acetone, TPA (1 nmol), in 20 μL acetone, or DBM + TPA (1 nmol) in 20 μL acetone. Five hours laters, the mice were killed by cervical dislocation and ear punches were weighed. Data are expressed as the mean ± SE.

*Statistical difference from the TPA treatment group 2 ($P < 0.05$) as determined by the Student'S t test.

Table II. Inhibitory Effect of Topical Application of DBM on TPA-induced Ttumor Promotion in Skin of CD-1 Mice Previously Initiated with DMBA

Weeks of TPA Promotion	*Group 1 TPA (5 nmol) + Acetone*		*Group 2 TPA (5 nmol) + DBM (3 μmol)*		*Group 3 TPA (5 nmol) + DBM (10 μmol)*	
	Tumors per mouse	*% of mice with tumors*	*Tumors per mouse*	*% of mice with tumors*	*Tumors per mouse*	*% of mice with tumors*
8	5.1±1.1	83	1.3±0.8* (74.5%)	24 (71.1%)	0* (100%)	0 (100%)
12	15.5±2.0	93	4.6±1.5* (70.3%)	52 (37.3%)	0.5±0.3* (96.8%)	24 (74.2%)
16	19.5±2.3	93	6.8±1.9* (65.1%)	66 (29.0%)	1.3±0.4* (93.3%)	47 (49.5%)

Female CD-1 mice (7-8 weeks old; 40 mice for the positive control group; all others were 30 mice per group), The mice were treated topically with a single dose 200 nmol of DMBA. One week later, the mice were treated topically with 200 μL acetone, TPA (5 nmol), or TPA (5 nmol) together with test compound in 200 μL acetone twice a week for 20 weeks. Skin tumors in diameter greater than 1 mm were counted and recorded.

Data are expressed as the mean±SE.

*Statistical difference from the TPA treatment group 1 ($P < 0.05$) as determined by the Student's t test. Data in parentheses are percent of inhibition.

The Protective Effect of Topical Aapplication of DBM on Mirex-induced Skin Tumors Promotion in Mice Pre-treated with DMBA

Mirex is a non-TPA type tumor promoter (*12,13*). Female CD-1 initiated with a single dose of 200 nmol of DMBA and promoted with 0.1 µmol of mirex 3 times a week for 18 weeks developed an average of 11.5 skin tumors per mouse, and 80% of mice had skin tumors. Topical application of 10 µmol of DBM with 0.1 µmol of mirex 3 times a week for 18 weeks inhibited the mirex-induced average number of skin tumors per mouse by 62.6%, and percentage of mice bearing with tumors was decreased by 12.5% (Table III). The results indicate that DBM inhibits both TPA- and a non-TPA type tumor promotion in mouse skin (Tables II & III).

Table III. Inhibitory effect of DBM on mirex-induced Skin Tumor Promotion in CD-1 Mice Previously Treated with DMBA

Weeks of mirex promotion	*Group 1* *Mirex (0.1 µmol)*		*Group 2* *DBM (10 µmol) + mirex*	
	Tumors per mouse	*Percent of mice with tumors*	*Tumors per mouse*	*Percent of mice with tumors*
10	1.53±0.62	37	0.25±0.16* (83.7%)	15 (59.5%)
14	6.35±1.84	60	1.65±0.74* (74.0%)	40 (33.3%)
18	11.5±2.41	80	4.30±1.09* (62.6%)	70 (12.5%)

Female CD-1 mice (8-9 weeks old; 20 mice per group) were treated topically with a single dose 200 nmol of DMBA. One week later, the mice in group 1 were treated topically with mirex (0.1 µmol) in 200 µL acetone, or the mice in group 2 were treated topically with DBM (10 µmol) + mirex (0.1 µmol) in 200 µL acetone twice weekly for 18 weeks. Skin tumors with diameter greater than 1 mm were counted and recounted.

*Statistical difference from the mirex treatment group 1 ($P < 0.05$) as determined by the Student's t test.

Data in parenthesis are percent of inhibition.

The Protective Effect of Topical Application of DBM on UVB-induced Sunburn Lesions

Irradiation of 180 mJ/cm^2 of UV light to female SKH-1 mice once a day for 3 days resulted in formation of red skin lesions at 3 days after the last dose UV light irradiation. Irradiation of 180 mJ/cm^2 of UV to SKH-1 mice once a day for 3 days developed 237, 375, 329, 166, or 59 square mm of red colored lesions on the backs of mice at 3rd, 4th, 5th, 6th and 7th after last dose of UV light irradiation in the control acetone group of mice (Table IV). Both topical application of DBM (10 μmol) and a commercial sunscreen agent, PABA (10 μmol) markedly decreases the area of red color lesions. DBM gave better protection against UV light-induced red color sunburn lesions than that of the commercial sun screening agent, PABA at the concentrations tested.

Table IV. Inhibitory Effect of DBM and PABA on Ultraviolet Light (UV)-induced Skin Sunburn Lesions in SKH-1 Mice

Days after last UV treatment	*Area of sunburn (mm^3)*		
	Group 1 *Acetone*	*Group 2* *DBM*	*Group 3* *PABA*
3	237±24	0* (100.0%)	27±24* (88.6%)
4	375±49	10±9* (97.3%)	42±38* (88.8%)
5	329±63	8±7* (97.6%)	38±34* (88.4%)
6	166±21	0* (100.0%)	0* (100.0%)
7	59±9	0 (100.0%)	0* (100.0%)

Female SKH-1 mice (10 weeks old; 5 mice per group) were treated topically with 100 μL acetone, DBM (10 μmol) or PABA (10 μmol) in 100 μL acetone at 10 min prior to UV (180 mJ/cm^2) irradiation once a day for 3 days. The backs of mice developed red sunburn lesion (based the size of red area as expressed mm^2). Data are expressed as the mean±SE.

*Statistical difference from the acetone treatment group 1 ($P < 0.05$) as determined as the student's t test.

Data in parentheses are percent of inhibition.

The Protective Effect of DBM on UVB-induced Skin Tumor Promotion in SKH-1 Mice Previously Initiated with DMBA

Female SKH-1 mice (7-8 weeks old) initiated with a single dose 200 nmol of DMBA and promoted with 30 mJ/cm^2 UV twice a week for 34 weeks resulted in formation of an average 13.6 skin tumors per mouse and 100% of mice had skin tumors (Table V). Topical application of 10 μmol DBM at 10 min prior to each UV irradiation twice a week for 34 weeks decreased the number of skin tumors was to 1.2 tumors per mouse (91% inhibition). The percentage of mice with tumors was also reduced to 56% (44% inhibition). Topical application of 10 μmol PABA at 10 min prior to each UV irradiation twice a week for 34 weeks inhibited the number of tumors per mouse by 79.7%, and the percentage of mice with tumors was inhibited by 14%. The results indicate that both DBM and ABA protect against UV-induced skin tumor promotion, and DBM has a better protection against UV-induced skin tumor promotion than PABA under these conditions.

Table V. Inhibitory Effect of DBM and PABA on UV-induced Skin Carcinogenesis in SKH-1 Mice Previously Treated with DMBA

UVB Irradiation (weeks)	*Group 1* *Acetone*		*Group 2* *Dibenzoylmethane (DBM)*		*Group 3* *Aminobenzoic acid (PABA)*	
	Tumor per mouse	*% of mice with tumors*	*Tumor per mouse*	*% of mice with tumors*	*Tumor per mouse*	*% of mice with tumors*
21	0.50±0.15	33	0.13±0.06* (74.0%)	17 (48.5%)	0.13±0.06* (74.0%)	10 (69.7%)
27	4.07±0.68	90	0.50±0.12* (87.7%)	43 (52.2%)	1.10±0.22* (73.0%)	55 (38.9%)
34	13.6±1.48	100	1.20±0.25* (91.2%)	56 (44.0%)	2.76±0.44* (79.7%)	86 (14.0%)

Female SKH-1 mice (7-8 weeks old; 30 mice per group) were treated topically with a single dose of DMBA. One week later, the mice were treated topically with 200 μL acetone, DBM (10 μmol), or PABA (10 μmol) in 200 μL acetone 10 min prior to each UVB (30 mJ/cm^2) irradiation twice a week for 34 weeks. Skin tumors in diameter greater than 1 mm were counted and recorded. Data are expressed as the mean±SE.

*Statistical difference from the acetone treatment group 1 ($P < 0.05$) as determined as the Student's t test.

Data in parentheses are percent of inhibition.

The Protective Effect of DBM on Complete UV Skin Carcinogenesis in SKH-1 Mice

The protective effect of DBM and PABA on UV-induced complete skin carcinogenesis also was examined and the results were shown in Table VI. Irradiation of 30 mJ/cm^2 UV to female SKH-1 mice twice a week for 34 weeks resulted in formation of 6 skin tumors per mouse and 90% of mice had skin tumors. Topical application 10 μmol DBM or 10 μmol PABA at 10 min prior each UV irradiation twice a week for 34 weeks inhibited the number of skin tumors per mouse by 95.9% and 88.4%, respectively. The percentage of mice with skin tumors was inhibited by 80% and 48%, respectively (Table VI). The results suggest that DBM had a better protective action on UV-induced complete skin carcinogenesis under these conditions.

Table VI. Inhibitory Effect of DBM and PABA on UV-induced Skin Carcinogenesis in SKH-1 Mice

UVB Irradiation (weeks)	*Group 1 Acetone*		*Group 2 Dibenzoylmethane (DBM)*		*Group 3 Aminobenzoic acid (PABA)*	
	Tumor per mouse	*% of mice with tumors*	*Tumor per mouse*	*% of mice with tumors*	*Tumor per mouse*	*% of mice with tumors*
21	0.17±0.07	17	0* (100%)	0 (100%)	0.07±0.05* (58.8%)	7 (58.8%)
27	1.43±0.38	43	0.07±0.08* (95.1%)	7 (83.7%)	0.17±0.07* (88.1%)	17 (60.5%)
34	6.03±1.12	90	0.25±0.11* (95.9%)	18 (80.0%)	0.70±0.16* (88.4%)	47 (47.8%)

Female SKH-1 mice (7-8 weeks old; 30 mice per group) were treated topically with 200 μL acetone, DBM (10 μmol), or PABA (10 μmol) in 200 μL acetone 5 min prior to each UVB (30 mJ/cm^2) irradiation twice a week for 34 weeks. Skin tumors in diameter greater than 1 mm were counted and recorded. Data are expressed as the mean±SE.

*Statistical difference from the acetone treatment group 1 ($P < 0.05$) as determined as the Student's t test.

Data in parentheses are percent of inhibition.

Discussion

The results of the present study demonstrated that topical application of DBM inhibited TPA-induced skin inflammation and skin tumor promotion (Tables I & II) as well as inhibited mirex (a non-TPA-type tumor promoter)-induced skin tumor promotion (Table III). Topical application of DBM also strongly inhibited UV-induced skin sunburn lesions (Table IV), UV-induced skin tumor promotion (Table V) and complete UV skin tumorigenesis (Table VI). The mechanism of inhibitory actions of DBM on chemically- and UV-induced skin inflammation, sunburn lesions, and tumorigenesis are unknown. Green tea and its constituent EGCG also have been shown to inhibit TPA-induced skin inflammation, and tumor promotion (*14*), as well as to inhibit the mirex-induced skin tumor promotion in mice (*15*). Green tea and its constituents also have been shown to inhibit UV-induced skin sunburn lesions, tumor promotion and complete uv skin carcinogenesis (*16*). The steroidial anti-inflammatory agent, fluocinolone acetonide and also trans-retinoic acid inhibit TPA-induced skin tumor promotion. However, they have little or no effect on mirex–induced skin tumor promotion in mice (*13*). Feeding 0.5% DBM in the diet to Sprague-Dawley rats at 2 weeks after a single dose of DMBA treatment inhibited DMBA-induced the average number of mammary tumors per rat and greatly reduced average mammary tumor size per rat (*17*). The data also indicated that feeding DBM in the diet to Sprague-Dawley rats inhibited mammary tumor development during the post-initiation period (promotion phase). The protective effect of DBM against free radical DNA damage and the ability of DBM to screen UVA light (*8,18*) could explain part of the mechanism of inhibitory action of DBM on chemical- and UV-induced skin tumorigenesis. Further study of the effect of DBM on various enzumatic and signal transduction pathways is needed to explain its inhibitory action on the post-initiation period (promotion phase). DBM could be proven a valuable tool for preventing chemical- and UV-induced carcinogenesis.

References

1. Shibata, S. In *Food Phytochemicals for Cancer Prevention II. Teas, Spices, and Herbs*, Ho, C.-T.; Osawa, T.; Huang, M.T.; Rosen, R.T. (Eds), ACS Symp. Ser. 547, American Chemical Society: Washington, DC 1994, pp 309-321.
2. Huang, M.T.; Smart, R.C.; Wong, C.Q.; Conney, A.H. *Cancer Res.* **1988**, *48,* 5941-5946.
3. Huang, M.T.; Newmark, H.H.; Frenkel, K. J. *Cell. Biochem. Suppl.* **1997**, *27*, 26-34.

4. Ireson, C.; Orr, S.; .Jones, D.J.L.; Verschoyle, R.; Kim, C.K.; Luo, J.L.; Howells, L.; Plummer, S.; Jukes, R.; Williams, M.; Steward, W.P.; Gescher, A. *Cancer Res.* **2001**, *61*, 1058-1064.
5. Dinkova-Kostova, A.T.; Talalay, P. *Carcinogenesis* **1999**, *20*, 911-914.
6. Wang, C.Y.; Lee, M.S.; Zukowski, K. *Mutat. Res.* **1991**, *262*, 189-193.
7. Singletary, K.; MacDonald, C. *Cancer Lett.* **2000**, *155*, 47-54.
8. Damiani, E.; Greci, L.; Parsons, R.; Knowland, J. *Free Radic. Biol. Med.* **1999**, *26*, 809-861.
9. Huang, M.T.; Lou, Y.R.; Xie, J.G.; Ma, W.; Lu, Y.P.; Zhu, B.T.; Newmark, H.; Ho, C.-T. *Carcinogenesis* **1998**, *19*, 1697-1700.
10. Lin, C.C.; Lu, Y.P.; Lou, Y.P.; Ho, C.-T.; Newmark, H.H.; MacDonald, C.; Singletary, K.W.; Huang, M.T. *Cancer Lett.* **2001**, *168*, 125-132.
11. Singletary, K.W.; MacDonald, C.; Iovinelli, M.; Fisher, C.; Wallig, M. *Carcinogenesis* **1998**, *19*, 1039-1043.
12. Kim, T.W.; Smart., R.C. Carcinogenesis **1995**, *16*, 2199-2204.
13. Meyer, S.A.; Kim, T.W.; Moser, G.J.; Monteiro-Riviere, N.A.; Smart., R.C. Carcinogenesis **1994**, *15*, 47-52.
14. Huang, M.T.; Ho, C.T.; Ferraro, T.; Finnegan-Olive; Lou, Y.R.; Wang, Z.Y.; Mitchell, J.M.; Laskin, J.D.; Newmark, H.; Yang, C.S.; Conney, A.H. *Carcinogenesis* **1992**, *13,* 947-954.
15. Wang, Z.Y.; Huang, M.T.; Ferraro, T.; Wong, C.Q.; Lou, Y.R.; Reuhl, K.; Iatropoulos, M.; Yang, C.S.; Conney, A.H. *Cancer Res.* **1992**, *52*, 1162-1170.
16. Suganuma, M.; Okabe, S.; Marino, M.W.; Sakai, A.; Sueoka, E.; Fujiki, H. *Cancer Res.* **1999**, *59*, 4516-4518.
17. Lou, Y.R.; Lu, Y.P.; Xie, J.G.; Zhu, B.T.; Thomas, P.E.; Newmark, H.L.; Huang, M.T. *Proc. Am. Associ Cancer Res.* **1999**, *40*, 652.
18. Journe, F.; Marguery, M.C.; Rakotondrazafy, J.; Ei, S.F.; Bazex, J. *Acta Derm. Venerol.* **1979**, *79*, 211-213.

Chapter 18

Inflammatory Response in the Pathogenesis of Atherosclerosis and Its Prevention by Rosmarinic Acid, a Functional Ingredient of Rosemary

Yuji Naito[1], Shigenori Oka[2], and Toshikazu Yoshikawa[1]

[1]First Department of Medicine, Kyoto Prefectural University of Medicine, Kyoto 602–8566, Japan
[2]Research and Development Center, Nagase Company, Ltd., Kobe 651–2241, Japan

Recent evidence suggests a role for the inflammatory response in the pathogenesis of atherosclerosis with the adhesion of circulating monocytes to the endothelium at site of injury. Leukocytes adhere and immigrate into the subendothelial space in response to chemoattractants and other activating molecules, which are mediated by adhesion molecules located on leukocyte/endothelial cells. Oxidatively modified low-density lipoprotein is thought to play a key role in these reactions. We recently found that the expression of adhesion molecules was upregulated by oxidized lipoprotein or inflammatory cytokines, and that the increased expression was inhibited by α-tocopherol as well as by functional ingredients of food factors such as rosmarinic acid. Rosmarinic acid has potent free radical scavenging and anti-inflammatory activities, and its administration reduced the serum levels of lipid peroxides and inhibited the progression of atherosclerosis in apolipoprotein E-deficient mice without affecting the serum level in cholesterol. These anti-inflammatory properties of this food factors suggest that they may have potential benefits in atherosclerosis.

There is considerable evidence that inflammatory response induced by oxidized low-density lipoprotein (oxLDL) contribute to the development of atherosclerosis. OxLDL or their metabolites have been found in atherosclerotic lesions in both human and animal models (*1*). OxLDLs have been shown to stimulate endothelial cells to express several proteins that contribute to atherosclerosis, including monocyte chemotactic protein-1 (MCP-1), macrophage-colony-stimulating factor (M-CSF), vascular cell adhesion molecule-1 (VCAM-1), and intracellular adhesion molecule1 (ICAM-1) (*2,3*). OxLDL is avidly taken up by macrophages, resulting in foam cell formation (*4*).

The significant role of adhesion molecules or macrophages in the process of atherosclerosis was recently confirmed by molecular biological techniques, in which knockout of ICAM-1 gene (*5*) or administration with monoclonal antibody against the receptor M-CSF (*6*) significantly inhibited the progression of atherosclerosis in apolipoprotein E-deficient mice. The expression of adhesion molecules ICAM-1 and VCAM-1 was upregulated by oxLDL or inflammatory cytokines, and that the increased expression was inhibited by α-tocopherol (*7*). Rosemary is one of the world's best-known spices, and it has also been universally used throughout the history for its health benefits. The dried extracts of rosemary contain caffeic acid, chlorogenic acid, rosmarinic acid, carnosol, carnosic acid, and ursolic acid. Rosmarinic acid is a major phenolic ingredient of rosemary (*8*). In this study, we investigated the antioxidative and anti-inflammatory activities of rosmarinic acid *in vitro*, and effects of its administration on inhibiting of progression of atherosclerosis in apolipoprotein E-deficient mice.

Free Radical scavenging activity

Superoxide and hydroxyl radical scavenging activities were measured by the electron paramagnetic resonance (EPR) spin trapping method. Following previous reports (*9,10*), superoxide and hydroxyl radicals generated by the hypoxanthine-xanthine oxidase enzyme system and the Fenton system, containing $FeSO_4$ and hydrogen peroxide, respectively, were trapped by 5,5-dimethyl-1-pyrroline-N-oxide (DMPO). Rosmarinic acid inhibited the signal intensity of DMPO-OOH (spin adduct trapping superoxide) as well as that of DMPO-OH (spin adduct trapping hydroxyl radical) in a concentration-dependent manner with IC_{50} concentrations of 0.62 μM for DMPO-OOH and 15 μM for DMPO-OH.

Inhibition of LDL oxidation

Human LDL was incubated at 37°C with 5 mM each azo-compound, 2, 2'-azobis-(2-amidinopropane)hydrochloride (AAPH) or 2,2'-azobis(2,4-dimethylvaleronitrile) (AMVN), in the absence or presence of different concentrations of rosmarinic acid. Lipid peroxides were determined by ferrous oxidation in xylenol orange assay (FOX-assay). Rosmarinic acid significantly inhibited the increase in lipid peroxides induced by AAPH in concentrations of 1 and 10 μM, and slightly inhibited those induced by AMVN at a dose of 10 μM.

Effects of rosmarinic acid on adhesion molecule expression induced by oxLDL

The LDL (d=1.019 – 1.063) was isolated from the serum of healthy human donors by density-gradient ultracentrifugation, dialyzed with phosphate buffered saline containing EDTA, and stored at 4°C. Lipoprotein concentrations were expressed as protein content. OxLDL was prepared by incubating LDL with 10 μM $FeSO_4$ at 37°C for 30 min. The oxidation of LDL produced 50 – 100 nM hydroperoxide per mg protein of LDL. Enzyme immunoassay (EIA) was used to assess the adhesion molecule expression on the human aortic endothelial cells (HAEC) monolayer. Confluent HAEC monolayers were pretreated with and without rosmarinic acid for 1 h, and then HAEC were stimulated with oxLDL (100 μg/ml). Rosmarinic acid significantly inhibited the increase in the ICAM-1 expression in a concentration-dependent manner (Fig.1). VCAM-1 expression was also increased by stimulation of oxLDL and the increase was significantly inhibited by rosmarinic acid in a concentration-dependent manner.

Effect of rosmarinic acid on monocyte adhesion to HAEC

The HAEC monolayers prepared in 48-well plates were stimulated with interleukin-1β (IL-1β, 20 u/ml) for 4 h in the presence or absence of rosmarinic acid. Subsequently, HAEC were washed with Hanks buffered salf solution, and monocytes (U937 cells) were added to each well and incubated at 37°C for 30 min. U937 cell adhesion was determined by visual counting under a phase-contrast microscope. The adherence of monocytes to HAEC exposed to IL-1β was siginificantly increased compared to that of unstimulated HAEC. Figure 2 shows the effect of rosmarinic acid on the adherence of monocyte to IL-1β-stimulated HAEC. The treatment of HAEC with rosmarinic acid significantly reduced the adherence of monocyte on HAEC in a concentration-dependent manner.

Rosmarinic acid attenuates development of atherosclerosis in apolipoprotein E-deficient mice

The *ex vivo* effect of rosmarinic acid on the development of atherosclerosis in apolipoprotein E-deficient mice, in relation to plasma cholesterol and lipid peroxide levels, was investigated. Apolipoprotein E-deficient mice (4-week-old) were divided into two groups fed for 6 weeks via their drinking water with the following: control group and rosmarinic acid group (0.04 % solution, 1.52 mg/kg/day). The aortic sections were made and stained with Oil-red-O, and counter-stained with hematoxylin. Average lesion sizes of 7-9 sections were measured by quantitating the lesion-covered areas on the aortic vessel walls (NIH image 1.62 program; National Institute of Health).

Aortic atherosclerotic lesion areas were reduced in mice that consumed 1.52 mg of rosmarinic acid /kg/day compared to mice on the control diet. Figure 3 shows the photomicrographs of typical atherosclerotic lesion of the aortic arch of apolipoprotein E-deficient mice after treatment. Rosmarinic acid inhibited plasma lipid peroxide levels in apolipoprotein E-deficient mice without affecting the total cholesterol levels in plasma, indicating that the anti-atherosclerotic properties of rosmarinic acid may be due, in part, to its antioxidative action which inhibits the increase in lipid peroxides.

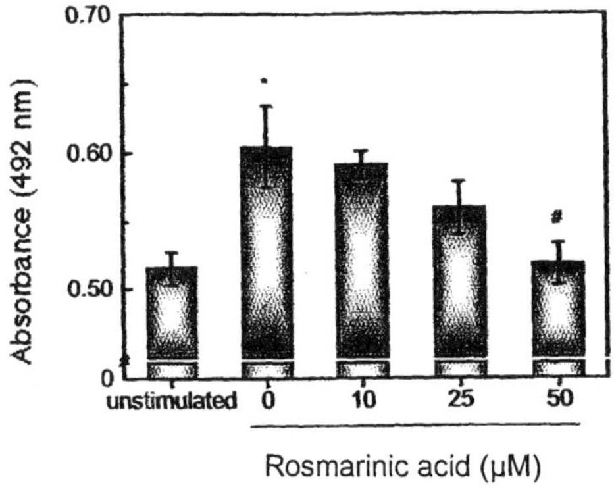

*Figure 1. Effect of rosmarinic acid on ICAM-1 expression stimulated with oxLDL. Confluent HAEC were incubated with ox-LDL (100 μg/mL) in the absence or presence of rosmarinic acid at 37 C for 6 h. The expression of ICAM-1 on the cell surface was measured using EIA. *p<0.05 vs. unstimulated group, and #p<0.05 vs. stimulated group without rosmarinic acid.*

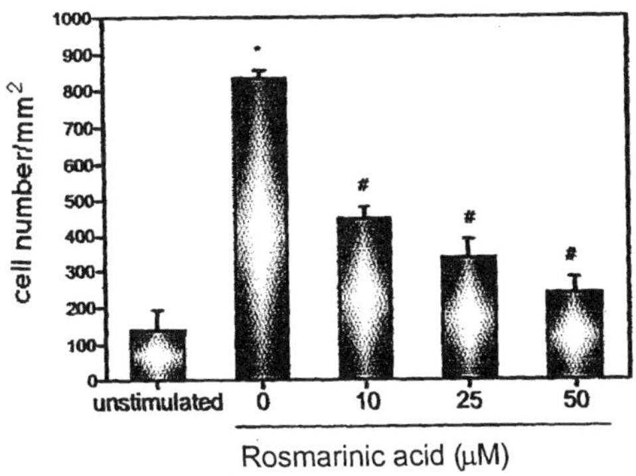

*Figure 2. Effect of rosmarinic acid on monocyte adhesion on HAEC stimulated with IL-1β (20 U/ml) for 4 h was incubated with non-stimulated monocytes (U937) for 30 min. *p<0.001 vs. unstimulated group, and #p<0.01 vs. stimulated group without rosmarinic acid.*

Conclusions

The antioxidative and anti-inflammatory effects of rosmarinic acid were confirmed. The anti-atherosclerotic effect of rosmarinic acid could be attributed to its potent scavenging effect on oxygen radicals, inhibitory effect on LDL oxidation, and inhibitory effect on monocyte-endothelial interaction. These results indicate that ingredients from natural plants that modulate oxidative stress or inflammation may benefit the development of novel strategies to treat atherosclerosis.

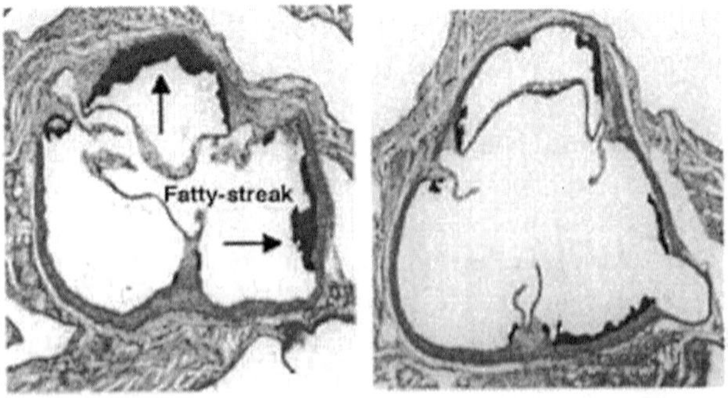

(a) (b)

Figure 3. Photomicrographs of typical atherosclerotic lesion of the aortic arch of apolipoprotein E-deficient mice after treatment with control water(a) and rosmarinic acid (b).

References

1. Yla-Herttuala, S. *Ann N.Y. Acad. Sci.* **1999**, *874*, 134-137.
2. Liao, L.; Starzyk, R.M. and Granger, D.N. *Arterioscler. Thromb. Vasc. Biol.* 1997, *7*, 437-444.
3. Steinberg, D. *Circulation* **1997**, *95*, 1062-1071.
4. Parthasarathy, S.; Steinberg, D. and Witztum, J.L. *Annu. Rev. Med.* **1992**, *43*, 219-225.
5. Collins, R.G., Velji, R.; Guevara, N.V.; Hicks, M.J.; Chan, L. and Beaudet, A.L. *J. Exp. Med.* **2000,** *191*, 189-194.
6. Murayama, T.; Yokode, M.; Kataoka, H.; Imabayashi, T.; Yoshida, H.; Sano, H.; Nishikawa, S. and Kita, T. *Circulation* **1999,** *99*, 1740-1746.
7. Yoshida, N.; Manabe, H.; Terasawa, Y.; Nishimura, H.; Enjo, F.; Nishino, H. and Yoshikawa, T. *Biofactors* **2000**, *13*, 279-288.
8. Cuvelier, M-E.; Richard, H. and Bersef, C. *JAOCS* **1996**, *73*, 645-652.
9. Miyagawa, H.; Yoshikawa, T.; Tanigawa, T.; Yoshida, N.; Sugino, S. and Kondo, M. *J. Clin. Biochem. Nutr.* **1988,** *5,* 1-7.
10. Tanigawa, T. *J. Kyoto Pref. Univ. Med.* **1990**, *99*, 133-143.

Chapter 19

Inhibitory Effects of Oral Administration of an Extract of Orange Peel in the Diet on Azoxymethane-Induced Formation of Aberrant Crypt Foci and Colon Tumor in CF-1 Mice

Wei Ding[1], Yue Liu[1], Robert T. Rosen[2], Geetha Ghai[2], and Mou-Tuan Huang[1]

[1]**Department of Chemical Biology, Susan Lehman Cullman Laboratory for Cancer Research, Ernest Mario School of Pharmacy, Rutgers, The State University of New Jersey, Piscataway, NJ 08854–8020**
[2]**Center for Advanced Food Technology, Rutgers, The State University of New Jersey, 65 Dudley Road, New Brunswick, NJ 08901–8520**

Orange peel possesses antioxidant and anti-inflammatory activity and preventive cancer activity. We have evaluated the effect of an extract of orange peel on azoxymethane (AOM)-induced formation of aberrant crypt foci and colon tumor in CF-1 mice. An extract of orange peel contains approximately 30% polymethoxyflavones. Female CF-1 (6 weeks old) that were s.c. injected with AOM (5, 10, 10, and 10 mg/Kg body weight) once every 4 days resulted in formation of an average of 5.2 aberrant crypt foci (ACF) per colon and 37 aberrant crypt (AC) per colon at 24 weeks after the first dose of AOM treatment. Feeding 0.2% orange peel extract in the AIN 76A diet to mice starting at 2 weeks before the first dose of AOM until the end of the experiment inhibited AOM-induced formation of the number of ACF per colon and AC per colon by 48% and 66% respectively. Feeding 0.2% norhydroxyguaiaretic acid (NDGA), an inhibitor of lipoxygenase, in the AIN 76A diet to mice during both the initiation and promotion phases inhibited the number of AOM-induced formation of ACF per colon and AC per colon by 48% and 75% respectively. Mice developed an average of 0.52 colon tumors per mouse and 44% of mice had colon tumors after 37 weeks of the first dose of AOM injection. The number of AOM-induced colon tumors was decreased by 44% or 48%, when 0.2% orange peel in AIN 76A diet or 0.2% nordihydroxguaiaretic acid in AIN 76A diet was used to replace the control AIN 76A diet. Feeding 0.2% orange peel diet or 0.2% nordihydroxyguaiaretic acid diet also decreased colon tumor incidence by 34% or 39%, respectively.

Introduction

Orange peel is a source rich in flavonoids. Monomethoxyflavones and polymethoxyflavones are the major constituents of orange peel extract. From a pharmacological point of view, the polymethoxyated flavones have a wide biological activity and cancer preventive activity. Some polymethoxyflavones have been reported to have antioxdant and anti-inflammatory activities (*1,2*). A polymethoxyflavone, nobiletin, extracted from orange peel, is shown to inhibit expression of inducible nitric oxide synthase and has a suppressive effect on generation of the superoxide radical (O_2^-) and nitric oxide (NO) (*1,2*). Citrus nobiletin also inhibits phorbol ester-induced inflammation, oxidative stress, and tumor promotion in mouse skin (1). Feeding citrus nobiletin in the diet to rats inhibits AOM-induced formation of ACF in colon epithelium (*3*). Some polymethoxyflavones have anti-mutagenic activity (*4,5*), anti-proliferation activity on tumor cells (*6,7*), anti-promotion activity in mouse epidermis and colon of epithelium (*1*), anti-invasion activity (*8*), anti-adhesive effect on platelets (*9,10*), and cancer preventive effect (*11*). Polymethoxyflavones have anti-leukemia activity (*12*) and differentiating activity (*13*). The polymethoxyflavone, nobiletin has been shown to have anti-ulcer effect (*14*), and protective effect on aflatoxin B-induced cytotoxicity and binding to DNA (*15*). Here we report that an extract of orange peel that contained approximately 30% polymethoxyflavones inhibited AOM-induced formation of ACF and colon tumors.

Material and Methods

Materials

Azoxymethane, nordihydroxyguaiaretic acid and methylene blue were purchased from Sigma-Aldrich Fine Chemicals (St Louis, MO). Acetone and 10% formalin-phosphate buffer were obtained from Fisher Scientific (Springfield, NJ).

Animals

Female CF-1 mice (4-6 weeks old) were purchased from Charles River Laboratories (Wilmington, MA). The animals had free access to food and water throughout the experiment. The mice (initially fed the control AIN 76A diet for 4 days after arrival at the laboratory) were either continued on the same diet (control) or fed a 0.2% orange peel extract in AIN 76A diet or 0.2% nordihydroxguaiaretic acid (NDGA) in AIN 76A diet until the end of the experiment. AIN 76A diet and 0.2% orange peel in AIN 76A diet and 0.2% nordihydroxyguaiaretic acid in AIN 76A diet were purchased from Research Diets, Inc. (New Brunswick, NJ).

Quantification of Aberrant Crypt Foci

Female CF-1 mice (5-6 weeks old; 10-30 mice per group) were giving a s.c. injection of AOM (5, 10, 10, 10 mg/kg) once a week (total 4 injections). The test compounds in the diet were given to mice at 2 weeks before the first AOM injection, during, and continuing until the end of the experiment (initiation + post-initiation period). At 24 weeks after the first dose of AOM injection, the mice were killed and colons (from anus to caecum) were removed, opened longitudinally, rinsed with normal saline solution, was stapled on a plastic sheet. The colon samples were placed in a 10% neutral buffered formalin solution for 24 hours. The entire colon was stained with 0.2% methylene blue dissolved in phosphate buffer saline (PBS) solution for 20 minutes. The whole mount of colon samples was examined in a light microscope magnification. Only ACF meeting the criteria, with crypts of increased size with a thicker and deeply stained epithelial lining and an increased pericryptal zone compared with normal crypts, were chosen.

Study on AOM-induced Formation of Colonic Tumor in CF-1 Mice

Female CF-1 mice were received s.c, injection with AOM (5, 10, 10, and 10 mg of AOM/Kg) at 6 weeks of age once every 4 days (total 4 injections and total 35 mg of AOM). The mice were given AIN 76A diet or test compound in AIN 76A diet at 2 weeks before the first dose of AOM, and continuing until the end of the experiment. Colon samples were removed, opened longitudinally, rinsed with normal saline solution, was stapled on a plastic sheet. The colon samples were stored in a 10% neutral buffered formalin. Colon tumors were counted and recorded.

Results

Chemical Composition of an Extract of Orange Peel

Orange peel extract is a crude product containing approximately 30% polymethoxylated flavones. The chemical structures of major compounds are shown in Figure 1. They include 5,6,7,8,3',4'-hexamethoxyflavone (nobiletin), 5,6,7,8,4'-penta-methoxyflavone (tangeretin), 5,6,7,3',4'-penta-methoxyflavone (sinensetin), 5,7,8,4'-tetra-methoxyflavone, 3,5,6,7,8,3',4'-heptamethoxyflavone, 5,7,8,3',4'-pentamethoxyflavone. Other bioactive compounds include the monohydroxylated analogs of the polymethoxylated flavones. Also present in large quantity are peel waxes.

Analysis was accomplished using a gradient reversed-phase system (Zorbax C-18 column, MacMod Analytical, Chadds Ford, PA). versus a standard of tangeretin (5,6,7,8,4'-pentamethoxyflavone) obtained from Apin Chemicals Ltd (Abingdon, Oxon, UK). The wavelength used for detection was 302 nm. Response factors for all compounds versus tangeretin were assumed to be equal. Orange peel extract was enriched from crude cold-pressed peel oil solids, a byproduct of the orange juice industry.

Inhibitory Effect of an Extract of Orange Peel on AOM-induced Formation of ACF in CF-1 Mice

The possible pathway of chemically-induced formation of aberrant crypt foci and subsequently developing to colon adenoma and adenocarcinoma in CF-1 mouse is shown in Figure 2. Female CF-1 mice were injected s.c. with AOM developed an average of 5.2 ACFs per colon and 37 ACs per colon at 24 weeks

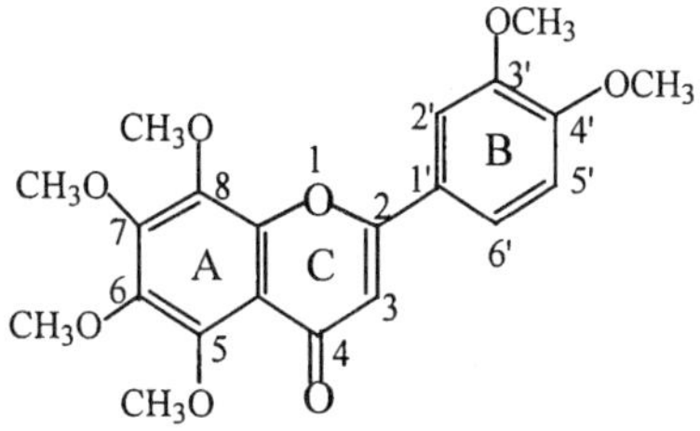

5,6,7,8,3',4'-Hexamethoxyflavone
(Nobeletin)

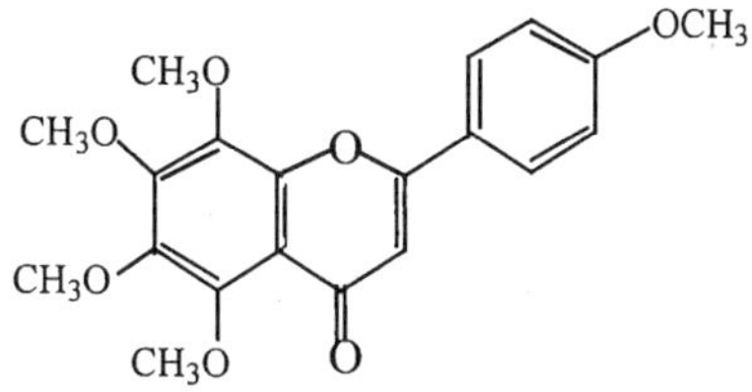

5,6,7,8.4'-Pentamethoxyflavone
(Tangeletin)

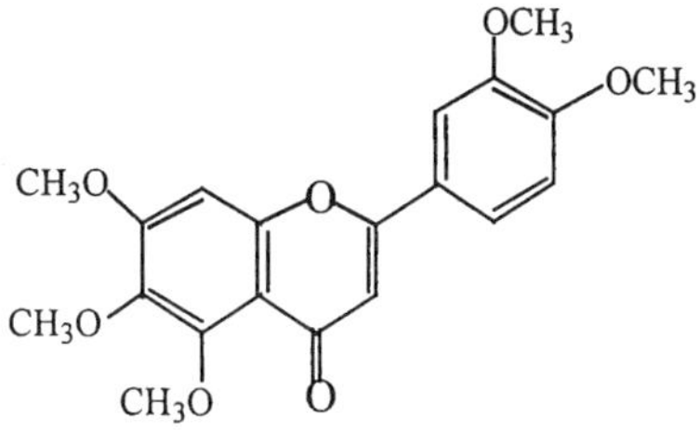

5,6,7,3',4'--Pentamethoxyflavone
(Sinensetin)

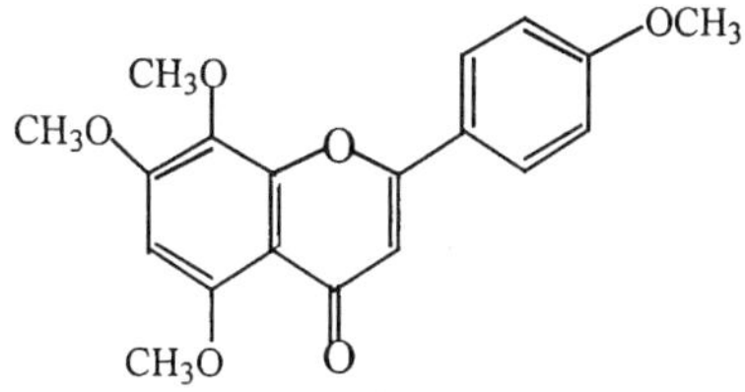

5,7,8,4'-Tetramethoxyflavone

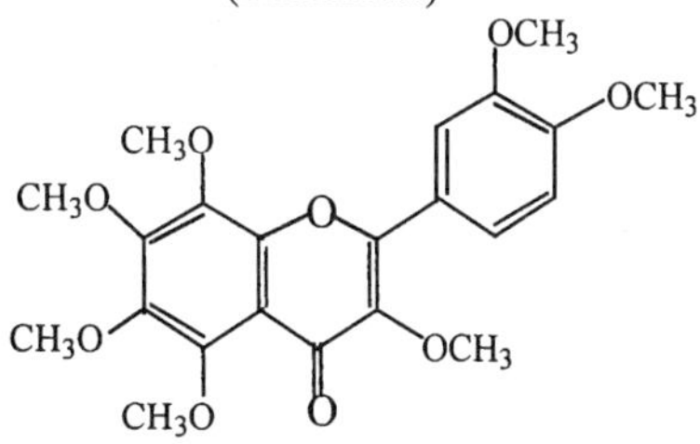

3,5,6,7,8,3'4'-Heptamethoxyflavone

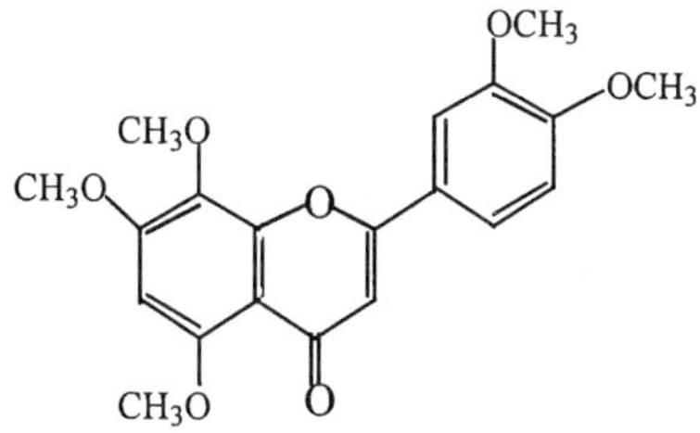

5,7,8,3'4'-Pentamethoxyflavone

Figure 1. Chemical structures of some polymethoxyflavones in orange peel extract.

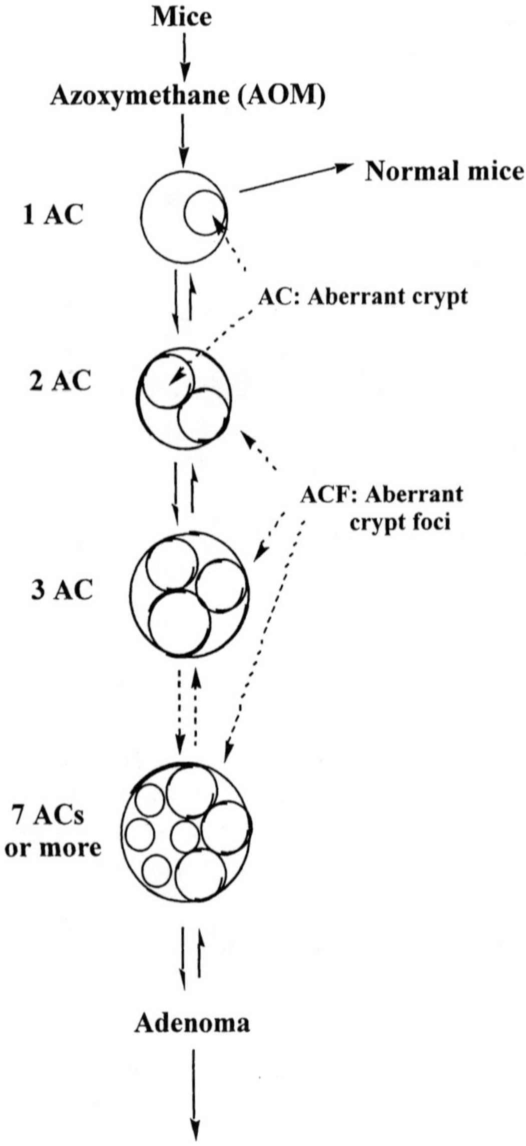

Figure 2. The possible pathway for azoxymethane-induced formation of aberrant crypt foci and colon tumor in CF-1 mice.

after the first dose of AOM injection (Table I). Feeding with 0.2% orange peel extract in AIN 76A diet to mice starting at 2 weeks before the first dose of AOM and continuing until the end of the experiment inhibited the number of AOM-induced ACFs per colon by 48%, and the number of AOM-induced ACs per colon by 66% (Table I). Feeding 0.2% nordihydroxyguaiaretic acid in AIN 76A diet to mice at 2 weeks before the first dose of AOM injection and continuing until the end of the experiment inhibited the number of ACFs per colon by 48%, and the number of AOM-induced ACs per colon by 75% (Table I). It is interesting that both feeding 0.2% orange peel extract diet and 0.2% nordihydroxyguaiaretic acid diet to mice had the smaller ACF size in comparison with the ACF size in the control group diet (Table I).

Inhibitory Effect of an Extract of Orange Peel on AOM-induced Formation of Colon Tumors in CF-1 Mice

Female CF-1 mice were s.c. injected with AOM (5, 10, 10, and 10 mg/Kg body weight) starting at 6 weeks of age once every 4 days resulted in formation of an average of 0.52 colon tumors per mouse and 44% of mice had colon tumor at 37 weeks after the first dose of AOM injection. Feeding 0.2% orange peel extract or 0.2% nordihydroxyguaiaretic acid in the diet to mice inhibited the number of AOM-induced colon tumor per mouse by 44% or 48%, respectively. Colon tumor incidence was reduced by 34% or 39%, respectively (Table II).

Discussion

The results of the present study demonstrate that feeding 0.2% orange peel in the diet to mice starting at 2 weeks before carcinogen injection, during, and continuing to end of the experiment (initiation period + promotion period) inhibited the number of AOM-induced formation of ACFs per colon, colon tumor per mouse and colon tumor incidence. The mechanism of the inhibitory action of orange peel on AOM-induced formation of ACF, colon tumor and colon tumor incidence is unknown. However, it is believed that antioxidant and anti-inflammatory property of polymethoxyflavones may play an important role on the carcinogenic pathways. Among polymethoxyflavones, nobiletin has been studied in more detail. Nobiletin may contribute the important role on anti-carcinogenic and anti-tumor promoting activity of orange peel. Topical application of citrus nobiletin to the back of mice inhibits phorbol ester-induced skin inflammation, oxidative stress, and tumor promotion in mice (*1*). Citrus nobiletin suppresses free radical generation and has anti-inflammatory activity (*2*). Feeding citrus nobiletin in the diet to rats inhibits azoxymethane induced

Table I. Inhibitory Effect of Oral Administration of Orange Peel Extract (OPE) on Azoxymethane (AOM)-induced Formation of Aberrant Crypt Foci in CF-1 Mice

Formation of ACF	*Control diet + Vehicle*	*Control diet + AOM*	*0.2% OPE diet + AOM*	*0.2% NDGAdiet + AOM*
ACF/colon	0	5.2±1.2	2.7±0.9	2.7±0.9
(% inhibition)	-	-	(48%)	(48%)
AC/colon	0	37±5.9	12.6±2.8	9.4±2.2
(% inhibition)	-	-	(66%)	(75%)
AC/ACF	0	7.1	4.7	3.5
(% inhibition)	-	-	(34%)	(51%)
1AC-ACF/colon	0	15.0±2.5	6.4±1.4	6.8±1.5
2AC-ACF/colon	0	5.5±1.2	2.0±0.3	1.0±0.3
3AC-ACF/colon	0	1.0±0.4	0.2±0.2	0.2±0.2
4AC-ACF/colon	0	1.0±0.4	0.2±0.2	0
5AC-ACF/colon	0	0.2±0.2	0	0
6AC-ACF/colon	0	0.3±0.3	0.2±0.2	0
7AC-ACF/colon	0	0.2±0.2	0	0

Female CF-1 mice were given AIN 76A diet , 0.2% orange peel extract in AIN 76A diet (0.2% OPE diet), or 0.2% nordihydroguaiaretic acid in AIN 76A diet (0.2% NDGA diet) starting at 2 weeks before the first dose of AOM. The mice received s.c. injection with AOM (5, 10, 10, 10 mg of AOM per kg of body weight) in saline once every 4 days starting at 2 weeks after 0.2% OPE diet or 0.2% NDGA diet. The mice were killed at 24 weeks after the first dose of AOM treatment. Colon samples were removed and stained with methylene blue and AACF were counted under microscope as described in the Materials and Methods section.

Table II. Inhibitory Effect of Oral Administration of Orange Peel Extract (OPE) on Azoxymethane (AOM)-induced Formation of Colon Tumors in CF-1 Mice

Measurement	*Control diet + Vehicle*	*Control diet + AOM*	*0.2% OPE diet + AOM*	*0.2% NDGA diet + AOM*
Number of mice per group	15	27	17	11
Body weight	51.3±1.9	46,7±1.9	46.7±2.2	45.8±2.1
Colon tumors per mouse (% inhibition)	0	0.52±0.12	0.29±0.11 (-44%)	0.27±0.14 (-48%)
Colon tumor incidence (% inhibition)	0	44%	29% (-34%)	27% (-39%)

Female CF-1 mice were injected s.c. with saline or AOM in saline (5, 10, 10 and 10 mg of AOM/Kg body weight) starting at 6 weeks of age once every 4 days (total 4 injections and total 35 mg of AOM). The mice were given AIN 76A diet in the control groups during the whole period. Both 0.2% orange peel extract in AIN 76A diet or 0.2% nordihydroxyguaiaretic acid in AIN 76 A diet were given to mice at 2 weeks before the first dose of AOM, and continuing until the end of the experiment. The mice were killed at 37 weeks after the first dose of AOM injection. The colon samples were removed and stored in a 10% formalin phosphate buffer. The colon tumors were counted and recorded.

formation of aberrant crypt foci in colon epithelium of rats (*3*). Citrus flavones have anti-mutagenic activity (*4,5*) and anti-proliferation activity (*6,7*).

Feeding 0.2% orange peel in the diet to mice inhibits the proliferation of ACF (see Table I). Our results suggest that orange peel may inhibit proliferation of ACF. In addition, citrus flavones also have several other biological activities, anti-invasion activity (*8*), anti-adhesive effect on platelets (*9,10*), cancer preventive activity (*1,3,11*), anti-leukemia activity (*12*) and cell differential activity (*13*). It is believed that the ortho position of 3′,4′-dimethoxy in C ring and the ortho position of 3-methoxy and 4 position of keto group in B ring are important for antioxidant and anti-inflammatory activity. Thus, sinensetin and nobiletin may be expect to have potent antioxidant and anti-inflammatory activity and cancer chemopreventive activity. Further study is need to confirm this hypothesis. Orange peel contains several polymethoxyflavones and its activity may be result from a combination of several polymethoxyflavones. Orange peel has been widely used as a food additive and food flavor. Intake more orange peel in daily food may be to have health benefit. Human chronic trial on the effect of orange peel on human colon pre-neoplastic tumors is under investigating.

References

1. Murakami, A.; Nakamura, Y.; Torik., K.; Tanaka, T.; Koshiba, T.; Koshimizu, K.; Kuwahara, S.; Takahashi, Y.; Ogawa, K.; Yano, M.; Tokuda, T.; Nishino, H.; Mimaki, Y.; Saahida, Y.; Kitanaka, S.; Ohigashi, H. *Cancer Res.* **2000**, *60*, 5059-5066.
2. Murakami, A.; Nakamura, Y.; Ohto, Y.; Yano, M.; Koshiba, T.; Koshimizu, K.; Tokudo, H.; Nishino, H.; Ohigashi, H. *Biofactors* **2000**, *12*, 187-192.
3. Kohno, H.; Yoshitomi, S-I.; Tsukio, Y.; Murakami, A.; Koshimizu, K.; Yano, M.; Tokuda, H.; Nishino, H.; Ohigashi, H.; Tanaka, T. *Life Sci.* **2001**, *69*, 901-913.
4. Calomme, M.; Pieters, L.; Vlietinck, A.; Vanden, B.D. *Planta Med.* **1996**, *62*, 222-226.
5. Miyazawa, M.; Okuno, Y.; Fukuyama, M.; Naakamura, S-I.; Kosaka, H. *J. Agric. Food Chem.* **1999**, *47*, 5239-5244.
6. Kandaswami, C.; Perkins, E.; Drzewiecki, G.; Soloniuk, D.S.; Middleton, Jr., E. *Anticancer Drugs* **1992**, *3*, 525-530.
7. Ito, A.; Ishiwa, J.; Sat, T.; Minaki, V.; Sashida, Y. *Ann NY Acad. Sci.* **1999**, *878*, 632-634.
8. Bracko, M.; Vyncke, B.; Opdenakker, G.; Foidart, J.M.; De Pestel, G.; Mareel, M. *Clin. Exp. Metastasis* **1991**, *9*, 13-25.

9. Sempinska, E.; Kostka, B.; Krolikowska, M.; Kalisiak, E. *Pol. J. Pharmacol. Pharm.* **1977**, *29*, 7-10.
10. Robbins, P.C. *Int. J. Vitam. Nutr. Res.* **1988**, *58*, 418-421.
11. Iwase, Y.; Takemura, Y.; Ju-ichi, M.; Yano, M.; Ito, C.; Furukawa, H.; Mukainaka, T.; Kuchide, M.; Tokuda, H.; Nishino, H. *Cancer Lett.* **2001**, *163*, 7-9.
12. Mak, N. K.; Wong-Leung, Y. L.; Chan, S. C.; Wen, J.; Leung, K. N.; Fung, M. C. *Life Sci,* **1996**, *58*, 1269-1276.
13. Kawai, S.; Tomono, Y.; Katase, E.; Ogawa., K.; Yano, M. *J. Agric. Food Chem.* **1999**, *47*, 128-135.
14. Takase H.; Yamamoto, K.; Hirano, H.; Saito, Y.; Yamashita, A. *Jpn. J. Pharmacol.* **1994**, *66*, 139-147.
15. Schwartz, A.Z.; Rate, W. R. *J. Environ. Pathol. Toxicol,* **1994**, *2*, 1021-1028.

Chapter 20

Tea Extracts Modulate a Glucose Transport System in 3T3-L1 Adipocytes

Takashi Furuyashiki[1], Sayaka Terashima[1], Hironobu Nagayasu[1], Atsushi Kaneko[1], Iwao Sakane[2], Takami Kakuda[2], Kazuki Kanazawa[1], Gen-ichi Danno[1], and Hitoshi Ashida[1,*]

[1]Department of Biofunctional Chemistry, Faculty of Agriculture, Kobe University, Nada-ku, Kobe 657–8501, Japan
[2]Central Research Institute, Ito En Ltd., Haibara-gun, Shizuoka 421–0516, Japan

In adipocytes, the excess uptake of glucose causes accumulation of fat and an increase in the cell size. It is considered that suppression of this uptake by food factors can reduce the risk of obesity. In this study, we investigated whether various tea extracts affect glucose transport in 3T3-L1 adipocytes. Green, black, and oolong tea extracts decreased 3-*O*-methylglucose (3-OMG) uptake under the insulin stimuli condition. The decrease in 3-OMG uptake by green tea extracts showed dose- and time-dependency. Green tea extracts also suppressed the translocation of glucose transporter (GLUT) 4 to the plasma membrane without altering phosphorylation of insulin receptor. These results indicated that tea extracts modulate a glucose transport system by reducing GLUT4 translocation.

In adipose tissue, glucose is used as a substrate of lipogenesis and as a source of energy. The excess intake of glucose causes accumulation of fat, and then leads to obesity. High concentrations of diet-derived triacylglycerols and free fatty acids may contribute to insulin resistant state by promoting insulin secretion from pancreatic β-cells (*1*) and impairing insulin signaling (*2*). Insulin resistance caused by obesity leads to non-insulin dependent diabetes mellitus (NIDDM) (*3*). Thus, impairment of the glucose transport system is concerned with obesity and NIDDM.

In mammalian cells, glucose cannot be transported across the plasma membrane without mediating the hexose transport system. There are two transport systems: facilitative glucose transporters (GLUTs) (*4*), and Na^+-dependent transporters (*5*). GLUTs consist of 9 isoforms, and each isoform has tissue-specific localization. Muscle and adipose tissue express GLUT1 and GLUT4. GLUT1 is probably the best studied glucose transporter and is located on the plasma membrane of the cell in many tissues including muscle, adipose tissues, brain, red blood cells and blood-tissue barriers, among others (*6*). On the other hand, GLUT4 is specifically expressing in muscle and adipose tissue and called insulin sensitive transporter (*7*). GLUT4 is located on endoplasmic reticulum in a steady state, and immediately translocated to the plasma membrane after insulin stimuli through the phosphorylation pathway mediating with insulin receptor (IR) and insulin receptor substrate (IRS), followed by phosphatidylinositol 3-kinase (PI3-K) and Akt (*8*).

In the nutritional field, it is very interesting and meaningful to decrease glucose uptake by food factors in order to prevent obesity. It has already been reported that some food components affect the glucose transport system. For instance, phloretin (*9*) and genistein (*10,11*), which are natural polyphenols, inhibit glucose transport in rat adipocytes and HL-60 cells. Quercetin inhibits tyrosine kinase of insulin receptor in its SH-domains without any effect on autophosphorylation of the receptor protein (*12*), suggesting that this inhibition may modulate GLUT4 translocation.

Tea contains polyphenols such as catechins and its polymeric theafravins, the latter in black tea. Tea components serve as anti-carcinogens (*13*), and anti-mutagens (*14*) among others. Recently, it has reported that green tea extracts reduce the risk of obesity in mice and rats (*15,16*). In addition, oolong tea is traditionally reported to have anti-obesity and hypolipidaemic actions (*17*). There is, therefore, a possibility that tea extracts modulate glucose metabolism in adipose tissue.

The 3T3-L1 cell line is fibroblasts and differentiates adipocytes. Since this cell line expresses both GLUT1 and GLUT4 (*18*), it is suitable for studying glucose transport and insulin signaling *in vitro*. In this study, we investigated whether tea extracts modulate the glucose uptake and GLUT4 translocation process by insulin stimulation in 3T3-L1 adipocytes. The results showed that the extracts of green, black, and oolong tea decreased insulin-stimulated glucose uptake in 3T3-L1 adipocytes, and green tea extracts suppressed GLUT4 translocation to the plasma membrane without altering an initial insulin signaling.

Materials and Methods

Materials

Murine 3T3-L1 cells were purchased from Dainippon Pharmaceutical Co. Ltd. (Osaka, Japan). Dulbecco's modified Eagle's medium (DMEM) was obtained from Nissui Pharmaceutical Co. Ltd (Tokyo, Japan). Calf serum and fetal bovine serum (FBS) were purchased from Gibco BRL Life Technologies, Inc. (Gaithersburg, MD) and Sigma Chemical Co. (St. Louis, MO), respectively. 3-*O*-Metyl-D-[1-^{3}H]-glucose was from DuPont/NEN Research Products (Boston, MA). Green tea extracts (*Sen-cha, Gyokuro* and *Ban-cha*), black tea extracts (*Uva*, *Nuwara Eliya* and *Dimbula*) and oolong tea extracts (*Tekkannon*, *Shikisyu* and *Suisen*) were products of Itoen Ltd. (Tokyo, Japan). Polyclonal anti-GLUT4 and anti-insulin receptor β-subunit (IRβ) antibodies were purchased from Santa Cruz Biotechnology, Inc. (Santa Cruz, CA). Anti-phosphotyrosine (PY20) antibody was from Transduction Laboratories Ltd. (San Diego, CA). Secondary antibodies to goat IgG and rabbit IgG were from Wako Pure Chemical Industries, Ltd. (Osaka, Japan) and Amarsham Pharmacia Biotech Ltd. (Tokyo, Japan), respectively. All other chemicals and reagents used in this study were analytical grade.

Cell Culture

Murine 3T3-L1 preadipocytes were grown and passaged in DMEM containing 10% calf serum. For adipocyte differentiation, 2 days after confluent state, cells were cultured in DMEM containing 10% FBS, 10 μg/ml insulin, 0.25 μM dexamethazone, 0.5 mM 3-isobutyl-1-methylxantine, and 100 μM ascorbic acid 2-phosphate as an accelerator of differentiation (*19*). After 2 days, the medium was changed to DMEM containing 10% FBS, 10 μg/ml insulin, and 100 μM ascorbic acid 2-phosphate, and cells were cultured for additional 3 days. Then, the medium was changed to the same fresh medium without insulin and ascorbic acid 2-phosphate. Thereafter, the cells were maintained with replacement of the medium every 2-3 days. The cells exhibited > 90% adipocyte phenotype 9-11 days after differentiation induction and used for experiments. Before each experiment, the cells were serum starved in DMEM containing 0.2% bovine serum albumin for 18 h.

Glucose Uptake Assay

Mature 3T3-L1 adipocytes on 35 mm dishes were treated with tea extracts in 1 ml of Krebs-Ringer phosphate-HEPES buffer (KRH: 50 mM HEPES, pH 7.4, 137 mM NaCl, 4.8 mM KCl, 1.85 mM $CaCl_2$, and 1.3 mM $MgSO_4$,) and insulin stimulation was performed for 15 min at 100 nM. To start uptake, 3-OMG was added at a final concentration of 6.5 mM (0.5 μCi/dish). After 30 seconds, the uptake was stopped by washing 4 times with ice-cold KRH containing 0.3 mM phloretin, and the cells were solubilized with 0.5 % sodium dodecyl sulfate (SDS) solution. The radioactivity incorporated into the cells was counted by a liquid scintillation counter. Non-specific uptake was measured in the presence of 0.3 mM phloretin.

Preparation of The Plasma Membrane Fractions

For preparation of the subcellular fractions, 3T3-L1 adipocytes were cultured on 100 mm dishes, and three dishes were used for one set of each treatment. The cells were incubated with tea extracts for 15 min, and then stimulated with insulin for 15 min at 100 nM. The cells were washed twice with ice-cold Tris/EDTA (TE) buffer (10 mM Tris-HCl, pH 7.4, 5 mM EDTA, 1 mM PMSF) containing 250 mM sucrose and scraped off. The cells were homogenized with 3 ml of ice-cold TE/sucrose buffer with 15 strokes of a motor-driven Teflon pestle in a 5-ml glass homogenization vessel. The homogenate was centrifuged at 16,000 X *g* for 20 min. The resulting pellet was resuspended in the same buffer, and homogenized with 10 strokes under the same condition as described above. The homogenate was applied to a sucrose cushion (1.12 M sucrose in the TE buffer) and centrifuged at 100,000 X *g* for 1h. The middle layer was collected and resuspended in TE buffer, and centrifuged at 30,000 X *g* for 45 min. The pellet was resuspended in TE/sucrose buffer, and referred as the plasma membrane fraction. To check the purity of plasma membrane fractions, the activity of 5′-nucleotidase as a maker enzyme for plasma membrane was determined by the method of by Clancy and Czech (*20*). This fraction was stored at –80 °C until use.

Western Blot Analysis

An aliquot of proteins prepared from 3T3-L1 adipocytes was separated by SDS-polyacrylamide gel electrophoresis (SDS-PAGE), and transferred to a PVDF membrane. The membranes were blocked with 5% non-fat dry milk in Tris-buffered saline/Tween 20 (TBST) (10 mM Tris-HCl, pH8.0, 150 mM NaCl, and 0.06% Tween 20) for 1h at room temperature. The membranes were washed 4 times with TBST for 5 min each, and then incubated with anti-GLUT4 antibody (1:1000), anti-PY20 (1:1000) or anti-IRβ (1:1000) for 1h at room temperature. The membrane were washed 4 times with TBST for 5 min each and incubated with secondary antibodies conjugated with horseradish peroxidase for 20 min. Specific immune complexes were visualized with a enhanced chemiluminescence detection kit (Amarsham Pharmacia Biotech).

Immunoprecipitation

Mature 3T3-L1 adipocytes on 100 mm-dish were incubated with green tea extracts for 15 min, and then stimulated with insulin for 15 min at 100 nM. The cells were washed twice with PBS, and lysed in modified radioimmunoprecipitation (RIPA) buffer (50 mM Tris-HCl, pH 8.0, 150 mM NaCl, 1.0% Nonidet-P40, 0.5% sodium deoxycholate, 0.1% SDS, 1 mM Na_3VO_4, 10 mg/ml leupeptin, 50 mM NaF, and 1 mM PMSF). The cells were allowed to stand on ice for 1 h to allow lysis, and centrifuged at 18,000 X *g* for 20 min. An aliquot of proteins (500 μg) of the cell lysate was incubated with anti-IRβ antibody overnight, and incubated with protein A/G agarose beads for another 1 h, and the beads were collected and washed 4 times with RIPA buffer. The immunoprecipitates were separated by SDS-PAGE, and subjected to Western blot analysis to detect phosphorylated IRβ subunit using anti-PY20 antibody.

Results

Tea Extracts Decreased Insulin Stimulated 3-OMG Uptake in 3T3-L1 Adipocytes

The effects of nine tea extracts on 3-OMG uptake in 3T3-L1 adipocytes in the presence or absence of insulin was investigated. In control cells, insulin increased 3-OMG uptake by 298 ± 2% compared with basal uptake. All tea extracts significantly decreased insulin stimulated 3-OMG, especially *Sen-cha, Uva, Tekkannon,* and *Shikishu* extracts decreased by 156 ± 1, 155 ± 21, 180 ± 3 and 165 ± 17%, respectively. On the other hand, oolong tea extracts increased the basal uptake (Figure 1). The suppressive effect of *Sen-cha* extracts on insulin stimulated 3-OMG uptake was dose-dependent; *Sen-cha* extracts significantly decreased uptake at a concentration of 10 μg/ml, and this decrease was dose-dependent (Figure 2). Insulin increased glucose uptake to 361 ± 36% compared with the basal level. When *Sen-cha* extracts were added to the cells for 15 min

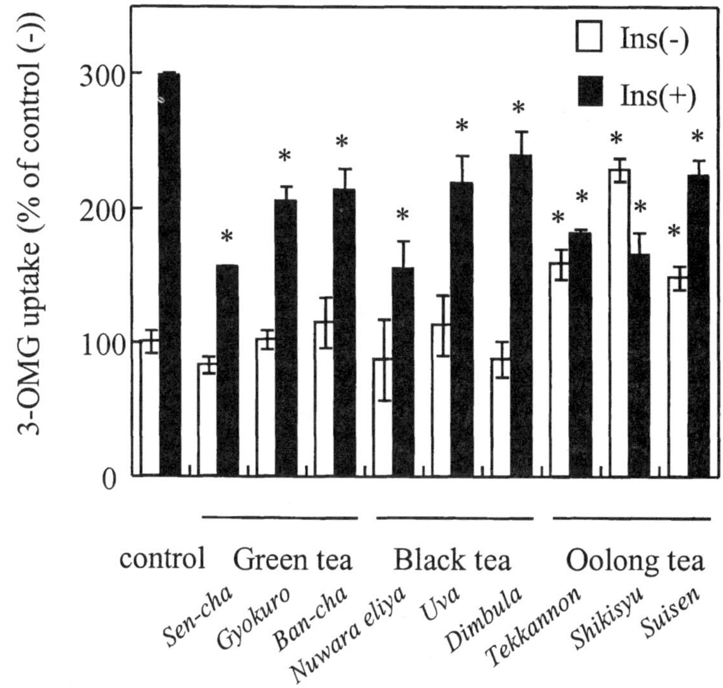

Figure 1. Effect of tea extracts on 3-OMG uptake in 3T3-L1 adipocytes in the absence or presence of insulin. 3T3-L1 cells were differentiated to adipocytes, and serum starved for 18h. The cells were treated with various tea extracts for 15 min and stimulated with 100 nM insulin for additional 15min. Uptake of 3-OMG to the cells were measured as described in Materials and Methods. Data are expressed as percent of the basal value from control cells, and represented as means ± S.D. (n=3). Asterisks indicate significant difference from corresponding control (p<0.01, Student t-test).

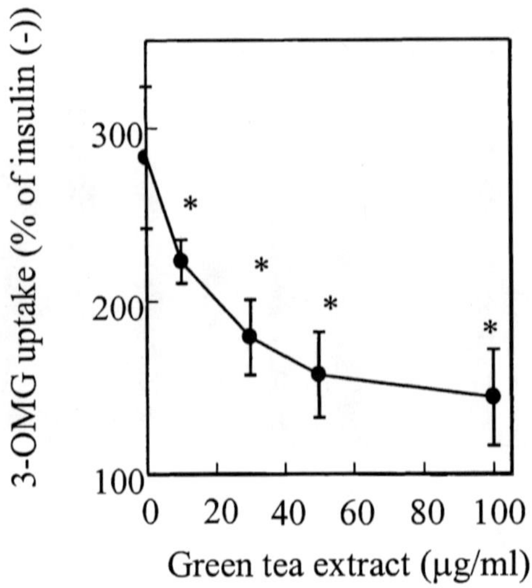

Figure 2. Green tea extracts decreased 3-OMG uptake dose-dependently. 3T3-L1 cells were differentiated to adipocytes, and serum starved for 18 h. The cells were treated with various concentration of Sen-cha extract for 15 min and stimulated with 100 nM insulin for additional 15min. Each cells were subjected to 3-OMG uptake assay as described in Materials and Methods. Data are expressed as percent of the basal value from control cells, and represented as means ± S.D. (n=3). Asterisks indicate significant difference from control (p<0.05, Student t-test).

and further 15 min with insulin, 3-OMG uptake became 147 ± 13%. In the case of simultaneous cotreatments with *Sen-cha* extracts and insulin for 15 min, the uptake was 197 ± 19%. These suppressive effects of *Sen-cha* extracts on glucose uptake were also observed in the post-treatments; When *Sen-cha* extracts were added to cells for 1 and 5 min during insulin stimuli, the uptake became 255 ± 26 and 207 ± 39%, respectively. These results suggested that tea extracts strongly suppress insulin stimulated 3-OMG uptake before and after treatment with insulin.

Tea Extracts Inhibited GLUT4 Translocation to The Plasma Membrane

Since various tea extracts decreased insulin stimulated 3-OMG uptake in 3T3-L1 adipocytes, we examined whether green tea extracts affect GLUT4 translocation from endoplasmic reticurum to plasma membrane. The plasma membrane fraction was prepared as described in the Experimental procedures, and the 5′-nucleotidase activity was measured to check the purity of subcellular fractions. The activity of 5′-nucleotidase in the plasma membrane fraction was 43-folds higher than that of the low-density microsome fraction containing endoplasmic reticurum. As shown in Figure 3, GLUT4 protein translocated to the plasma membrane was dramatically increased by insulin stimuli in control cells. On the other hand, green tea extracts decreased the amounts of GLUT4 protein in the plasma membrane fraction from the cells treated with insulin, indicating that green tea extracts inhibited GLUT4 translocation.

Effect of Sen-cha Extracts on Phosphorylation of IRβ

To study whether insulin signaling transmits to the cells after treatment with tea extracts, the autophosphorylation of IRβ was examined. The total cellular IRβ levels, a protein of about 95 kDa, remained unchanged. IRβ was phosphorylated by insulin stimuli in control cells and *Sen-cha* extracts treated cells as well (Figure 4). These results demonstrated that *Sen-cha* extracts did not affect the function of insulin receptor.

Discussion

In this study, the effects of various tea extracts on the glucose transport and on the translocation of GLUT4 in 3T3-L1 adipocytes was examined. All tea extracts decreased insulin stimulated 3-OMG uptake and the ethyl acetate fraction of *Sen-cha* extracts, which contains tea polyphenols abundantly, showed

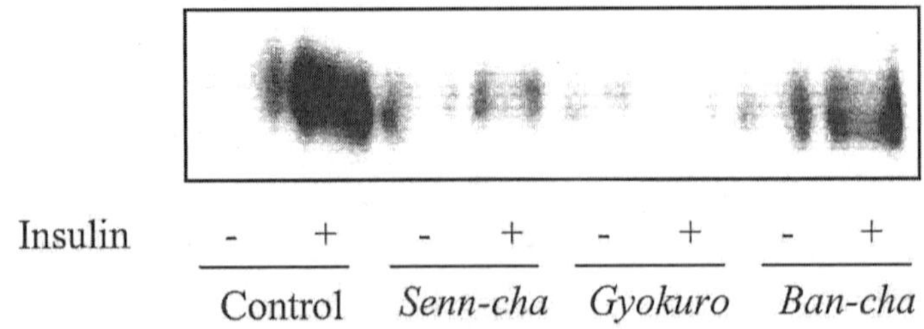

Figure 3. Green tea extracts inhibited insulin-induced GLUT4 translocation. 3T3-L1 cells were differentiated to adipocytes, and serum starved for 18 h. Green tea extracts were treated to the cells at 50 μg/ml for 15 min and stimulated with 100 nM insulin for additional 15 min. Translocation of GLUT4 to the plasma membrane was detected by Western blot analysis as described in the Materials and Methods section.

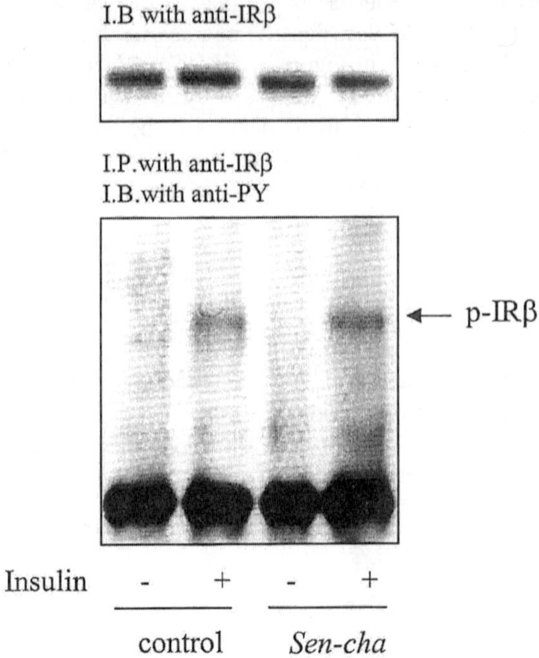

Figure 4. Sen-cha extracts did not alter phosphorylation of insulin receptor β-subunit. 3T3-L1 cells were differentiated to adipocytes, and serum starved for 18 h. Sen-cha extracts were treated to the cells at 50 μg/ml for 15 min and stimulated 100 nM insulin for additional 15 min. The levels of IRβ were detected by Western blot analysis. Phosphorylated IRβ was also detected by Western blot analysis using anti-PY20 antibody, after IRβ was immunoprecipitated with anti-IRβ antibody.

a strong suppression of insulin stimulated glucose transport (data not shown). These results suggested that the suppressive effect on 3-OMG uptake was caused by tea polyphenols such as catechins. Tea extracts contain not only catechins but also other beneficial compounds such as theaflavins, caffeine, theanine, and some pigments. Theaflavins showed an intensive effect on the suppression of insulin stimulated 3-OMG uptake (date not shown), suggesting that various components in teas may additively or synergistically act with each other. Here, the question is arisen whether these components act intracellularly. The intracellular concentrations of various flavonoids have been reported in HL-60 and Jurkat cells (*21*). This study assumes that catechins may be incorporated into 3T3-L1 adipocytes and show their suppressive effect.

GLUT4 translocation and insulin receptor phosphorylation, a part of sequential glucose transport signals, in adipocytes are elucidated as follows: when insulin is bound to its receptor, which consists of two α-subunits and two β-subunits, the receptor complex causes autophosphorylation by itself, and undergoes a series of intracellular transphosphorylation reactions (*22*). In the downstream signaling, IRS-1 is phosphorylated, PI3-K and Akt are activated, and finally GLUT4 is translocated (*8*). However, the activation of PI3-K by stimulation with interleukin-4 or by an engagement of certain integrins does not induce GLUT4 translocation (*23,24*). In this study, green tea extracts suppressed GLUT4 translocation to the plasma membrane (Figure 3) without altering the phosphorylation of IRβ (Fig. 4). These results suggest that the modulation of glucose uptake by green tea extracts through GLUT4 translocation may be due to altering the activation PI3-K and/or Akt, since certain flavonoids such as quercetin and myricetin are potent inhibitor of PI3-K (*25*).

In this study, green, black, and oolong tea extracts modulated the glucose transport system through translocation of GLUT4, and these results may be relevant for prevention of obesity and NIDDM. In rat brown adipose tissue, green tea polyphenols and caffeine are effective in stimulating thermogenesis (*26*). Green tea catechins also inhibit acetyl-CoA carboxylase, a rate-limiting enzyme in lipogenesis (*27*). It is reported that oolong tea and catechins reduce the risk of obesity (*16-18*), and catechins also modulate the plasma cholesterol level in cholesterol-fed rats (*28*). It is, therefore, suggested that tea extracts and their components are beneficial for prevention of obesity and NIDDM.

References

1. Milburn, J. L. Jr.; Hirose, H.; Lee, Y. H.; Nagasawa, Y.; Ogawa, A.; Ohneda, M.; BeltrandelRio, H.; Newgard, C. B.; Johnson, J. H.; Unger, R. H. *J. Biol. Chem.* **1995,** *270*, 1295-1299.

2. Boden, G.; Chen, X. *J. Clin. Invest.* **1995,** *96*, 1261-1268.
3. Orci, L.; Unger, R. H.; Ravazzola, M.; Ogawa, A.; Komiya, I.; Baetens, D.; Lodish, H. F.; Thorens, B. *J. Clin. Invest.* **1990,** *86*, 1615-1622.
4. Carruthers, A. *Physiol. Rev.* **1990,** *70*, 1135-1176.
5. Hediger, M. A.; Rhoads, D. B. *Physiol. Rev.* **1994,** *74*, 993-1026.
6. Gould, G. W.; Holman, G. D. *Bichem. J.* **1993,** *295*, 329-341.
7. Suzuki, K.; Kono, T. *Proc. Natl. Acad. Sci. USA* **1980,** *77*, 2542-2545.
8. Czech, M. P.; Corvera, S. *J. Biol. Chem.* **1999,** *274*, 1865-1868.
9. Whitesell, R. R.; Gliemann, J. *J. Biol. Chem.* **1979,** *254*, 5276-5283.
10. Smith, R. M.; Tiesinga, J. J.; Shah, N.; Smith, J. A.; Jarett, L. *Arch. Biochem. Biophys.* **1993,** *300*, 238-246.
11. Vera, J. C.; Reyes, A. M.; Carcamo, J. G.; Velasquez, F. V.; Rivas, C. I.; Zhang, R. H.; Strobel, P.; Iribarren, R.; Scher, H. I.; Slebe, J. C.; Golde, D. W. *J. Biol. Chem.* **1996,** *371*, 8719-8724.
12. Shisheva, A.; Shechter, Y. *Biochemistry* **1992,** *31*, 8059-8063.
13. Yang, C. S.; Wang, Z. Y. *J. Natl. Cancer Inst.* **1993,** *85*, 1038-1049.
14. Okuda, T.; Mori, K.; Hayatsu, H. *Chem. Pharm. Bull. (Tokyo)* **1984,** *32*, 3755-3758.
15. Sayama, K.; Lin, S.; Zheng, G.; Oguni, I. *In Vivo* **2000,** *14*, 481-484.
16. Kao, Y. H.; Hiipakka, R. A.; Liao, S. *American J. Clin. Nutr.* **2000,** *72*, 1232-1234.
17. Han. L.; Takaku, T.; Kimura, Y.; Okuda, H. *Int. J. Obesity* **1999,** *23*, 98-105.
18. Rosen, O. M.; Smith, C. J.; Fung, C.; Robin, C. S. *J. Biol. Chem.* **1978,** *253*, 7579-7583.
19. Ono M.; Aratani Y.; Kitagawa I.; Kitagawa Y. *Exp Cell Res* **1990,** *187*, 309-314.
20. Clancy, B. M.; Czech, M. P. *J. Biol. Chem.* **1990,** *265*, 12434-12443.
21. Park, J. B.; Levine, M. *J. Nutr.* **2000,** *130*, 1297-1302.
22. Pessin, J. E.; Saltiel, A. R. *J. Clin. Invest.* **2000,** *106*, 165-169.
23. Isakoff SJ.; Taha C.; Rose E.; Marcusohn J.; Klip A.; Skolnik EY. *Proc. Natl. Acad. Sci. USA* **1995,** *92*, 1024710251.
24. Guilherme, A.; Czech, M. P. *J. Biol. Chem.* **1998,** *273*, 33119-33122.
25. Agullo G.; Gamet-Payrastre L.; Manenti S.; Viala C.; Remesy C.; Chap H.; Payrastre B. *Biochem. Pharmacol.* **1997,** *53*,1649-1657.
26. Dulloo, A.G.; Seydoux, J.; Girardier, L.; Chantre, P.; Vandermander, J. *Int. J. Obese.* **2000,** *24*, 252-258.
27. Watanabe, J.; Kawabata, J.; Niki, R. *Biosci. Biotechnol. Biochem.* **1998,** *62*, 532-534.
28. Muramatsu, K.; Fukuyo, M.; Hara, Y. *J. Nutr. Sci. Vitaminol.* **1986,** *32*, 613-622.

Chapter 21

Suppression of Cytochrome P4501 a Subfamily in Mouse Liver by Oral Intake of Polysaccharides from Mushrooms, *Lentinus edodes* and *Agaricus blazei*

Hitoshi Ashida[1,2,*], Takashi Hashimoto[2], Yuji Nonaka[1], Itsuko Fukuda[1,2], Kazuki Kanazawa[2], Gen-ichi Danno[1,2], Ken-ichiro Minato[3], Sachiko Kawakami[2,4], and Masashi Mizuno[2]

[1]Department of Biofunctional Chemistry, Faculty of Agriculture and [2]Division of Life Science, Graduate School of Science and Technology, Kobe University, Nada-ku, Kobe 657–8501, Japan
[3]Miyagi Agricultural College, Sendai 982–0215, Japan
[4]The Tottori Mycological Institute, Kogoke, Tottori 689–1125, Japan

Mushrooms have been consumed as flavorful and medicinal foods for millenniums. Mushroom polysaccharides possess antitumor activity through the stimulation of cytokine productions from immunocytes. On the other hand, lipopolysaccharide suppresses the expression of various hepatic cytochrome P450s (CYPs) through the production of cytokines such as tumor necrosis factor (TNF)-α. In this study, lentinan prepared from *Lentinus edodes* and polysaccharides from *Agaricus blazei* (ABPS) were intraperitoneally injected to female BALB/c mice, and the effects of these polysaccharides on the expression of CYPs were investigated in the liver. Both polysaccharides down-regulated the activity and level of constitutive and 3-methylcholanthrene-inducible CYP1A accompanied by the TNF-α production. When lentinan was orally administered to mice, down-regulation of the level and activity of CYP1A through the suppression of DNA binding activity of aryl hydrocarbon receptor also occurred. These results suggest that the mushroom polysaccharides such as lentinan and ABPS have an anti-carcinogenic activity, since the down-regulation of CYP1A is considered to prevent the metabolic activation of procarcinogens.

Mushrooms have been valued as flavorful foods and medicinal substances for thousands of years. Their extracts are widely used as nutritional supplements and touted as benefits for health, because they are claimed to exhibit antitumorigenic, antiviral, antibiotic, anti-inflammmatory, hypoglycemic, hypocholesterolemic, and hypotensive activities (reviewed in *1*). Particularly, the antitumor activity of mushroom polysaccharides has enthusiastically been researched. Lentinan (β-1,3-D-linked-glucan with β-1,6 branches), which was purified from *Lentinus edodes*, shows an antitumor activity (*2*) through immunomodulatory effects: the release of cytokines (*3, 4*) and the stimulation of phagocytosis (*5*). *Agaricus blazei* also contains polysaccharides (ABPS) showing immunomodulatory and antitumor activities (*6-9*).

Lentinan and ABPS stimulate the release of tumor necrosis factor (TNF)-α and nitric oxide (NO) from macrophages (*9-10*). NO is known as a bioregulatory agent in a wide variety of biological functions such as control of blood pressure, platelet aggregation, cytotoxicity of macrophages, and carcinogenesis (*11-13*). Thus, NO is likely to be associated with the antitumor activity of the mushroom polysaccharides.

Meanwhile, TNF-α is recognized as a factor inducing cell death to tumor cells (*14*). It is involved in hepatic inflammation induced by infectious stimuli such as lipopolysaccharide (LPS), a Gram-negative bacterial endotoxin (*15*). Inflammatory signaling by LPS down-regulates the expression of cytochrome P450s (CYPs), a class of drug- and xenobiotic-metabolizing enzymes (*16, 17*). Suppression of CYP activity contributes to prolonged duration and intensifying pharmaceutical actions (*18*) and to prevent carcinogenesis because the CYP1A subfamily, which is mainly expressed in the liver and induced by xenobiotics such as polyaromatic hydrocarbons, metabolically activates procarcinogens. LPS suppressed the expression of CYP1A, which was induced by the treatment with 3-methylcholanthrene (MC), benzo(*a*)pyrene, and β-napthoflavone, through the production of certain cytokines such as TNF-α and interleukin-1β (*19, 20*). However, little information is available about the suppressive effects of mushroom-derived polysaccharides on CYP1A expression.

In this study, the effects of lentinan and ABPS on the expression of constitutive or inducible CYPs were investigated in the liver of BALB/c mice. After intraperitoneal injection, both polysaccharides down-regulated the activity and the level of CYP1A accompanied by the release of TNF-α from peritoneal macrophages. In addition, oral administered lentinan also down-regulated the activity and level of CYP1A.

Materials and Methods

Reagents and Preparation of Lentinan and ABPS

Lentinan and ABPS were prepared according to the previous reports (*2, 7*). MC and LPS were purchased from Nacalai Tesque (Kyoto, Japan) and Difco Laboratories (Detroit, MI), respectively. All other chemicals were of the highest quality commercially available.

Animals and Treatment

All animal treatments in this study conformed to the "Guidelines for the care and use of experimental animals, in Rokkodai Campus, Kobe University". Female BALB/c mice (Japan SLC, Shizuoka, Japan), body weight 16-20 g, were housed in aluminum cages in a temperature-controlled (25 ± 4°C) room with 60 ± 5% humidity and a 12 h light-dark cycle. In Experiment I, a total of 16 mice were divided into 4 groups (Figure 1): lentinan (10 mg/kg body weight), ABPS (200 mg/kg body weight) or 200 μl of saline (0.85% NaCl, vehicle control) was intraperitoneally injected to mice four times every other day, and the last group was received LPS (0.25 mg/kg body weight) as a positive control twice every other day. One hour after the final administration of the polysaccharides, two mice in each group received a single intraperitoneal injection of MC (10 mg/kg body weight) or the remaining two mice received 200 μl of corn oil (vehicle control). In Experiment II, 4 mice were divided into 2 groups: lentinan (10 mg/kg body weight) or 200 μl of saline (0.85% NaCl, vehicle control) were orally administered to mice four times every other day. One hour after the final administration of the polysaccharides, one of the mice in each group received a single intraperitoneal injection of MC (10 mg/kg body weight) and the other received 200 μl of corn oil (vehicle control). All mice were killed 18 h after MC treatment.

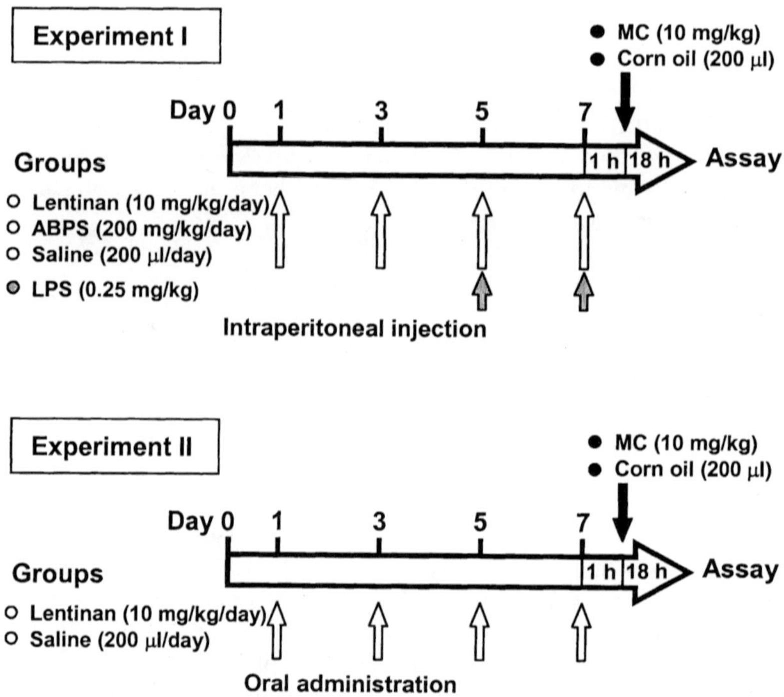

Figure 1 Experimental designs of animal treatment with polysaccharides. Detail of animaltreatment was described in Materials and Methods. Abbreviations: ABPS, polysaccharides from Agaricus blazei; LPS, lipopolysaccharide; MC, 3-methylcholanthrene.

Preparation of Subcellular Fractions of The Liver

The livers were perfused with ice-cold 1.15% KCl and homogenized with 4 volumes of the same solution using a Potter-type Teflon-glass homogenizer. The homogenate was centrifuged at 750×*g* for 10 min at 4°C, and the supernatant was centrifuged at 10,000×*g* for 10 min at 4 °C. The supernatant was further centrifuged at 100,000×*g* for 70 min at 4 °C, and then the pellet was suspended in 0.1 mM Tris-HCl, pH 7.4, containing 20% glycerol and 1 mM phenylmethylsulfonylfluoide (PMSF) as the microsomal protein fraction. The pellet of the 750×*g* centrifugation step was washed twice with buffer A (10 mM Tris-HCl, pH 7.9, 10 mM KCl, 1.5 mM $MgCl_2$, 0.1% Nonidet P-40, 5 μg/ml aprotinin, 20 μg/ml leupeptin, 0.5 mM dithiothreitol and 1 mM PMSF) containing 1% Triton X-100 and once with Triton X-100 free-buffer A to obtain nuclei under the same centrifugation conditions. The pellet was then suspended in extraction buffer (10 mM Tris-HCl, pH 7.9, 25% glycerol, 0.42 M NaCl, 5 μg/ml aprotinin, 20 μg/ml leupeptin, 0.5 mM dithiothreitol and 1 mM PMSF) and homogenized. The homogenate was rotated at 4 °C for 1 h, and the supernatant was collected as the nuclear protein fraction following the centrifugation at 17,000×*g* for 20 min.

Measurement of Activity and Level of CYPs

Ethoxyresorufin *O*-deethylation (EROD) activity was measured according to a previous report (*21*) with slight modifications. Briefly, aliquots of the microsomal protein were incubated at 37 °C for 20 min in 0.1 M potassium phosphate buffer (pH 7.4) with 250 μM β-NADPH and 5 μM ethoxyresorufin. The formed resorufin was measured spectrofluorometically at excitation and emission wavelengths of 530 and 585 nm, respectively. Ethoxycoumarin *O*-deethylation (ECOD) activity was measured as given in a previous report (*22*) with slight modifications. In brief, aliquots of the microsomal protein were incubated at 37 °C for 30 min in 0.1 M potassium phosphate buffer (pH 7.4) with 250 μM β-NADPH and 20 μM 7-ethoxycoumarin. The formed hydroxycoumarin was extracted with chloroform followed by extraction with 0.1 M NaCl/0.01 M NaOH, and determined spectrofluorometically in the water phase at excitation and emission wavelengths of 366 and 452 nm, respectively. Spectrophotometric analysis of the total CYP contents in hepatic microsomal protein was performed as described previously (*23*). CYP1A was detected by Western blotting analysis as follows. Aliquots of the microsomal protein (10 μg protein) were separated by 10% SDS-PAGE and transferred onto the poly(-vinylidene difluoride) membranes followed by blocking with 10% fetal bovine serum in Tris-buffered saline/Tween 20 (TBST) buffer (10 mM Tris-HCl, pH

8.0, 150 mM NaCl and 0.06% Tween 20) at room temperature for 30 min. The membranes were washed several times with TBST buffer and incubated with goat polyclonal antibody to CYP1A (Daiichi Pure Chemicals, Tokyo, Japan) as a primary antibody for 1 h. The membranes were washed again with TBST buffer and incubated with a secondary antibody to goat IgG conjugated with horseradish peroxidase (Wako Pure Chemicals Industries, Osaka, Japan) for 30 min. After washing the membranes with TBST buffer, the specific immune complexes were visualized with a enhanced chemiluminescence detection kit (Amersham Pharmacia Biotech, Tokyo, Japan).

Electrophoretic Gel Mobility Shift Assay (EMSA)

DNA binding activity of nuclear proteins to xenobiotic responsive element (XRE) was measured using EMSA as described previously (*24*).

Measurement of The TNF-α and NO Production from Peritoneal Macrophages

Isolated peritoneal macrophages were cultured for 24 h, and the released TNF-α and NO in the cultured medium were determined by L929 killing assay and the Griess assay, respectively, as described previously (*10*).

Results and Discussion

Experiment I:
Intraperitoneal Injection of Mushroom Polysaccharides

Suppressive Effects of Lentinan and ABPS on CYPs

Since LPS is known to down-regulate CYPs (*16, 17*), the effects of lentinan and ABPS on constitutive and inducible CYPs were investigated in the liver of corn oil- and MC-injected mice, respectively. In the saline-dosed mice, MC expectedly increased the total CYP contents, ECOD (reflecting CYP1A) activity and EROD (reflecting broad-spectrum CYP) activity by 1.6-, 1.5- and 3.0-fold, respectively, in comparison with the constitutive level (Figure 2). Lentinan and ABPS suppressed the MC-incduced total CYP contents, although they did not affect the constitutive contents (Figure 2A). LPS as a positive control markedly down-regulated both the constitutive and the MC-induced CYP contents.

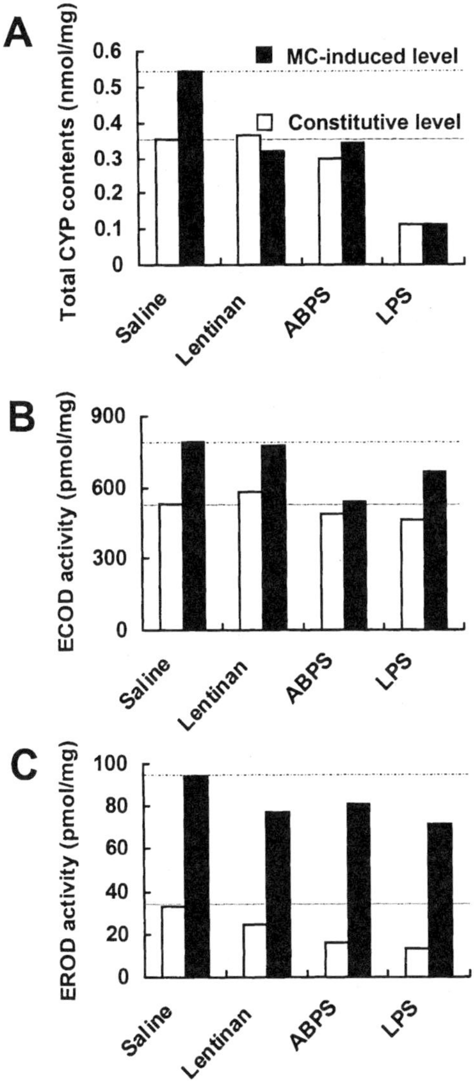

Figure 2 Effects of i.p.-injected polysaccharides on the level and activity of cytochrome P450s (CYPs). Mice were intraperitoneally administered polysaccharides and /or MC as described in Figure 1. (A) Microsomal proteins were prepared from the liver, and the total CYP contents and (B) the ethoxycoumarin O-deethylation (ECOD) and (C) ethoxyresorufin O-deethylation (EROD) activities were measured as described in Materials and Methods.

Regarding the ECOD activity, polysaccharides did not affect the constitutive activity, but ABPS and LPS suppressed the MC-induced activity (Figure 2B). In the case of the EROD activity, all of polysaccharides down-regulated both the constitutive and MC-induced activities (Figure 2C). These results suggest that lentinan and ABPS decreased both the constitutive and the MC-induced CYP1A activities. In addition, lentinan and ABPS partially reduced the MC-induced total CYPs but not the constitutive ones, while LPS drastically reduced the content of CYPs. Thus, the suppressive mechanism of the expression and the activity of CYPs by mushroom polysaccharides are different from that by LPS.

Mushroom Polysaccharides Stimulate The Production of TNF-α in Peritoneal Macrophages *Ex Vivo*

Various kinds of cytokines down-regulate the expression of multiple CYPs including MC-induced CYP1A (*19, 25*). LPS down-regulates CYP1A1 and CYP1A2 through TNF-α production (*26, 27*). To determine whether cytokines are involved in down-regulation of the CYP1A by mushroom polysaccharides, the TNF-α level in plasma and TNF-α production from peritoneal macrophages of mice were investigated. TNF-α was not detected in plasma even from LPS-dosed mice (data not shown). Probably, TNF-α may disappear in plasma, because LPS markedly but transiently increased TNF-α in plasma 1 to 2 h after administration (*28*). When the TNF-α production was determined in the 24 h-cultured medium of peritoneal macrophages from polysaccharides-dosed mice, *in vivo* treatment with lentinan and ABPS significantly increased the TNF-α production from macrophages of both corn oil- and MC-injected mice (Table). These results suggest the possibility that mushroom polysaccharides induce the TNF-α production, and a transient increase in TNF-α may be associated with the down-regulation of CYP1A.

Since NO is also produced from macrophages after LPS stimulation. NO is also one of the immune responses simultaneous with an induction of TNF-α and involved in LPS-caused down-regulation of CYP1A (*29*). Thus, the production of NO was measured in the culture medium of peritoneal macrophages under the *ex vivo* system. Lentinan and ABPS rather slightly decreased the NO production from peritoneal macrophages as shown in Table I, while MC alone increased the production. Moreover, lentinan and ABPS did not affect the expression of inducible NO synthase (data not shown). On the other hand, LPS is known to up-regulate both the TNF-α production and NO synthesis (*30*). Thus, lentinan and ABPS cause down-regulation of CYP1A with a different mechanism from that of LPS inducing inflammatory stimuli.

Table I. Effects of lentinan and ABPS on the release of TNF-α and NO from peritoneal macrophages of mice injected polysaccharides

	TNF-α (pg/hr/10⁶ cells)		*Nitrite (pmol/hr/10⁶ cells)*	
Treatment	*Corn oil*	*MC*	*Corn oil*	*MC*
Saline	0.06	n.d	4.33	5.87
Lentinan	1.82	0.50	3.27	5.07
ABPS	3.98	1.51	2.13	4.40

Mice were intraperitoneally administered polysaccharides and/or MC as described in Fig. 1. The peritoneal macrophages were collected and cultured for 24 h. The released TNF-α and NO from the macrophages into the culture medium were determined as described in Materials and Methods.

n.d., not detected

Experiment II:
Oral Administration of Mushroom Polysaccharides

Suppressive Effects of Oral Administered Lentinan on CYPs

In Experiment I, it was demonstrated that intraperitoneally injected lentinan down-regulates the expression of CYPs. To further investigate the effects of lentinan as a food component on the CYP expression, mice were orally administered lentinan and the activities of EROD and ECOD were measured in the liver (Figure 1). The oral administration of lentinan down-regulated the EROD activity in MC-treated mice and slightly decreased the constitutive activity (Figure 3A). Lentinan also slightly suppressed ECOD in both corn oil- and MC-dosed mice (Figure 3B). These results indicated that orally administrated lentinan down-regulates CYPs, particularly CYP1A, which is induced by xenobiotics including polyaromatic hydrocarbons and heterocyclic amines, and the results from post-oral administration (Figure 3) are almost consistent with the results from intraperitoneal administration (Figures 2B and 2C).

Effects of Lentinan on Aryl Hydrocarbon Receptor (AhR)

The Western blotting analysis showed that orally administered lentinan also decreased the protein levels of CYP1A in the liver of both corn oil- and MC-treated mice in comparison with the saline control (Figure 4A). Since the

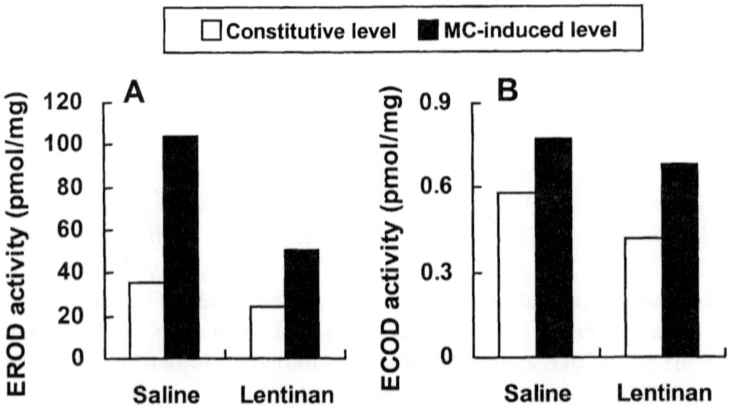

Figure 3 Effects of p.o.-administered lentinan on the EROD and ECOD activities. Mice were orally administered lentinan and intraperitoneally injected MC as described in Figure 1. The EROD and ECOD activities were measured in hepatic microsomal proteins.

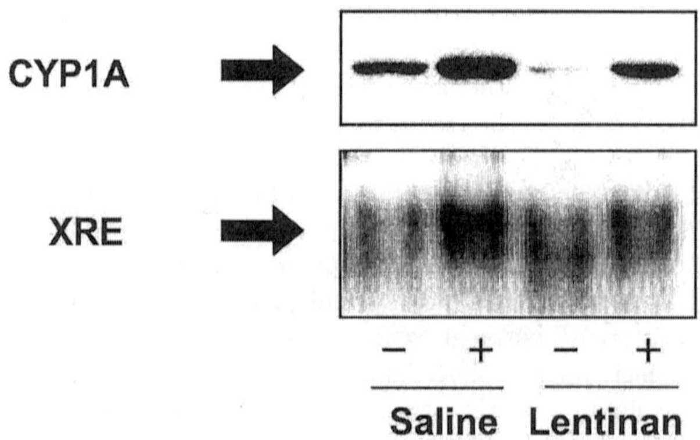

Figure 4 Effects of p.o.-administered lentinan on the aryl hydrocarbon receptor (AhR) binding activity to xenobiotic responsive element (XRE) and the expression level of CYP1A. Mice were orally administered lentinan and intraperitoneally administered MC as described in Figure 1. Nuclear and microsomal proteins, which were prepared from the livers of the mice, were used for en electrophoretic gel mobility shift assay to determined the AhR binding activity to XRE and for Western blotting analysis to determine the expression level of CYP1A, respectively

expression of CYP1A is mainly mediated by the interaction between AhR and XRE, the binding activity of nuclear proteins to XRE was determined by EMSA. Lentinan decreased the MC-activated binding activity to XRE (Figure 4), indicating that down-regulation of MC-induced CYP1A by lentinan was dependent upon the suppression of AhR activation. The suppressive effect of lentinan is unlikely due to the antagonism of AhR, because AhR favors hydrophobic compounds that have van der Waals dimensions of 14×12×5 Å (*31*), while lentinan has a large molecular weight of approximately 400,000 Da. Moreover, it seems difficult for such a large molecule to be transported into the cells. Therefore, cytokines or other factors influenced by mushroom polysaccharides may indirectly down-regulate the AhR activation. One possible mechanism of the down-regulation of CYPs by lentinan is the activation of TNF-α/NF-κB signaling pathway: Lentinan stimulates immunocytes and induces the production of TNF-α, and the released TNF-α subsequently activates a pleiotropic transcriptional factor NF-κB (*15*) through the autocrine and/or paracrine mechanisms. The activated NF-κB interacts with AhR (*32*), resulting in the down-regulation of CYPs. Therefore, NF-κB may be involved in the lentinan-induced down-regulation of CYPs.

Conclusion

The results in this study demonstrated that glucan type polysaccharides lentinan and ABPS from *L. edodes* and *A. blazei*, respectively, down-regulated CYPs, particularly CYP1A, in the liver through the TNF-α production from macrophages and AhR/XRE binding activity. Antitumor and anticarcinogenic abilities of lentinan and ABPS are shown in Figure 5. Lentinan and ABPS increased TNF-α production in mice, and TNF-α is involved in the down-regulation of CYP1A through the suppression of AhR. The TNF-α production is also concerned with the antitumor activities of these polysaccharides, because TNF-α is recognized as a cell death-inducing factor in transplanted murine tumors (*14*). We suggest the down-regulation of CYPs as a novel mode for anti-carcinogenic activity of the polysaccharides. Xenobiotics including procarcinogens are metabolized by CYPs (phase I enzymes), conjugated by phase II enzymes and finally excreted. During the process, procarcinogens such as polyaromatic hydrocarbons and heterocyclic amines are metabolized to their ultimate carcinogenic forms by CYPs. Therefore, the down-regulation of CYPs is advantageous for prevention of carcinogenesis, because lowered CYPs gradually metabolize procarcinogen, and ultimate carcinogen formed are enough to conjugate by phase II enzymes. From the viewpoint of chemotherapy, the down-regulation of CYPs is also advantageous for suppression of cancer, because it prolongs the duration and intensifies the pharmaceutical actions in

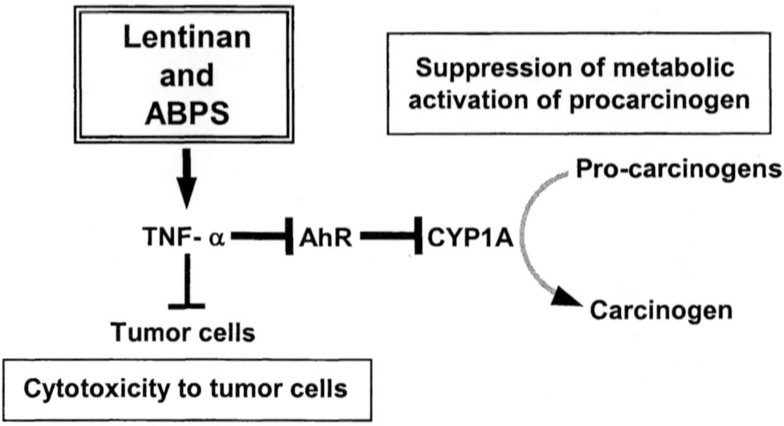

Figure 5 Antitumor and anticarcinogenic abilities of lentinan and ABPS.

patients (*18*). This study supplies important information about cancer prevention by mushroom polysaccharides through down-regulation of CYPs, although further studies are needed to elucidate the precise mechanism of the suppression. We propose that intake of mushrooms in the diet will help the prevention of cancer caused by xenobiotics.

References

1. Borchers, A. T.; Stern, J. S.; Hackman, R. M.; Keen, C. L.; Eric Gershwin, M. E. *Proc. Soc. Exp. Biol. Med.* **1999,** *221*, 281-293.
2. Chihara, G.; Hamuro, J.; Maeda, Y.; Arai, Y.; Fukuoka, F. *Cancer Res.* **1970,** *30*, 2776-2781.
3. Fruehauf, J. P.; Bonnard, G. D.; Herberman, R. B. *Immunopharmacology* **1982,** *5*, 65-74.
4. Kerékgyártó, C.; Virág, L.; Tankó, L.; Chihara, G.; Fachet, J. *Int. J. Immunopharmacol.* **1996,** *18*, 347-353.
5. Abel, G.; Szollosi, J.; Chihara, G.; Fachet, J. *Int. J. Immunopharmacol.* **1989,** *11*, 615-621.
6. Itoh, H.; Ito, H.; Amano, H.; Noda, H. *Jpn. J. Pharmacol.* **1994,** *66*, 265-271.
7. Mizuno, M.; Morimoto, M.; Minato, K.; Tsuchida, H. *Biosci. Biotechnol. Biochem.* **1998,** *62*, 434-437.
8. Mizuno, M.; Minato, K.; Ito, H.; Kawade. M.; Terai, H.; Tsuchida, H. *Biochem. Mol. Biol. Int.* **1999,** *47*, 707-714.
9. Sorimachi, K.; Akimoto, K.; Ikehara, Y.; Inafuku, K.; Okubo, A.; Yamazaki, S. *Cell Struct. Funct.* **2001,** *26*, 103-108.
10. Minato, K.; Mizuno, M.; Ashida, H.; Hashimoto, T.; Terai, H.; Tsuchida, H. *Int. J. Medicinal Mushrooms* **1999,** *1*, 265-272.
11. Marletta, M. A. *Trends Biochem. Sci.* **1989,** *14*, 488-492.
12. Moncada, S.; Palmer, R. M. J.; Higgs, E. A. *Pharmacol. Rev.* **1991,** *43*,109-142.
13. Ohshima, H.; Bartsch, H. *Mutat. Res.* **1994,** *305*, 253-264.
14. Carswell, E. A.; Old, L. J.; Kassel, R. L.; Green, S.; Fiore, N.; Williamson, B. *Proc. Natl. Acad. Sci. U.S.A.* **1975,** *72*, 3666-3670.
15. Bradham, C. A.; Plumpe, J.; Manns, M. P., Brenner, D. A.; Trautwein. C. *Am. J. Physiol.* **1998,** *275*, G387-G392.
16. Morgan, E. T. *Mol. Pharmacol.* **1989,** *36*, 699-707.
17. Morgan, E. T. *Biochem. Pharmacol.* **1993,** *45*, 415-419.
18. Walter-Sack, I.; Klotz, U. *Clin. Pharmacokinet.* **1996,** *31*, 47-64.
19. Abdel-Razzak, Z.; Corcos, L.; Fautrel, A.; Campion, J. P.; Guillouzo, A. *Mol. Pharmacol.* **1994,** *46*, 1100-1110.

20. Calleja, C.; Eeckhoutte, C.; Larrieu, G.; Dupuy, J.; Pineau, T.; Galtier, P. *Biochem. Biophys. Res. Commun.* **1997,** *239*, 273-278.
21. Burke, M. D.; Thompson, S.; Elcombe, C. R.; Halpert, J.; Haaparanta, T.; Mayer, R. T. *Biochem. Pharmacol.* **1985,** *34*, 3337-3345.
22. Jacobson, M.; Levin, W.; Poppers, P. J.; Wood, A. W.; Conney, A. H. *Clin. Pharmacol. Ther.* **1974,** *16*, 701-710.
23. Omura, T.; Sato, R. *J. Biol. Chem.* **1964,** *230*, 2379-2385.
24. Ashida, H.; Fukuda, I.; Yamashita, T.; Kanazawa, K. *FEBS Lett.* **2000,** *476*, 213-217.
25. Abdel-Razzak, Z.; Loyer, P.; Fautrel, A.; Gautier, J.-C.; Corcos, L.; Turlin, B.; Beaune, P.; Guillouzo, A. *Mol. Pharmacol.* **1993,** *44*, 707-715.
26. Monshouwer, M.; McLellan, R. A., Delaporte, E.; Witkamp, R. F.; van Miert, A. S. J. P. A. M.; Renton, K. W. *Biochem. Pharmacol.* **1996,** *52*, 1195-1200.
27. Paton, T. E.; Renton, K. W. *Biochem. Pharmacol.* **1998,** *55*,1791-1796.
28. Shedlofsky, S. I.; Tosheva, R. T.; Snawder, J. A. *Biochem. Pharmacol.* **2000,** *59*, 1295-1303.
29. Stadler, J.; Trockfeld, J.; Schmalix, W. A.; Brill, T.; Siewert, J. R.; Greim, H.; Doehmer, J. *Proc. Natl. Acad. Sci. U.S.A.* **1994,** *91*, 3559-3563.
30. Chen, F.; Sun, S. C.; Kuh, D. C.; Gaydos, L. J.; Demers, L. M. *Biochem. Biophys. Res. Commun.* **1995,** *214*, 985-992.
31. Waller, C. L.; McKinney, J. D. *Chem. Res. Toxicol.* **1995,** *8*, 847-858.
32. Tian, Y.; Ke, A,; Denison, M. S.; Rabson, A. B.; Gallo, M. A. *J. Biol. Chem.* **1999,** *274*, 510-515.

Antioxidants

Chapter 22

Antioxidants in Processed Garlic: Tetrahydro-β-carboline Derivatives in Aged Garlic Extract

Nagatoshi Ide, Makoto Ichikawa, Kenjiro Ryu, Jiro Yoshida, Takashi Sasaoka, Shin-ichiro Sumi, and Hiromichi Sumiyoshi

Healthcare Research Institute, Wakunaga Pharmaceutical Company, Ltd., 1624, Shimokotachi, Koda-cho, Takata-gun, Hiroshima 739–1195, Japan

A variety of biological activities, including antioxidant effects and reduction of cardiovascular disease risk factors, have been previously reported using fresh and processed garlic (*Allium sativum* L.). In this chapter, antioxidant effects of 1,2,3,4-tetrahydro-β-carboline derivatives (THβCs) in aged garlic extract (AGE) will be discussed. In *in vitro* assay systems, these compounds have shown strong hydrogen peroxide scavenging activities. Among the four compounds identified in AGE, (1S, 3S)-1-methyl-1,2,3,4-tetrahydro-β-carboline-1,3-dicarboxylic acid was found to be stronger than the common antioxidant, ascorbic acid. These alkaloids also inhibited AAPH-induced lipid peroxidation and LPS-induced nitrite production from murine macrophages. In chemical analyses using liquid chromatography mass spectrometry (LC-MS), these compounds were not detected in raw garlic, but the contents increased during the natural aging process of garlic. Our data demonstrate that not only organosulfur compounds but also these four alkaloids may contribute to the antioxidant activities of AGE, and suggesting that processing procedure such as natural aging process could play an important role in influencing medicinal functions of foodstuffs.

Garlic (*Allium sativum* L.) has been considered a valuable healing agent by people of many different cultures for thousands of years. Even today, it is commonly used for its medical benefit through the world, especially Eastern Europe and Asia. It has been considered that the medicinal and beneficial properties may be attributed to specific constituents found in garlic and its extracts, and many studies suggest that organosulfur compounds are responsible for the biological activities (*1*). Organosulfur compounds in garlic are converted into a variety of compounds depending on the processing procedure. Therefore, different processing procedures result in various kinds of garlic products with varying chemistry. Among the many commercial garlic products, aged garlic extract (AGE) is uniquely manufactured by a more than 10-months natural aging process. It has been previously reported that AGE shows a variety of biological activities including antioxidant (*2-4*), cancer-preventing (*5*), anti-atherogenic (*6*) and anti-platelet aggregation (*7, 8*). The extract contains unique and bioactive organosulfur compounds, *S*-allylcysteine (SAC) and *S*-allylmercaptocysteine (SAMC).

SAC is one of major water-soluble compounds in processed garlic. The compound is formed by the transformation of γ-glutamyl-*S*-allylcysteine through an enzymatic process. The bioavailability of this compound has been well established in animals and it has been shown to be evenly absorbed and distributed systemically (*9*). The reported effects of SAC include: inhibition of LDL oxidation (*10*), inhibition of oxidized LDL-induced endothelial cell injury (*3*) and nuclear factor kappa B activation in T lymphocytes, macrophages and endothelial cells (*11-13*). SAC also directly scavenges reactive oxygen species in cells and cell free systems (*14, 15*), regulates nitric oxide availability from macrophages and endothelial cells, and protects neuronal damage in rat brain ischema (*16*).

SAMC is also a unique compound, which is formed by the reaction between allicin (allyl 2-propenethiosulfinate) and cysteine during processing. SAMC has been reported to inhibit LDL oxidation (*10*), *tert*-butyl hydroperoxide-induced chemiluminescence in liver microsomal fraction (2) and liver injury induced by acetaminophen (*17*).

More recently, non-sulfur fructosyl arginine, a Maillard reaction product, was isolated from AGE and was found to inhibit LDL oxidation (*18*), inhibit oxidized LDL-induced endothelial cell injury (*18*) and directly scavenging reactive oxygen species in cells and cell free systems (*18, 19*).

This chapter discusses the antioxidant effects of 1,2,3,4-tetrahydro-β-carboline derivatives (THβCs) in AGE; 1-methyl-1,2,3,4-tetrahydro-β-carboline-

3-carboxylic acids (MTCC; **1a/b**) and 1-methyl-1,2,3,4-tetrahydro-β-carboline-1,3-dicarboxylic acid (MTCdiC; **2a/b**) in both diastereoisomers. Also, the changes in concentrations of the alkaloids during the natural aging process of garlic using liquid chromatography mass spectrometry (LC-MS) will be described.

Materials and Methods

Aged Garlic Extract (AGE). AGE was manufactured under a license issued by the Ministry of Health and Welfare of Japan, and formulated as follows: sliced raw garlic (*Allium sativum* L.) was dipped into the aqueous ethanol, and extracted for more than 10 months at room temperature (*2*). AGE used for these experiments contained SAC in the range of 1.6-2.4 mg/g (calculated as dry weight)(*20*).

Cell Lines. Murine macrophage cell line (J774.A) was obtained from Japan Health Sciences Foundation (Tokyo, Japan). J774.A was grown in Dulbecco's modification of Eagle's medium (DMEM) with 10% foetal bovine serum. The media was supplemented with 200 U/mL penicillin and 0.2 mg/mL streptomycin. Cells were incubated at 37°C in a humidified 5% CO_2 atmosphere for 3-4 days before experimental use. Viability of cells used throughout the experiments was always greater than 95% as determined by trypan blue exclusion.

AGE Fractionation. AGE fractionation was performed according to the method of Ryu et al. (*19*). AGE was partitioned between ethyl acetate and water. The water layer (AGE-P) was dialyzed against distilled water at 4°C for 3 days to give fraction-1 [F-1; Mw: <1000] and fraction-2 [F-2; Mw: >1000]. F-2 was chromatographed on DEAE TOYOPEAL 650M (Tosoh, Tokyo, Japan) to give fraction-3 (F-3; sugars) and fraction-4 (F-4; proteins). F-1 was subjected to reversed-phase column chromatography on MCI gel CHP20P (Mitsubishi Chemical, Tokyo, Japan) with aqueous methanol (MeOH) in stepwise gradient mode. MeOH eluate was further fractionated on Si gel eluting with the gradient mixtures of $CHCl_3$-MeOH, and given subfractions were chromatographed on reversed-phase HPLC using MeOH/water (1:9, v/v) as eluent.

Mass Spectrometric Analysis of Tetrahydro-β-carboline Derivatives. Chromatographic separation for LC-MS was performed on a Capcell Pak C18UG120 (75 mm x 2.0 mm i.d., 3 μm) (Shiseido, Tokyo, Japan). Gradient elution was performed using HP-1100 binary pump (Hewlett-Packard, CA,

USA). Solvent A was 0.05% TFA in water, solvent B was 0.05% TFA in water/acetonitrile (1:1, v/v) and the linear gradient was programmed as following; t=0 min 20% solvent B, t=20 min 60% solvent B, t=30 min 100% solvent B. The flow rate was 0.2 mL/min and injection volume was 5 μL, respectively. The mass spectrometric detector was an ion trap mass spectrometer LCQ (Thermoquest, CA, USA) equipped with atmospheric pressure chemical ionization (APCI). An optimal condition of the APCI source parameter was obtained at the following values: sheath gas flow rate was 60 (arbitrary unit defined by the software), vaporizer temperature was 450°C, discharge current was 5 μA, capillary voltage was 3V, capillary temperature was 150°C, scanning mode was positive and scan range was 100-300 amu. Analytical data were acquired using *Xcalibur* software (version 1.0 SR1). Fragmentation experiments (MS/MS) was performed in the trap with helium as the collision gas and the relative collision energy (RCE) was set at 35%.

Nuclear Magnetic Resonance Spectroscopy (NMR). ^{1}H- and ^{13}C-NMR and NOE experiments were performed on a JEOL JNM-ECP500 (JEOL, Tokyo, Japan) apparatus at 500 MHz and 125 MHz, respectively.

Synthesis of Reference Compounds. Synthesis of THβCs were according to the methods described before (*21, 22*), and assignment of NMR signals was confirmed by GROESY, H-H COSY, HMQC, and HMBC experiments.

H_2O_2 Scavenging Assay. The scavenging effects of obtained fractions or THβCs identified in aged garlic extract on hydrogen peroxide was determined according to the method of Okamoto et al. with slight modification (*23*). Briefly, 10 μL of 500 μM hydrogen peroxide, 10 μL of sample or H_2O as a control, 40 μL of 150 U/mL horseradish peroxidase, and 40 μL of 0.1% 2,2'-Azino-di-[3-ethyl-benzthiazoline-6-sulfonic acid] (ABTS) were added to 120 μL of 0.1 N phosphate buffer (pH 6.0). The solution was then incubated at 37°C for 15 min. Absorbance at 414 nm was measured using Multiskan Ascent (Labsystems, Helsinki, Finland).

AAPH-induced Lipid Peroxidation. 2,2'-azobis(2-amidinopropane) hydrochloride (AAPH) is a water-soluble and azo compound, which works as a radical initiator and causes lipid peroxidation. The effects of THβCs on AAPH-induced lipid peroxidation were determined according to the method described before (*14, 24*). Briefly, 1.4 mL of 50 mM linoleic acid-50 mM SDS micelles solution was added to the reaction vessel equipped with an oxygen electrode, kept at 37°C and stirred to saturate oxygen. Various concentrations of THβCs (0.1 and 1 mM) or H_2O as a control was added to the mixture, kept for 2 min, and 40 μL of 0.5M AAPH as a radical initiator were added to the system. The amounts of oxygen consumed in the mixture were monitored for 20 min, and compared with control.

Determination of Nitrite Production from Macrophages. The effects of THβCs on nitrite production from macrophages were determined according to the methods as described before (*4, 25*). Harvested J774.A cells ($2x10^5$/well) were incubated for 2 h in 96-well plates. After incubation, the media were removed, and cells were washed and incubated with 10-250 μM of THβCs in DMEM, and 10 μg/mL of LPS for 20 h at 37°C. Nitrite was determined in supernatant using the Griess Reagent System Kit according to the manufacture's instruction. This assay is based on converting nitrite into a deep purple azo compound using Griess Reagent. The intensity of color is proportional to the concentration of nitrite. Absorbance was measured at 540 nm with a 96-well plate ELISA reader (Labsystems, Helsinki, Finland). Nitrite solution included in the assay kit was used as a standard.

Statistical Analysis. Data were analyzed using the one-tailed Student's t-test (Microsoft Excel), and results were expressed as the mean ± SE. A *p* value of less than 0.05 was considered significant.

Result and Discussion

Oxidative modification of lipids, proteins and DNA by reactive oxygen species plays an important role in a wide range of common diseases including cardiovascular diseases, inflammatory condition, and neurodegenerative diseases (*26-28*). Under oxidant-stressed condition, peroxides such as hydrogen peroxide and lipid peroxide change cell functions and interactions with surrounding cells. In the cardiovascular field, for instance, hydrogen peroxide damages endothelial cell membranes, reduces cell viability and induces lipid peroxidation (*29*). Also hydrogen peroxide serve as an important second messenger in the activation of the transcription factor NF-κB, which is associated with expression of cell adhesion factors, vascular cell adhesion molecules-1 (VCAM-1), and intercellular cell adhesion molecules-1 (ICAM-1) (*30, 31*). Lipid peroxidation in endothelial cells changes the permeability of cell membranes and ion efflux. Lysophosphatidylcholine (Lyso PC), which is a lipid peroxide composed of oxidized LDL, can be a trigger of inflammation that leads to the release of inflammatory mediators such as reactive oxygen species and cytokines (eg. TNF-α and IL-6). All of these mediators and oxidative stress cause endothelial injury and dysfunction, foam cells formation and smooth muscle cell proliferation, and eventually lead to the formation of atherosclerotic lesion. In the present study, in order to further find the antioxidants, AGE was fractionated using hydrogen peroxide scavenging assay.

Identification of THβCs and H_2O_2 Scavenging Activities. Given fractions were added to the hydrogen peroxide scavenging assay. The strongest scavenging activities (100% scavenging at 0.1 mg/mL) were demonstrated by 50% MeOH and 100% MeOH eluates. Column chromatography on Si gel and reversed-phase HPLC were further repeated in two bioactive fractions. After these subfractions were analyzed using LC-MS and MS/MS, assumed compounds were synthesized, analyzed using LC-MS, MS/MS, ^{1}H- and ^{13}C-NMR, and these alkaloids were identified as bioactive compounds. Figure 1 shows THβCs identified in AGE; MTCCs (**1a/b**) and MTCdiCs (**2a/b**) in both diastereoisomers. Scavenging effects of MTCCs (**1a/b**) or MTCdiCs (**2a/b**) on hydrogen peroxide are shown in Figure 2. At 250 μM, (1R, 3S)- or (1S, 3S)-MTCC scavenges hydrogen peroxide 49.0% or 35.4%, respectively. However, scavenging activities of MTCdiCs (**2a/b**) are about 5 to 10 times stronger than MTCCs (**1a/b**). Especially, (1S, 3S)-MTCdiC (**2b**) has shown stronger activity than the common antioxidant, ascorbic acid. To elucidate the mechanism by which (1S, 3S)-MTCdiC (**2b**) scavenges hydrogen peroxide, we also analyzed the change of **2b** in the presence of hydrogen peroxide and peroxidase using LC-MS and MS/MS. The data showed **2b** was decarboxylated at 1 position and dehydrated between 1 and 2 position (data not shown), suggesting that this compound functions as an electron donor and scavenge hydrogen peroxide, and the presence of carboxyl group at 1 position may explain the difference in scavenging activity between **1a/b** and **2a/b**.

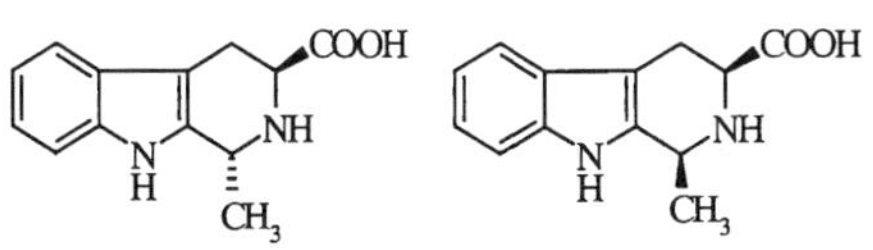

(**1a**): (1R, 3S)- (**1b**): (1S, 3S)-

1-methyl-1,2,3,4-tetrahydro-β-carboline-3-carboxylic acids (**MTCC; 1a/b**)

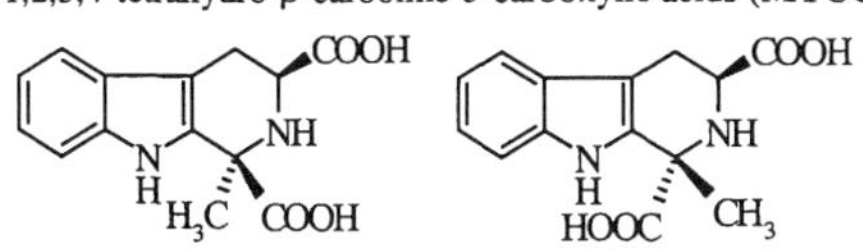

(**2a**): (1R, 3S)- (**2b**): (1S, 3S)-

1-methyl-1,2,3,4-tetrahydro-β-carboline-1,3-dicarboxylic acids (**MTCdiC; 2a/b**)

Figure 1. Chemical structures of 1,2,3,4-tetrahydro-β-carboline derivatives

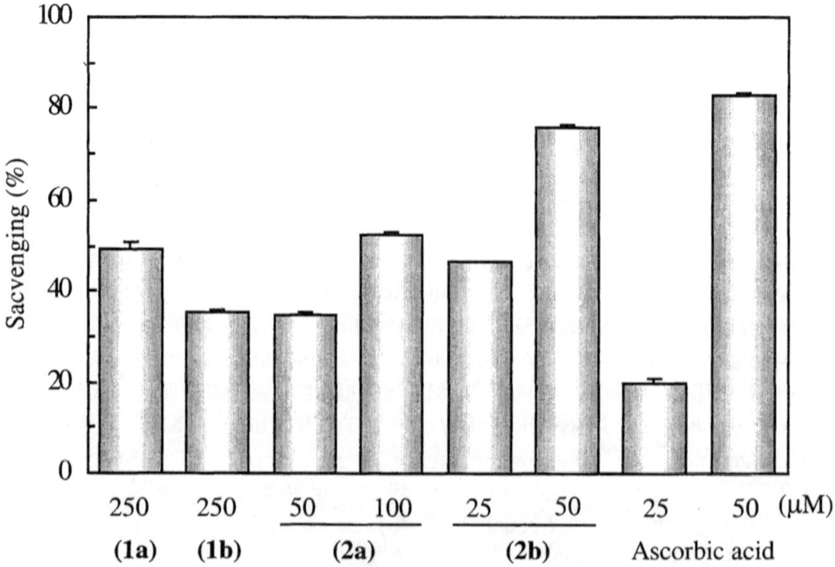

identified in aged garlic extract.

Figure 2. Effects of 1,2,3,4-tetrahydro-β-carboline derivatives identified in aged garlic extract on hydrogen peroxide. Data represent means ± SE of triplicate samples.

Effects of THβCs on AAPH-induced Lipid Peroxidation. Table I shows the effects of THβCs on AAPH-induced lipid peroxidation. In this experiment, the strongest hydrogen peroxide scavenger, (1S, 3S)-MTCdiC (**2b**) and its mono-carboxylate, (1S, 3S)-MTCC (**1b**) were used. Incubation of linoleic acid-SDS micelle solution with AAPH for 20 min resulted in a significant O_2 consumption and caused lipid peroxidation. Co-incubation with (1S, 3S)-MTCC (**1b**) or (1S, 3S)-MTCdiC (**2b**) inhibited AAPH-induced lipid peroxidation 30.7% or 28.6% at 1 mM and 10.3% or 10.0% at 0.1 mM. However, there was no difference between **1b** and **2b**, and the activities were not strong compared with the common antioxidant, butylhydroxytoluene (BHT). It has been previously reported that in THβCs the saturated feature of the A ring provides the antioxidant activity (*32*). This feature may be considered as one of the mechanisms by which used THβCs inhibited lipid peroxidation.

Effects of THβCs on Nitrite Production from Macrophages. The effects of four MTCCs (**1a/b**) and MTCdiCs (**2a/b**) on LPS-induced nitrite production from macrophages are shown in Figure 3. Exposure of LPS (10 μg/mL) to J774 cells resulted in a significant release of nitrites. Co-incubation of J774 cells with (1R, 3S)-MTCdiC (**2a**) or (1S, 3S)-MTCdiC (**2b**) resulted in a significant inhibition of nitrite release from macrophages at 50 and 100 μM or 10 to 100 μM, respectively, though MTCCs (**1a/b**) didn't inhibit it at 250 μM. The intracellular level of inducible nitric oxide synthase (iNOS) plays an important role in determining nitric oxide (NO) production rates in activated macrophages and several other cell types. In pathological condition, macrophages increase NO and superoxide anion productions resulting in the formation of peroxynitrite ($ONOO^-$), which can exert strong oxidant effects (*33, 34*). The high amounts of NO and /or $ONOO^-$ are associated with acute and chronic inflammation and atherosclerosis through cytotoxicity and injury to the surrounding cells and tissue. In this study, LPS-induced nitrite production from macrophages was measured. MTCdiCs (**2a/b**) exhibited inhibition at low concentrations. It was previously reported that AGE inhibited LPS-induced NO production (*4*). Another group also reported that carboline derivatives isolated from *Melia azedarach* suppress iNOS activity through the inhibition of NF-κB activation (*35*). These data suggest that MTCdiCs identified in AGE may reduce the iNOS activity in activated macrophages and inhibit NO production.

Changes in Concentrations of THβCs During the Natural Aging Process. In order to identify and quantify the compounds, LC-MS analyses were performed. LC-MS is a potent analytical method for the efficient analysis of minor compounds in complex materials. The excellent sensitivity and selectivity allowed specific detection of THβCs from coeluting compounds (*36*). Figure 4A and B show the changes in concentrations of **1a/b** and **2a/b** during the natural

Table I. Effects of Tetrahydro-β-carboline Derivatives Identified in Aged Garlic Extract on AAPH-induced Lipid Peroxidation

Sample	*Concentration (mM)*	*O_2 Consumption (μM ± SE)*	*Inhibition (%)*
Control	-	138.5 ± 2.16	-
(**1b**)	1	96.0 ± 5.12*	30.7
	0.1	124.2 ± 3.15*	10.3
(**2b**)	1	98.9 ± 5.40*	28.6
	0.1	124.6 ± 1.35*	10.0
BHT	0.1	42.5	69.3

Data represent means ± SE of repeated studies (n=4). Significant difference compared with control without samples (p<0.05). BHT: butylhydroxytoluene

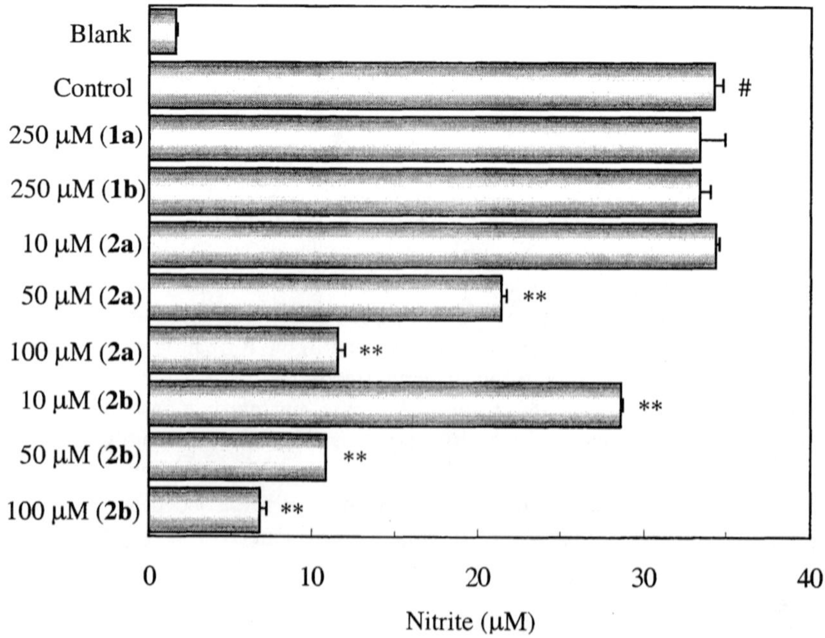

Figure 3. Effects of tetrahydro-β-carboline derivatives identified in aged garlic extract on LPS-induced nitrite production from macrophages. Data represent means ± SE of triplicate samples. Significant difference ($p<0.01$) compared with control without samples.

aging process. In raw garlic, all of these compounds were not detected since they were either not present or below the detection limit [(1R, 3S)-MTCC (**1a**): 74.5 ng/g; (1S, 3S)-MTCC (**1b**): 86.1 ng/g; (1R, 3S)-MTCdiC (**2a**): 1.67 μg/g; (1S, 3S)-MTCdiC (**2b**): 1.54 μg/g]. However, all of these alkaloids were formed from the beginning of the natural aging process, and remarkably increased between 4 and 10 months. MTCdiCs (**1a/b**) further increased in concentrations after 10 months of aging, while MTCCs (**2a/b**) plateaued at 10 months (Figure 4A).

It has been previously reported that the chemical formations of THβCs depend on storage time, pH, temperature and processing conditions. THβCs in fermented and maturated foodstuffs, such as beer and wine, are also believed to be related to the amount of aldehydes (*37-39*). Chemically, MTCCs (**1a/b**) and

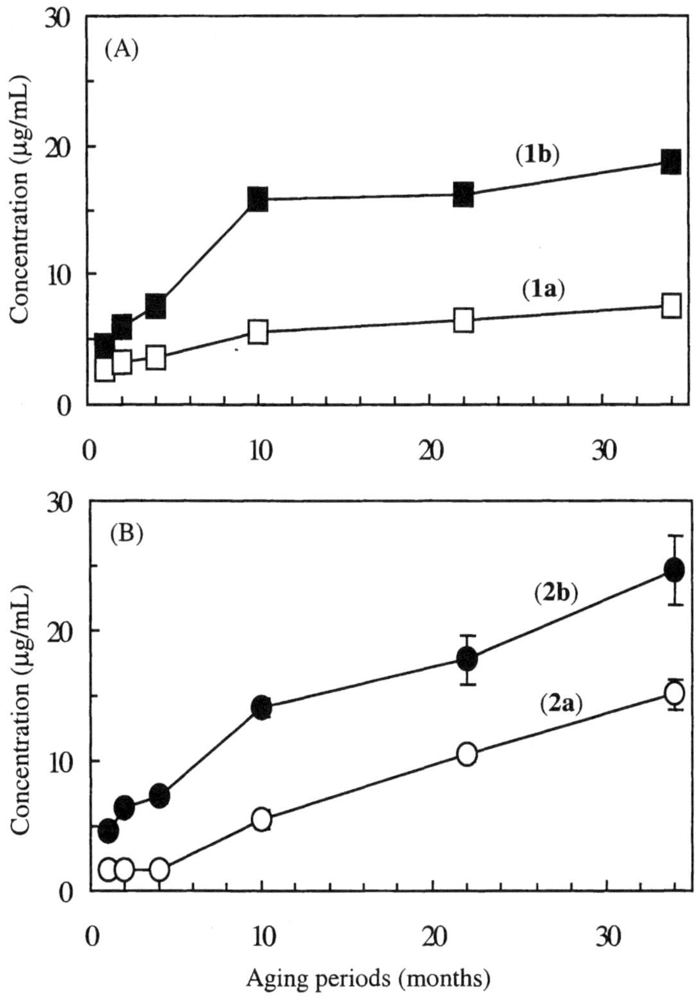

*Figure 4. Changes in concentration of MTCCs (**1a/b**; A) and MTCdiCs (**2a/b**; B) during the natural aging process. Samples prepared during the natural aging process of garlic were analyzed by LC-MS. Data represent mean ± SE of repeated studies (at least 3 times).*

MTCdiCs (**2a/b**) are synthesized by the condensation between tryptophan and acetaldehyde or pyruvic acid, respectively. It is expected that acetaldehyde, which is a precursor to form **1a/b**, comes from alcohol as previously reported (*38, 39*). While, in the natural aging process of garlic, two pathways are expected to form pyruvic acid for determining **2a/b** contents in AGE; one is the alliin-allicin pathway, and another is via the Maillard reaction process. The former is the most common pathway in garlic. When raw garlic is cut or processed, a major organosulfur compound in raw garlic, alliin (*S*-allylcysteine sulfoxide), is converted into allicin (allyl 2-propenethiosulfinate) by a C-S lyase called alliinase, and pyruvic acid is formed as a by-product (*40, 41*). In the later process, 3-deoxyglucosone is a key compound, which is well-known as a Maillard reaction product. The compound has been reported to cause C3/C3 cleavage and form the pyruvaldehyde in a model Maillard reaction system (*42*). MTCdiCs (**2a/b**) in processed garlic may be formed by the non-enzymatic reaction between tryptophan and pyruvic acid and/or pyruvaldehyde formed in these two expected pathways (Figure 5).

Conclusion

Antioxidant effects of four tetrahydro-β-carboline derivatives; 1-methyl-1,2,3,4-tetrahydro-β-carboline-3-carboxylic acid (MTCC; **1a/b**) and 1-methyl-1,2,3,4-tetrahydro-β-carboline-1,3-dicarboxylic acid (MTCdiC; **2a/b**) in both diastereoisomers in aged garlic extract (AGE) were discussed. Tetrahydro-β-carboline derivatives (THβCs) are formed through the Pictet-Spengler chemical condensation between tryptophan and aldehyde during food production, processing and storage. It has been previously reported that these compounds were identified and quantified in beer, wine, vinegar, sauce, soy sauce, fruit juice, chocolate and cocoa (*21, 36, 43, 44*). Reported biological effects of THβCs include antioxidant effects (*32, 45*), anti-platelet aggregation (*43*), and neuromodulation such as inhibiting monoamine oxidase (MAO), biogenic amine (serotonin) uptake/release and benzodiazepine receptor binding (*46, 47*). Our data indicate that not only organosulfur compounds but also these alkaloids may contribute to the antioxidant activities of AGE, suggesting that processing garlic, such as by natural aging, could play an important role in influencing medicinal functions of foodstuffs.

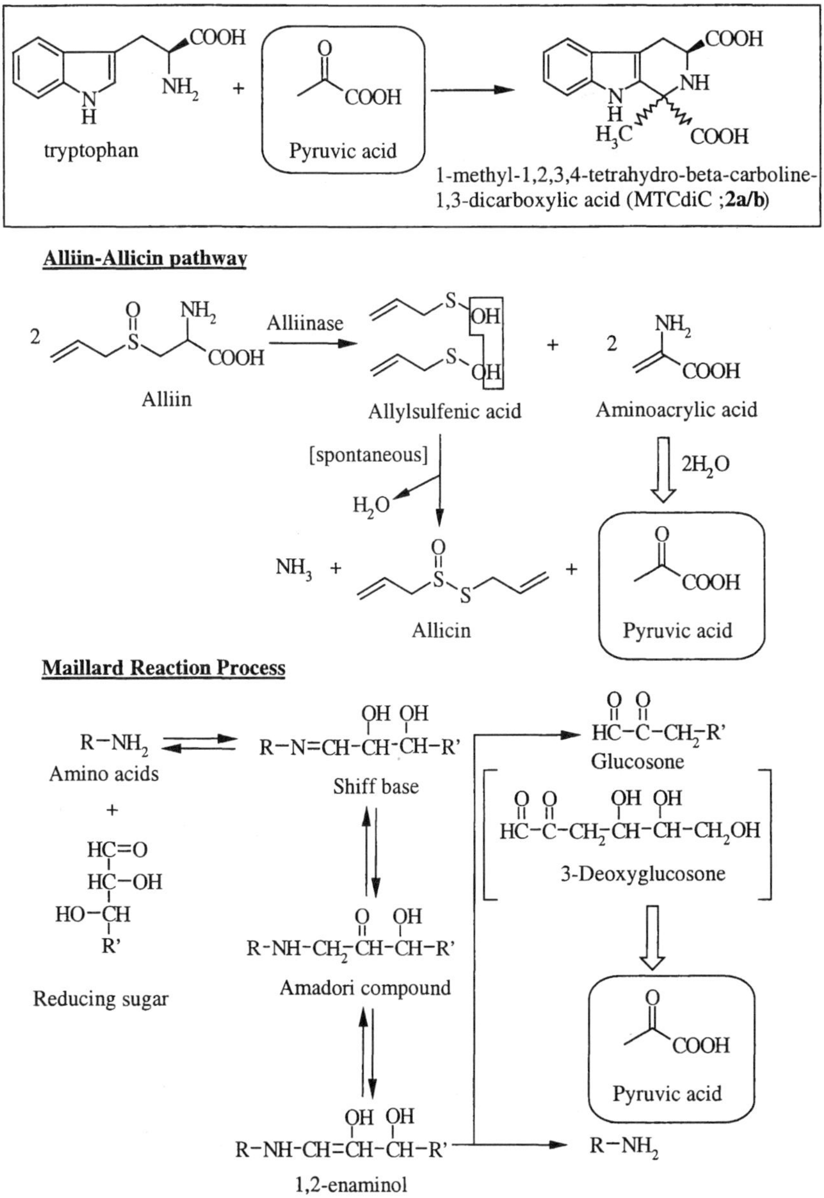

*Figure 5. Expected pathway to form 1-methyl-1,2,3,4-tetrahydro-β-carboline-1,3-dicarboxylic acids (**2a/b**) during the natural aging process of garlic.*

References

1. Block, E. *Angew Chem. Int. Ed. Engl.* **1992**, 31, 1135-1178.
2. Imai, J.; Ide, N.; Nagae, S.; Moriguchi, T.; Mastuura, H.; Itakura, Y. *Planta Med.* **1994**, 60, 417-420.
3. Ide, N.; Lau, B. H. S. *J. Pharm. Pharmacol.* **1997**, 49, 908-911.
4. Ide, N.; Lau, B. H. S. *Phytomed.* **1999**, 6, 125-131.
5. Amagase, H.; Milner, J. *Carcinogenesis* **1993**, 14, 1627-1631.
6. Efendy, J. L.; Simmons, D. L.; Campbell, G. R.; Campbell, J. H. *Atherosclerosis* **1997**, 132, 37-42.
7. Rahmann, K.; Billington, *J. Nutr.* **2000**, 130, 2662-2665.
8. Steiner, M.; Li, W. *J. Nutr.* **2001**, 131, 980S-984S.
9. Nagae, S.; Ushijima, M.; Hatono, S.; Imai, J.; Kasuga, S.; Matsuura, H.; Itakura, Y.; Higashi, Y. *Planta Med.* **1994**, 60, 214-217.
10. Ide, N.; Nelson, A.B.; Lau, B.H.S. *Planta Med.* **1997**, 63, 263-264.
11. Geng, Z.; Rong, Y.; Lau, B.H.S. *Free Radic. Bio. Med.* **1997**, 23, 345-350.
12. Ide, N.; Lau, B.H.S. *J. Nutr.* **2001**, 131, 1020S-1026S.
13. Kim, K.M.; Chun, S.B.; Koo, M.S.; Choi, W.J.; Kim, T.W.; Kwon, Y.G.; Chung, H.T.; Billiar, T.R.; Kim, Y.M. *Free Radic. Bio. Med.* **2001**, 30, 747-756.
14. Ide, N; Matsuura, H; Itakura, Y. *Phytother. Res.* **1996**, 10, 340-341.
15. Ide, N.; Lau, B.H.S. *Drug Dev. Ind. Pharm.* **1999**, 25, 619-624.
16. Numagami, Y.; Ohnishi, S.T. *J. Nutr.* **2001**, 131, 1100S-1005S.
17. Sumioka, I.; Matsuura, T.; Kasuga, S.; Itakura, Y.; Yamada, K. *Jpn. J. Pharmacol.* **1998**, 78, 199-207.
18. Ide, N.; Lau, B.H.S.; Ryu, K.; Matsuura, H.; Itakura, Y. *J. Nutr. Biochem.* **1999**, 10, 372-376.
19. Ryu, K.; Ide, N.; Matsuura, H.; Itakura, Y. *J. Nutr.* **2001**, 131, 972S-976S.
20. Moriguchi, T.; Saito, H.; Nishiyama, N. *Biol. Pharm. Bull.* **1996**, 19, 305-307.
21. Gutsche, B.; Herderich, M. *J. Agric. Food Chem.* **1997**, 45, 2458-2462.
22. Bobbitt, J.M.; Willis, J.P. *J. Org. Chem.* **1980**, 45, 1978-1984.
23. Okamoto, G.; Hayase, F; Kato, H. *Biosci. Biotech. Biochem.* **1992**, 56, 928-931.
24. Pryor, W.A. *J. Am. Chem. Soc.* **1988**, 110, 2224-2229.
25. Dirsch, V.M.; Kiemer, A.K.; Wagner, H; Vollmar, A.M. *Atherosclerosis* **1998**, 139, 333-339.
26. Spatz, L. Introduction, In *Biological consequences of oxidative stress*; Spatz, L.; Bloom, A eds., Oxford University Press, New York, NY, 1992; pp3-22.
27. Chabrier, P.E.; Demerle Pallardy, C.; Auget, M. *Cell. Mol. Life Sci.* **1999**, 55, 1029-1035.
28. Crawford, D.W.; Blankenhorn, D.H. *Atherosclerosis* **1991**, 89, 91-108.

29. Yamasaki, T.; Li, L.; Lau, B.H.S. *Phytother. Res.* **1994**, 8, 408-412.
30. Sen, C.K.; Packer, L. *FASEB J.* **1996**, 10, 709-720.
31. Geng, Z.; Rong, Y.; Lau, B.H.S. *Free Radic. Biol. Med.* **1997**, 23, 345-350.
32. Pari, K.; Sundari, C. S.; Chandani, S.; Balasubramanian, D. *J. Biol. Chem.* **2000**, 275, 2455-2462.
33. Ischiropoulos, H.; Zhu, L.; Beckman, J.S. *Arch Biochem. Biophys.* **1992**, 298, 446-451.
34. Rees, D.D.; Cellek, S.; Palmer, R.M.; Moncada, S. *Biochem. Biophys. Res. Commun.* **1990**, 173, 541-547.
35. Lee, B.G.; Kim, S.H.; Zee, O.P.; Lee, K.R.; Lee, H.y.; Han, J.W.; Lee, H.W. *Eur. J. Pharmacol.* **2000**, 406, 301-309.
36. Gutsche, B.; Herderich, M. *J. Chromatogr. A* **1997**, 767, 101-106.
37. Bosin, T.R.; Krogh, S.; Mais, D. *J. Agric. Food Chem.* **1986**, 34, 843-847.
38. Herraiz, T.; Ough, C.S. *J. Agric. Food Chem.* **1993**, 41, 959-964.
39. Herraiz, T.; Huang, Z.; Ough, C.S. *J. Agric. Food Chem.* **1993**, 41, 455-459.
40. *Garlic- the science and therapeutic application of Allium sativum L. and related species;* Lawson, L.D.; Koch, H.P., Lawson, L.D., eds.; Williams & Wilkins: Boltimore, MD, 1996; pp37-107.
41. *Garlic Science;* Matsuura, H.; Saito, H. eds.; Asakura Publishing Co.: Tokyo, 2000; pp93-122.
42. Wnorowski, A.; Yaylayan, V.A. *J. Agric. Food Chem.* **2000**, 48, 3549-3554.
43. Tsuchiya, H.; Sato, M.; Watanabe, I. *J. Agric. Food Chem.* **1999**, 47, 4167-4174.
44. Herraiz, T. *J. Agric. Food Chem.* **1996**, 44, 3057-3065.
45. Arutselvan, N.; Gopalan, S.; Kulkarni, V. G.; Balakrishna, K. *Arzneim.-Forsch./Drug Res.* **1999**, 49, 729-731.
46. McKenna, D. J.; Towers, G. H. N. *J. Psychoact. Drugs* **1984**, 16, 347-358.
47. Rommelspacher, H.; May, T.; Salewski, B. *Eur. J. Pharmacol.* **1994**, 252, 51-59.

Chapter 23

Liquid Chromatography–Mass Spectrometry Method for Fructosylarginine, an Antioxidant in the Aged Garlic Extract

Kenjiro Ryu[1,2], Nagatoshi Ide[2], Makoto Ichikawa[2], Kozue Ogasawara[2], and Robert T. Rosen[1]

[1]Center for Advanced Food Technology, Cook College, Rutgers, The State University of New Jersey, New Brunswick, NJ 08901–8020
[2] Healthcare Research Institute, Wakunaga Pharmaceutical Company, Ltd., 1624, Shimokotachi, Koda-cho, Takata-gun, Hiroshima 739–1195, Japan

A liquid chromatography-mass spectrometry (LC/MS) method for fructosylarginine (Fru-Arg) has been developed. Fru-Arg is an antioxidant isolated from aged garlic extract. Fru-Arg is less stable in basic conditions than in acidic or neutral conditions. The half-life of Fru-Arg was 2.6 and 20.5 hours at pH 12.8 and 11.0 respectively. No degradation was observed in a phosphate buffer of pH 4.0 or less within 24 hours. LC/MS method was developed for the direct determination of Fru-Arg in aged garlic extract using an amino column. The results were obtained by the LC/MS method without pre-treatment or extraction of the sample. This new method was demonstrated to be quite useful because of its high sensitivity and speed of analysis. A kinetic study was performed to study the decomposition of Fru-Arg at various pH.

Maillard reaction products in food are very important not only as the factors for flavor and color but also beneficial constituents for our health. The Maillard reaction is the reaction between amino (e.g. amino acids, peptides and proteins) and carbonyl compounds (e.g. sugars, acids and aldehydes). Since the discovery of the Maillard reaction, much research has been directed to reveal the whole sequence of this complicated reaction (*1,2*). Some researchers have also been attempting to understand the biological effects of these compounds including toxicity, digestibility and beneficial effects (*1,3*). It has been reported some Maillard reaction products have antimutagenic, antioxidant, antibiotic and anti-allergenic effects (*2*).

Fructosylarginine (*N*-α-(1-deoxy-D-fructos-1-yl)-L-arginine, Fru-Arg, chemical structure shown in Figure 1), is an Amadori compound which is the key intermediate in the Maillard reaction (*4*). Fru-Arg was previously isolated from aged garlic extract (AGE) in the course of searching for antioxidant constituents (*5*). Fru-Arg has a strong hydrogen peroxide scavenging activity and prevention effect against oxidized LDL-induced damage on endothelial cells. (*6*). It has been shown that Fru-Arg in AGE is generated by the Maillard reaction between arginine and glucose and increases during the aging process (*5*). Fru-Arg is also reported to be contained in red ginseng and to suppress the noradrenalin-induced hypertension in *in vivo* study (*7,8*).

In this study, to examine the chemical character of Fru-Arg, we studied its kinetic properties at various pH. This kinetic study showed this compound was labile under basic conditions.

Also, a liquid chromatography-mass spectrometry (LC/MS) method for Fru-Arg was developed. LC/MS is very useful analytical method especially in the biomedical and biochemical area because of its sensitivity and selectivity (*9*). Vinale et al reported the quantification method for the Amadori compound, fructosyllysine (*10*), however this is the first report concerning a LC/MS method for Fru-Arg.

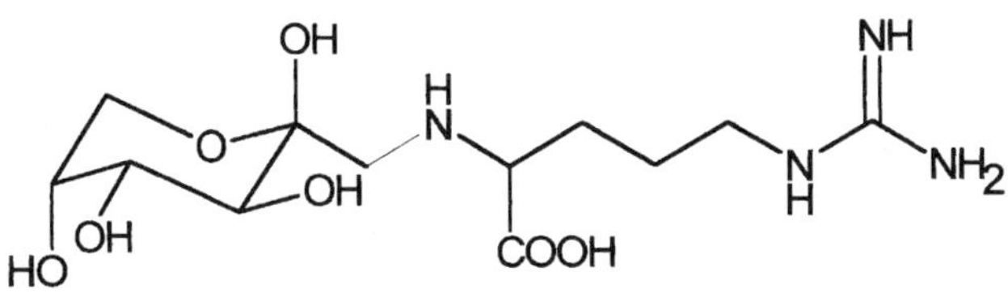

Figure 1. Chemical structure of fructosylarginine.

Materials

Acetonitrile and water solvents were HPLC grade and were obtained from Fisher (Pittsburgh, PA). Acetic acid (glacial), ammonium acetate, ammonium hydroxide and ethanol were purchased from Fisher (Pittsburgh, PA). Arginine, dipotassium phosphate, disodium phosphate, Dowex 50Wx8, glucose, glucose-$^{13}C_6$, monopotassium phosphate, monosodium phosphate, 2,3,5-triphenyl-2H-tetrazolium chloride and trisodium phosphate were purchased from Sigma-Aldrich (Milwaukee, WI). Aged garlic extracts were supplied by Wakunaga Pharmaceutical Co., Ltd. (Osaka, Japan). The detail description about the aged garlic extract has been published in the U.S. Pharmacopoeia as garlic fluidextract made by soaking sliced garlic in aqueous alcohol for a length of time sufficient to extract the constituents (*11*).

Methods

Synthesis and Purification

Fru-Arg was synthesized by the modified method previously reported (*7*). Arginine 8.7 g (50 mmol) and glucose 18 g (100 mmol) were added into glacial acetic acid 20 mL. The mixture were stirred and heated at 50 °C for 3 hours. After the reaction, the mixture was subjected to ion-exchange column chromatography Dowex50Wx8 in NH_4^+ form (Sigma-Aldrich, Milwaukee, WI). After flushing with 1 L of deionized water, crude Fru-Arg was eluted with 1 L of 0.2 M ammonium hydroxide. Crude Fru-Arg was refined using column chromatography with cellulose microcrystalline (Merck, Darmstadt, Germany) followed by Cosmosil 140C18-OPN (Nacalai Tesque, Tokyo, Japan). The purity of the refined Fru-Arg was more than 95% as determined by HPLC using UV detection at 195 nm. Confirmation of purity was obtained using ^1H and ^{13}C NMR. Fru-Arg-$^{13}C_6$, the internal standard, was synthesized in the same way as described above using glucose-$^{13}C_6$ (> 99 atom % ^{13}C).

Kinetic Study

0.2 M phosphate buffers in various pH were prepared by mixing 0.2 M monosodium phosphate, disodium phosphate and trisodium phosphate solution using a pH meter. The pH values of the phosphate buffer used were 2.1, 4.0,

6.0, 7.0, 7.4, 8.0, 9.0, 11.0, and 12.8. Fru-Arg was dissolved in 0.2 M phosphate buffer at pH 7.4 to make a 10.1 mg/mL solution. A 10 mL of aliquot of 0.2 M phosphate buffer was pre-incubated for 10 min at 37 °C. The experiments were performed at 37 °C and initiated by adding 100 μL of the Fru-Arg solution. A portion of 100 μL was taken from the reaction solution after 0, 1, 2, 4, 6, 8, 12, and 24 hours. The solution was added to 400 μL of the potassium-phosphate buffer (K_2HPO_4 17.7 g + KH_2PO_4 12.2 g/L in water, which was diluted and used as mobile phase in following HPLC analysis) which was ice-colded. The sample solutions were stored in the deep freezer (-85 °C) until analyzed. The pH value of these buffer solutions was checked before and after the reaction, and remained unchanged up to 24 hour. The HPLC analysis was performed with the same conditions as below. Detection was at 195 nm and there were no interfering peaks or components.

HPLC Analysis

HPLC method was previously reported (*5*). Two mL of AGE was applied into an ion exchange column containing 4 mL of Dowex 50Wx8 (NH_4^+ form) resin. After washing with 40 mL of water, the sample solution was eluted with 0.2 M ammonium hydroxide (20 mL). The effluent was appropriately diluted with 0.2 M ammonium hydroxide, if necessary. The HPLC system was a LC10VP (Shimadzu, Kyoto, Japan) with reaction coil heater: CRB-6A (Shimadzu, Kyoto, Japan). HPLC conditions were as follows, column: Shodex Asahipak NH2P-50 4E (Showa Denko K.K., Tokyo, Japan); mobile phase: acetonitrile-10 mM potassium-phosphate buffer (pH 6.7) (31:19, v/v), 1.0 mL/min; reaction solution: 2,3,5-triphenyl-2H-tetrazolium chloride 2.0 g/L in 100 mM sodium hydroxide-ethanol (1:1, v/v), 0.2 mL/min; reaction coil: 95 °C, 0.5 mm i.d. x 5 m; detection: absorbance at 480 nm; injection volume: 10 μL; column temperature: ambient.

LC/MS Analysis

One hundred μL of AGE was added into 400 μL of internal standard solution (Fru-Arg-$^{13}C_6$ approx. 100 μg/mL in 70 % ethanol). After shaking for 30 sec, the mixture was centrifuged at 14,000 rpm for 15 min. The supernatant was directly injected into the LC/MS. LC/MS conditions were as follows. The HPLC system was a Varian 9012 (Varian, Sugar Land, TX) and the mass spectrometer a VG Platform II (Micromass, Beverly, MA). Ionization mode: ESI positive (selected ion monitoring at *m/z* 337 for Fru-Arg and 343 for ^{13}C-labeled internal standard), source temperature: 135 °C, cone voltage: 25 V, column: Shodex Asahipak NH2P-50 2D (Showa Denko K.K., Tokyo, Japan); mobile phase: acetonitrile-50 mM ammonium acetate (75:25), flow rate: 0.2 mL/min; injection volume: 5 μL; column temperature: ambient. The column was rinsed with acetonitrile-50 mM ammonium acetate (40:60) after each analysis. The confirmation of identify was carried out at 50 V cone voltage. The *m/z* 112, 158 and 175 fragment ions were observed at a ratio to the protonated molecular ion (*m/z* 337) 56 %, 17 % and 29 % respectively.

Results and Discussion

Kinetic Study

The relationships between the time and the remaining Fru-Arg at the various pH values were plotted on the logarithmic graph. Each plot was linear. Figure 2 shows the results at pH 11.0 and 12.8. No degradation was observed at pH 4.0 or less. Half-life of Fru-Arg was more than 24 hours at pH 9.0 or less. These results indicated that the degradation reaction of Fru-Arg within the range of pH 6.0 to 12.8 followed pseudo-first order kinetics. Each straight slope drawn in figure 2 allows to calculate the apparent first-order rate constants, k_{obs}, at various pH. The relationship between k_{obs} and pH values is plotted in Figure 3. Obviously Fru-Arg is more labile in basic conditions than in neutral and acidic conditions. As a degradation product, arginine was detected by HPLC (data not shown). This indicated that beta-elimination occurred in the decomposition process. In basic condition, Amadori compounds preferentially undergo 2,3-enolizations rather than 1,2-enolizations (*4*). Thus, Fru-Arg might decompose into arginine and 1-deoxyglucosone via 2,3-enolization.

LC/MS Method

The LC conditions were confirmed based on a HPLC method reported previously (*5*). By replacing the modifier in mobile phase into with a volatile salt, the method became amenable for use in a mass spectrometer. Chromatograms of the aged garlic extract and Fru-Arg standard are shown in Figure 4. Due to the high selectivity of the mass spectrometer, any special preparation or purification of injected sample solutions was not necessary. Internal isotopically labeled standardization allowed not only the linear

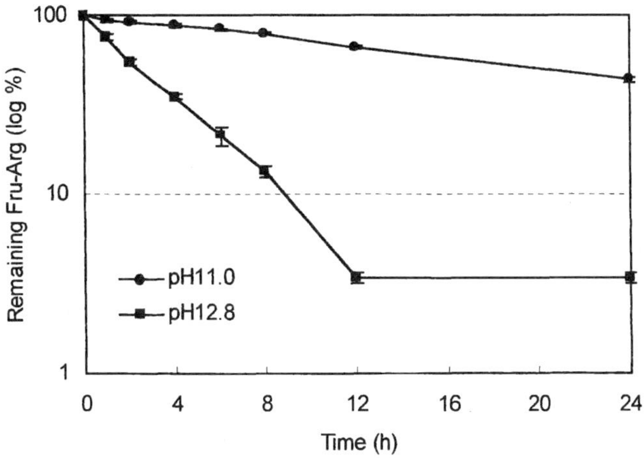

Figure 2. First-order plots for the degradation of Fru-Arg in pH 11.0 and 12.8. Each data represents the mean of triplicate studies with standard deviation.

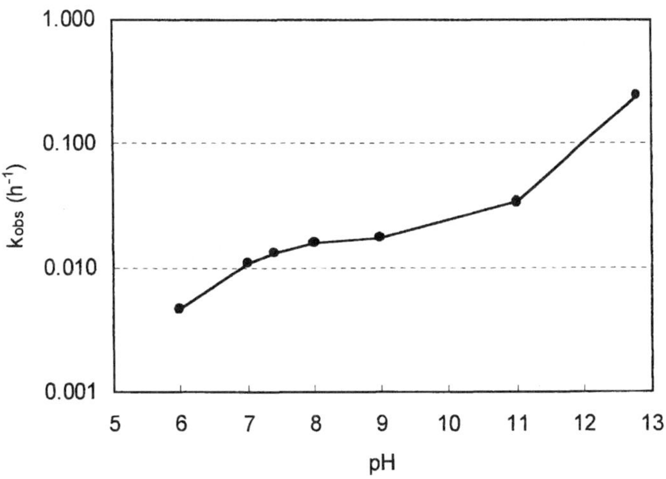

Figure 3. Rate-pH profile for the degradation of Fru-Arg in 0.2 M phosphate buffer solution at 37 °C.

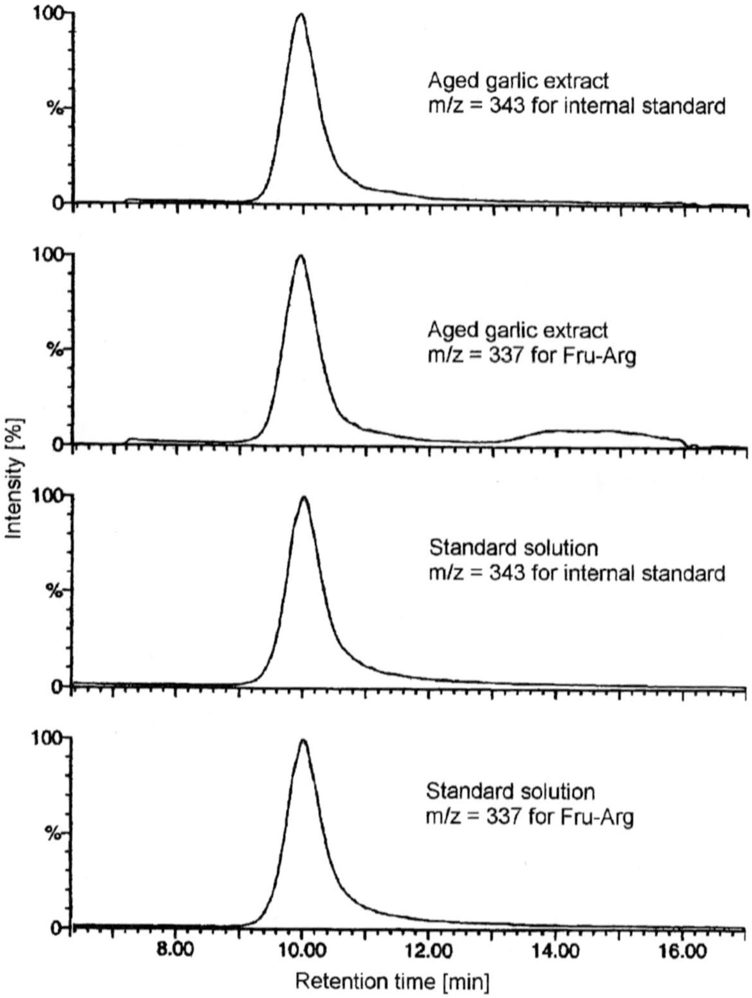

Figure 4. Typical chromatogram of the aged garlic extract (upper two plots) and Fru-Arg standard (bottom two plots).

response with the range 0.24 to 2.55 mM but also the reliable data that is not affected by ionization efficiency.

The change of Fru-Arg concentration in the garlic extract during aging process was determined by a new LC/MS method as well as HPLC method. These results corresponded with each other. Figure 5 shows the result by new LC/MS method. It tended to be slightly higher than the result from HPLC. This tendency suggests that the sample preparation with basic condition for HPLC method might cause some loss of Fru-Arg. As reported before, the concentration of Fru-Arg in garlic extracts increased during aging process. In this study it was demonstrated that the concentration of Fru-Arg remained increasing until 34 months and it seemed to reach the plateau.

The coefficient of variation for aged garlic extracts was 2.6 (n=7). The quantification limit has been set at 0.24 mM because the calibration curve lost its linearity at less than this concentration.

Conclusion

A kinetic study of Fru-Arg showed that this compound was less stable in basic conditions than neutral or acidic conditions. In phosphate buffer, half-life of Fru-Arg at pH 12.8 and 11.0 was 2.6 and 20.5 hours respectively. However Fru-Arg was rather stable in neutral and acidic condition. There was no degradation observed at pH 4.0 or less.

Using LC/MS, a quantitative method for Fru-Arg was developed. The results by LC/MS were quite similar with the results by HPLC method. This new LC/MS method does not require any special pre-treatment for injected sample and allowed high sensitive and less time-consuming quantification.

Acknowledgements

We acknowledge Dr. Chi-Tang Ho, (Rutgers University) for his helpful suggestions and advice. The authors also would like to thank Dr. Elaine Fukuda and Mr. Joseph Lech (Rutgers University) for their technical support.

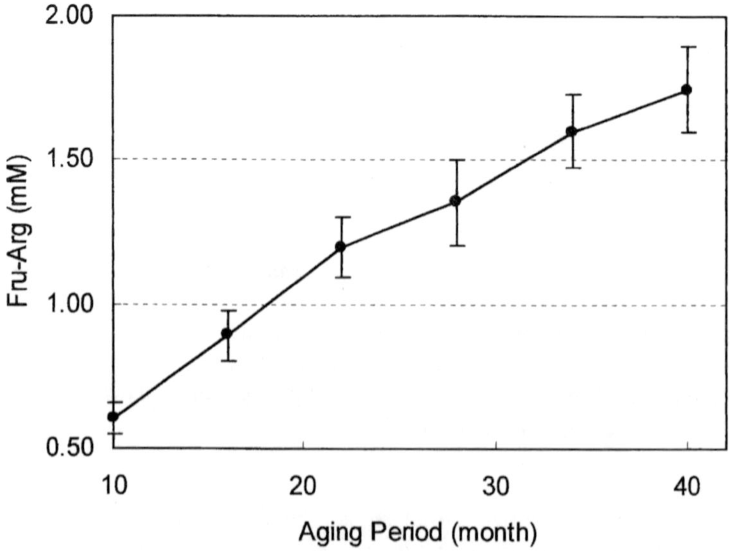

Figure 5. Change of Fru-Arg concentration in garlic extract during aging process determined by LC/MS. Each value represents the mean of triplicate studies. These data were corrected by adjusting the solid extract content 28 %. Fru-Arg concentration was less than quantification limit (0.24 mM) in 1,2 and 4 months old extracts.

References

1. Namiki, M. *Adv. Food Res.* **1988**, *32*, 115-184.
2. O'Brien, J.; Morrissey, P.A. *Crit. Rev. Food Sci. Nutr.* **1989**, *28*, 211-248.
3. Friedman, M. *J. Agric. Food Chem.* **1996**, *44*, 631-653.
4. Yaylayan, V.A.; Huyghues-Despointes, A. *Crit. Rev. Food Sci. Nutr.* **1994**, *34*, 321-369.
5. Ryu, K; Ide, N; Matsuura, H.; Itakura, Y. *J. Nutr.* **2001**, *131*, 972S-976S.
6. Ide N.; Lau B.H.S.; Ryu, K.; Matsuura, H.; Itakura, Y. *J. Nutr. Biochem.* **1999**, *10*, 372-376.

7. Matsuura, Y.; Zheng, Y.; Takaku, T.; Kameda, K.; Okuda, H. *J. Trad. Med.* **1994**, *11*: 256-263.
8. Kitao, T.; Kon, K.; Nojima, K.; Takaku, T.; Maeda, N.; Okuda, H. *J. Trad. Med.* **1995**, *12*: 294-295.
9. Gelpí E. *J. Chormatogr. A.* **1995**, *703*, 59-80.
10. Vinale, F.; Fogliano, V.; Schieberle, P.; Hofmann, T. *J. Agric. Food Chem.* **1999**, *47*, 5084-5092.
11. USP 24-NF19 supplement 3, pp 3135.

Chapter 24

Antioxidant Activity of Electrolized Sodium Chloride

Inhibitory Effect of Cathodic Solution Produced by the Electrolysis of a Dilute NaCl Solution on the Oxidation of Lipids and Lipid Related Compounds

Kazuo Miyashita, Eiichi Nara, Hiroaki Kubouchi, and Tetsuya Suzuki

Graduate School of Fisheries Sciences, Hokkaido University, Hakodate 041–8611, Japan

The cathodic solution prepared by the electrolysis of an NaCl solution showed a strong antioxidant activity on the aqueous oxidation of polyunsaturated fatty acid esters, squalene, vitamin A and β-carotene. Although the mechanism for the antioxidant effect of the cathodic solution has not been fully elucidated, the effect would be partly due to radical scavenging ability and/or alkaline molecules formed in the cathodic solution. On the other hand, the antioxidant activity of the cathodic solution has not been found on phosphatidylcholine, free fatty acids and α-tocopherol. The different effect of the cathodic solution on the oxidation of polar lipids may be correlated with the ionization of these lipids in the cathodic solution.

Oxidative deterioration of unsaturated lipids is one of the most important problems in the field of food chemistry, because lipid oxidation products not only cause undesirable flavors but also decrease the nutritional quality and safety of lipid-containing foods. In the course of investigation on the dietary effects of n-3 and n-6 polyunsaturated fatty acids, lipid peroxidation has also received considerable attention because of its possible contribution to the potential damage of biological systems. Therefore, inhibition of free radical autoxidation by antioxidants is of considerable practical importance in preserving polyunsaturated lipids from oxidative deterioration.

The solution produced in the cathodic compartment by electrolyzing a dilute solution of NaCl exhibits low dissolved oxygen and high dissolved hydrogen (*1*). These properties of the cathodic solution suggest that it is potentially useful for preventing the oxidation of polyunsaturated lipids and their related compounds in an aqueous systems. Furthermore, this solution is reported to have superoxide dismutase-like and catalase-like activities (*1*). However, this data has not yet been confirmed.

Lipid oxidation has been extensively studied in bulk fats and oils, and there is a fairly good understanding of the mechanisms and factors that affect oxidation in such systems (*2,3*). On the other hand, lipid oxidation is still not well understood in systems in which the fat is dispersed in an aqueous solution, although a large number of foods exist partially or entirely in the form of emulsion. Food emulsions are complex multicomponent heterogeneous systems, in which different molecular species interact with each other. Lipid oxidation in such systems is an interfacial phenomenon that is greatly influenced by the nature of the interface, dispersed components and water. However, understanding of the factors that affect lipid oxidation in an aqueous system is still fairly poor, and effective inhibition of oxidation in such systems is required (*3*). From this point of view, the inhibitory effect of the cathodic solution toward the oxidation of lipids in an aqueous system is very interesting and important subject for research.

In this chapter, the characteristic effect of the cathodic solution on the oxidation of some lipids in an aqueous system is described.

Ethyl Esters and Acylglycerols

When ethyl linoleate (1.0 mM) was oxidized in distilled water, NaCl solution and cathodic solution under the presence of $FeSO_4$ (1.0 mM) and ascorbic acid (20.0 mM), it was easily oxidized in distilled water and in the NaCl solution with about a 60% loss of the substrate after only 24 h of oxidation (Figure 1, (A)). On the other hand, in the cathodic solution, it was very stable to oxidation, more than 90% of the substrate remaining unchanged after more than 100 h of oxidation (*4*). The antioxidative activity of the cathodic solution toward ethyl linoleate oxidation was also confirmed by measuring the increase in total

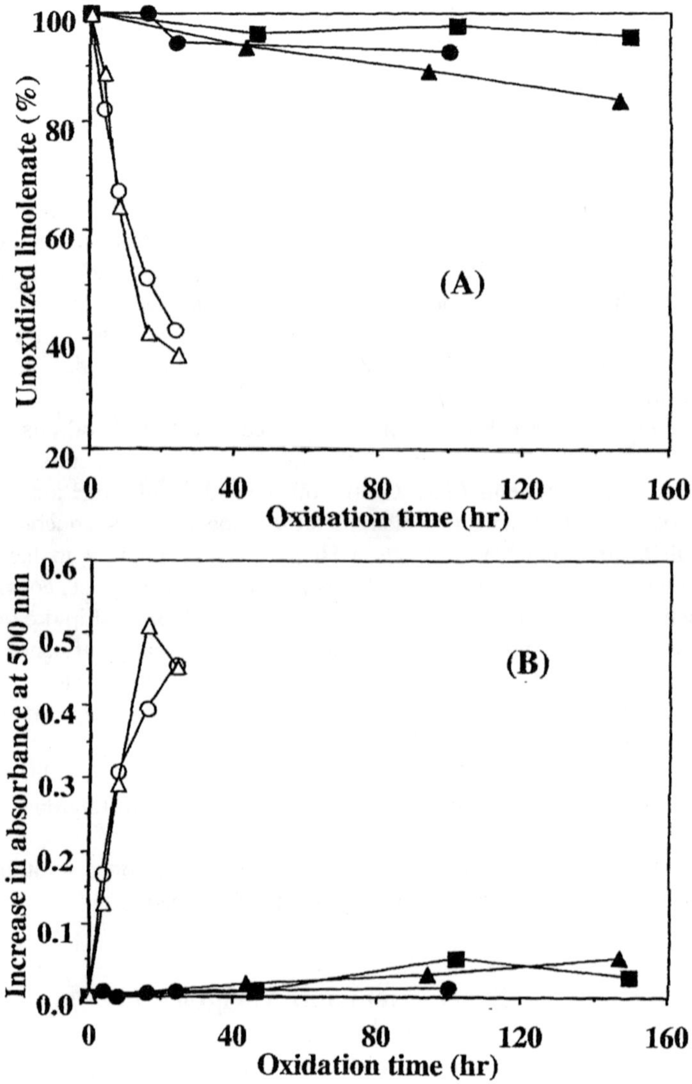

Figure 1. Oxidative stability of ethyl linoleate in an aqueous micelles. (A) Decrease in unoxidized linoleate. (B) Formation of peroxides.

(Reproduced with permission from reference 4. Copyright 1999 Japan Society for Bioscience, Biotechnology, and Agrochemistry.)

peroxides (*Figure 1*, (B)). The strong inhibiting effect of the cathodic solution on lipid oxidation was also apparent with the aqueous oxidation of ethyl docosahexaenoate (*4*).

Ethyl or methyl esters of polyunsaturated fatty acids are good models for lipid oxidation, however, fatty acids occur usually as esters of triacylglycerols, which are the main constituents of vegetable oils and food lipids. It is, therefore, necessary to evaluate the antioxidant activity of the cathodic solution on triacylglycerols. *Figure 2* shows the changes in the peroxide values of lipids extracted into chloroform/methanol from two kinds of soybean oil emulsions. Both emulsions were prepared by dispersing soybean oil triacylglycerols (10 wt%) with Triton X-100 (1 wt%) as an emulsifier in NaCl and cathodic solutions and the oxidation was induced by the addition of 1.0 mM of 2,2'-azobis (2-amidinopropane) dihydrochloride (AAPH). As shown in Figure 2, the increase in the peroxide value of soybean oil dispersed in the cathodic solution was lower than that in the NaCl solution, thus reflecting the antioixdant effect of the cathodic solution on soybean oil triacylglycerol in emulsion.

The antioxidant activity of the cathodic solution was also observed in the aqueous oxidations of three kinds of linoleoyl acylglycerols (*Figure 3*) (*5*). The oxidation of these acylglycerols was induced with AAPH (1.0 mM) and the stability was compared by measuring the decrease in the unoxidized linoleate during oxidation. Every acylglycerol showed higher oxidative stability in the cathodic solution than in the NaCl solution, but the effect of the cathodic solution was different for each of acylglycerol. When these acylglycerols were oxidized in the cathodic solution, trilinolein was most stable, followed by 1,3-dilinolein and 1-monolinolein, respectively, despite the equal mole concentrations of linoleate in these acylglycerols (2 mM). On the other hand, when each acylglycerol was dispersed in the NaCl solution, the difference in the oxidative stability among three kinds of acylglycerols was minor. The different antioxidant action of the cathodic solution on each acylglycerol was also confirmed by measuring the consumption of the dissolved oxygen concentration (*5*). This result suggests that the antioxidant effect of the cathodic solution on linoleoyl acylglycerol decreases with the increasing number of OH groups in acylglycerols. Because the OH groups in dilinolein and monolinolein were thought to ionize in the alkaline cathodic solution, it may be difficult for the cathodic solution to have an antioxidative effect on the ionized lipid molecule.

Squalene, Vitamin A and β-Carotene

Squalene is mainly distributed in the human skin surface (*6*) and has been thought to provide moisture and smoothness to skin. Squalene is also an efficient quencher of singlet oxygen and protects the lipids in the human skin surface (*7*).

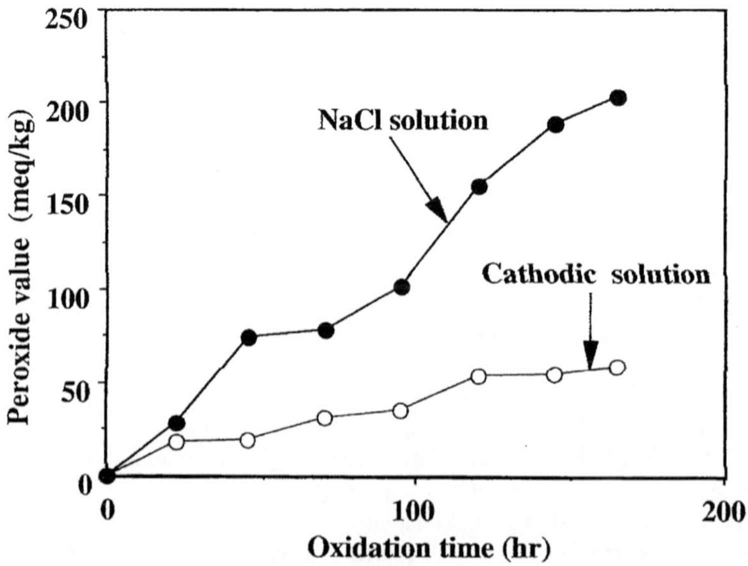

Figure 2. Oxidative stability of soybean oil triacylglycerol in an emulsion.

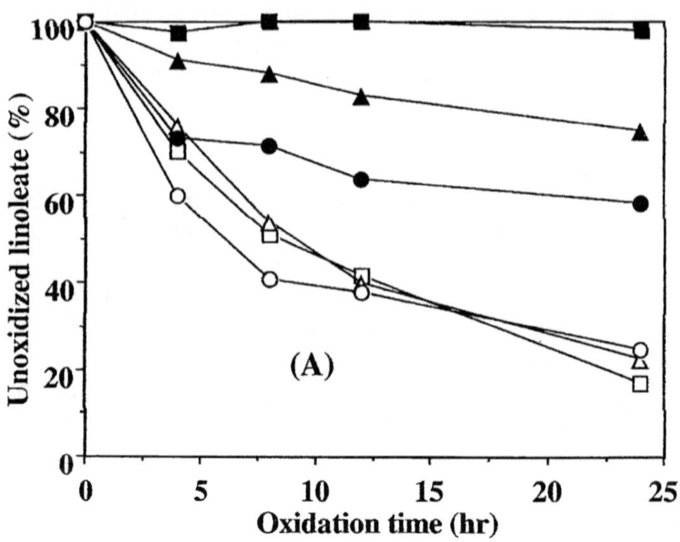

Figure 3. Oxidative stability of 1-monolinolein (circle), 1,3-dilinolein (triangle) and trilinolein (square) in the NaCl solution (open) and in the cathodic solution (solid).

(Reproduced with permission from reference 8. Copyright 2001 Japan Oil Chemist's Society.)

These physiological properties of squalene have encouraged its use in cosmetics and other products, but squalene is susceptible to oxidation because of its high degree of unsaturation. It is, therefore, necessary to develop an effective method for stabilizing this functional compound and the cathodic solution is potencially useful for this purpose.

Figure 4 shows the effectiveness of the cathodic solution in protection of squalene (*8*). When the oxidation of squalene dispersed in the cathodic and NaCl solutions was induced by 1.0 mM of AAPH (*Figure 4*, (A) and (B)), the rate of formation of total peroxides in the NaCI solution was much higher than that in the cathodic solution (Figure 4, (A)). The same result for the antioxidant effect of the cathodic solution was obtained by analyzing the decrease in the unoxidized squalene upon oxidation (Figure 4, (B)). The cathodic solution also inhibited the aqueous oxidation of squalene induced by 5.0 mM 2,2'-azobis (2,4-dimethyl-valeronitrile) (AMVN) (Figure 4, (C) and (D)), but the effect of the cathodic solution on AMVN-induced oxidation was weaker than that on AAPH-induced oxidation.

The cathodic solution exerted a radical scavenging effect on aqueous 1,1-diphenyl-2-picrylhydrazyl (DPPH) radical (*4*), so that the antioxidant effect of the cathodic solution on AAPH-induced oxidation would be in part due to the trapping of aqueous AAPH radicals by the cathodic solution. The radical scavenging effect of the cathodic solution may be derived from the reduction in activity caused by dissolved hydrogen formed just after preparation. The cathodic solution also had an inhibitory effect on AMVN-induced oxidation, although this effect was weaker than that on AAPH-induced oxidation (*Figure 4*). AMVN is a fat-soluble radical initiator and induces the oxidation of lipids in emulsion from the lipid droplet interior, but it was reported that AMVN also induced oxidation from the interface of water and the lipid phase (*9*). Therefore, the antioxidant action of the cathodic solution on AMVN-induced oxidation would be derived from its scavenging effect on the AMVN radical at the interface.

The strong antioxidant action of the cathodic solution on vitamin A palmitate and β-carotene (*8*), composed of isoprene units similar to that in squalene was also evident. Vitamin A has a regulation effect on cellular growth, differentiation (*10*), cell death (*11*) and induction of epidermal thickening in skin (*12*). β-Carotene is well known as not only a provitamin A, but also one of the dietary carotenoids with free radical scavenging effect (*13*), singlet oxygen quenching effect (*14*) and preventionof various types of cancer (*15-17*). Therefore, the cathodic solution may also stabilize physiologically active compounds in cosmetics, pharmaceuticals and functional foods.

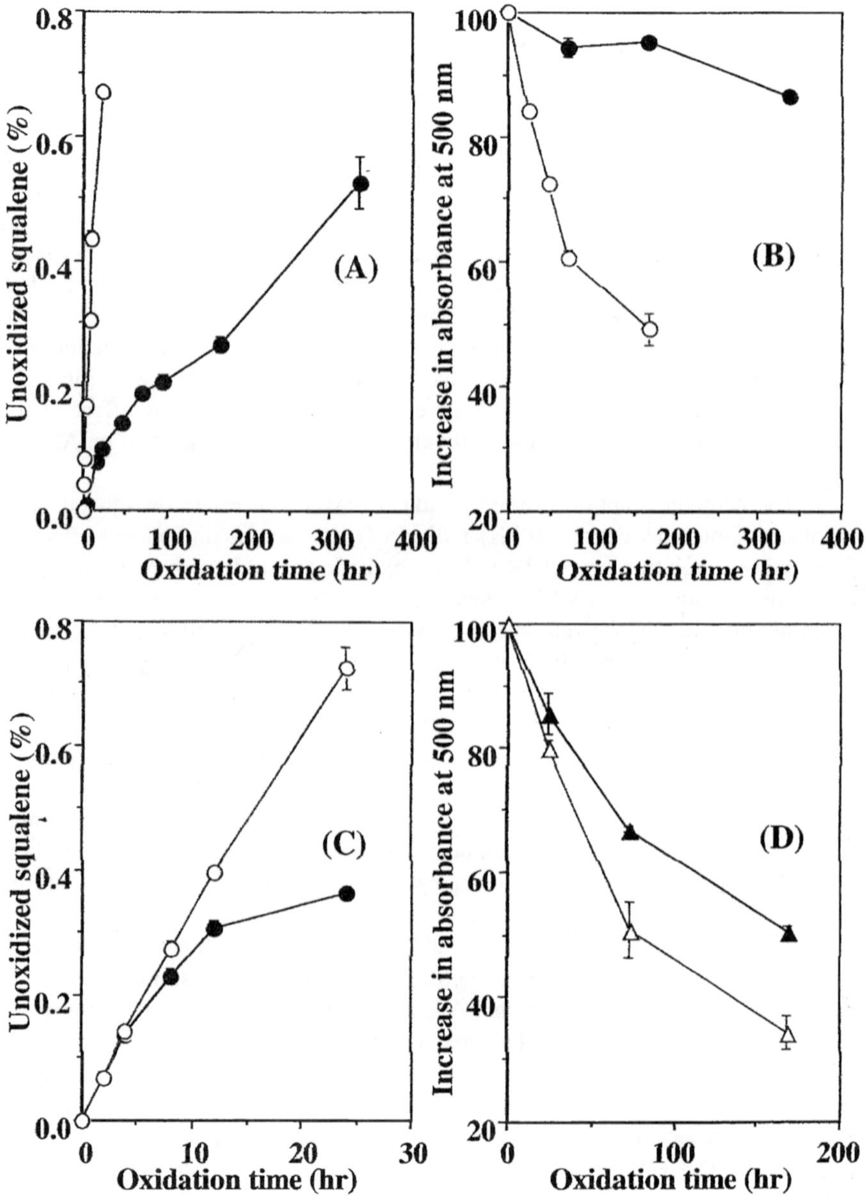

Figure 4. Oxidative stability of squalene in an emulsion under the presence of AAPH (A and B) or AMVN (C and D) as radical inducer. (A and C) Formation of peroxides. (B and D) Decrease in unoxidized squalene.

Antioxidant Effect of Cathodic Solution

The antioxidant activity of the cathodic solution may also arise from its low dissolved oxygen level. The cathodic solution just after electrolysis showed less than 4 mg/l of dissolved oxygen, but this value immediately increased to almost the same level as that found in distilled water after dispersing lipid in the cathodic solution (*4*). Therefore, it is apparent that the low dissolved oxygen level in the cathodic solution just after electrolysis did not contribute to the antioxidative activity of the cathodic solution.

Lipid peroxidation proceeds via a free radical chain reaction consisting of initiation, propagation and termination steps. The key event in initiation is the formation of a lipid radical. This can occur by abstraction of a hydrogen radical from the substrate lipid. The hydrogen abstraction is induced by the active oxygen or free radicals such as those generated from AAPH and AMVN. The resulting lipid free radicals react with oxygen to form peroxy radicals. In the propagation steps, peroxy radicals react with more substrate lipids to form lipid hydroperoxides. The most important mechanism for antioxidation is to break this chain reaction by reacting with free radicals to form nonradical products. Therefore, the most important factor responsible for the antioxidant activity of the cathodic solution is its scavenging ability toward free radicals, which could be expected from the high level of dissolved hydrogen with reducing potential in the cathodic solution.

Indeed, the cathodic solution just after electrolysis showed a high scavenging effect, but this effect disappered upon exposure to air (*4*). The decrease in the scavenging effect of the cathodic solution during incubation may have been due to the instability of hydrogen in an aqueous solution. To elucidate the relationship between the scavenging effect of the cathodic solution and its strong antioxidative property, the oxidative stability of ethyl docosahexaenoate (ethyl DHA) in the cathodic solution just after electrolysis was compared with that in the cathodic solution that had been incubated for 7 days (*Figure 5*). Although the scavenging effect of the cathodic solution on DPPH radicals disappeared after incubation, no significant difference in the antioxidant activity was apparent between the cathodic solution just after electrolysis and after incubation for 7 days (*4*), thus suggesting that the strong scavenging effect on free radicals found in the cathodic solution after electrolysis could not be the only reason for its strong antioxidant activity.

Antioxidant Activity of Alkaline Solution

The effects of the cathodic solution and two kinds of alkaline solutions on the oxidation of β-carotene are shown in *Figure 6*. Both cathodic solutions just

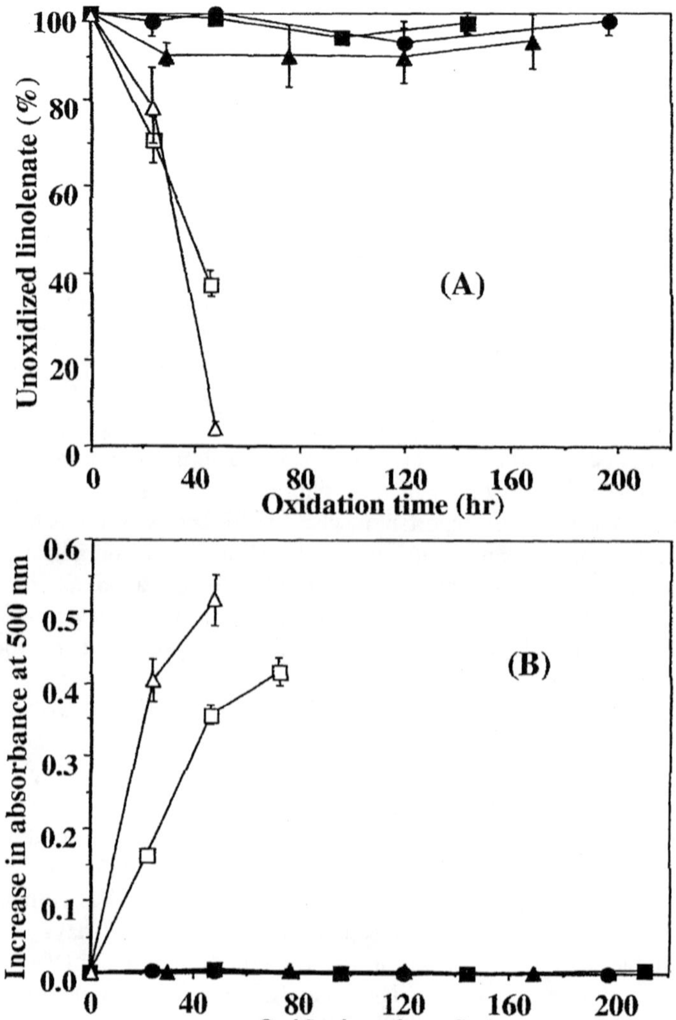

Figure 5. Oxidative stability of ethyl docosahexaenoate in super pure water (open triangle), NaCl solution (open circle),cathodic solution just after electrolysis (solid circle) and cathodic solution after incubation for 7 days (solid triangle). (A) Decrease in unoxidized linoleate. (B) Formation of peroxides.

(Reproduced with permission from reference 4. Copyright 1999 Japan Society for Bioscience, Biotechnology, and Agrochemistry.)

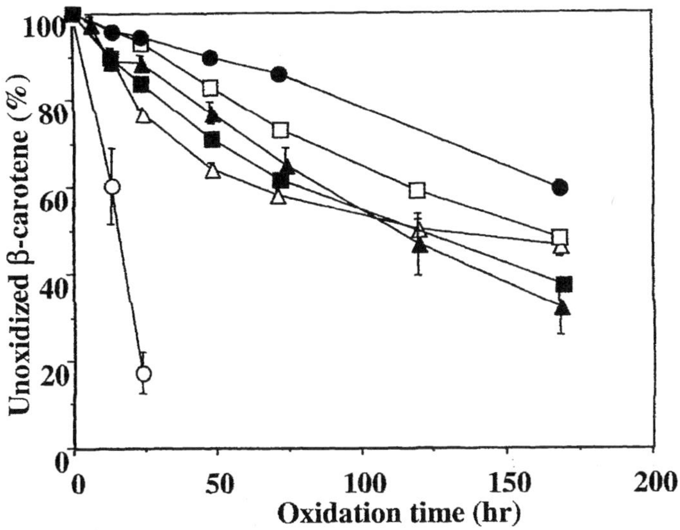

Figure 6. Oxidative stability of β-carotene in the NaCl solution (open circle), cathodic solution just after electrolysis (open square), cathodic solution after incubation for 7 days (solid square), NaOH solution just after preparation (open triangle), NaOH solution after incubation for 7days (solid triangle) and $NaHCO_3$ solution (solid circle). Reproduced from reference 8. Copyright 2001 Japan Oil Chemists' Society.

after electrolysis and after incubation for 7 days inhibited the autoxidation of β-carotene at the same level, although the radical scavenging effect of the cathodic solution was remarkably decreased by incubation for 7 days (Table I).

Table I. Analysis of pH and DPPH Radical Scavenging Effect (%) of Aqueous Solutions

Incubation time at 37°C	pH			
after preparation (h)	0	7	0	7
Super pure water	7.1	-	-	-
NaCl solution	7.0	-	0.0	-
Cathodic solution	12.1	11.0	58.3	19.4
NaOH solution	12.8	8.8	58.9	3.8
$NaHCO_3$ solution	8.3	-	0.4	-

Adapted from Reference 8.

Alkaline solutions of NaOH and $NaHCO_3$ showed the same antioxidant effetct on β-carotene as the cathodic solution (*Figure 6*). The NaOH solution just after preparation showed a strong and the same radical scavenging effect on the DPPH radical as the cathodic solution, however, the effect of NaOH solution after incubation for 7 days decreased, but remained strong (Table I). Furthermore, $NaHCO_3$ solution, which had no scavenging effect, also showed the strong antioxidant acitivity on β-carotene. These results suggest the similarity of the antioxidant activity of the cathodic solution and the alkaline solutions.

A main molecular species dissolved in the cathodic solution and in the NaOH solution is thought to be NaOH. By incubation for 7 days, a part of NaOH in the cathodic solution and in the NaOH solution would be changed to Na_2CO_3 and/or $NaHCO_3$ by absorption of CO_2 from air, suggesting the importance of an alkaline molecular species for the antioxidant action of the cathodic solution. Kajimoto et al. (18) also reported that the oxidative stability of soybean oil increased with increasing the amounts of NaOH, though the mechanism for the effect of NaOH still remains to be clarified.

Polar Lipids

In case of polar lipids, no antioxidant activity of the cathodic solution was observed. When soybean phosophatidylcholine (PC) (5.0 mM) was oxidized in aqueous monomers (dispersed with sodium deoxycholate), micelles (dispersed with Triton X-100) and liposomes in the presence of 1.0 mM AAPH (*Figure 7*), little antioxidant activity of the cathodic solution was observed in the increase in total peroxides (*Figure* 7, (A) and (B)) and the decrease in the total amount of linoleate (LA) and linolenate (LN) (*Figure* 7, (C) and (D)) (*5*). Furthermore, the analysis of the decrease in the oxygen consentration in the solution (*Figure* 7, (E) and (F)) showed the prooxidant effect of the cathodic solution. A prooxidant activity of the cathodic solution was also observed in the oxidation of linoleic acid and α-tocopherol (*5*). Linoleic acid and α-tocopherol were oxidized in both NaCl and cathodic solutions in the presence of AAPH, but the oxidation rates of linoleic acid and α-tocopherol in the cathodic solution were slightly and much higher than that in the NaCl solution, respectively.

Since these lipid molecules could be ionized in the cathodic solution, this would suggest difficulty in the antioxidant action of the cathodic solution on the ionized lipid molecule. Ingold and Puddington (*19*) reported that the rate of oxidation of lubricating oils containing carboxylic acids was increased by the presence of NaOH. They also reported that the bleaching action of NaOH must be the result of oxygen attack directed at or near conjugated double bounds with probable C-C bond cleavage (*19*).

Furthermore, it is well known that alkali acts as a catalyst for autoxidation of ascorbic acid, tocopherols and phenols (*20-24*). In these reactions, autoxidation begins from ionizing the substrate. Weissberger et al. (*20*) reported that autoxidation of ascorbic acid was dependent on the pH and the double-charged ion reacts 10^5 times faster than the single-charged ion, so that the lower oxidative stability of linoleic acid and α-tocopherol in the cathodic solution compared to the NaCl solution would be due to the ionization of these lipids and the promoting effect of alkaline species in the cathodic solution. In addition, alkaline saponification often causes destruction of tocopherols (*21,22*). In general, the alkaline saponification method containing pyrogallol is applied for the determination of tocopherols. Kawasaki (*24*) reported that oxidation of phenol was also very fast in an alkaline solution, and this oxidation involved ionization of phenol and the formation of the complex of ion and radical. Similar reactions may also occur in the oxidation of α-tocopherol in the cathodic solution.

Application of Cathodic Solution

Polyunsaturated fatty acids, such as linoleic acid, α-linolenic acid, arachidonic acid and docosahexaenoic acid have characteristic physiological activities and are essential for human health. However, when these polyunsaturated fatty acids are exposed to oxygen, they are oxidized to form complex oxidation products. Since autoxidation of unsaturated fatty acids decreases their biological availability in foods and produces offensive odors and

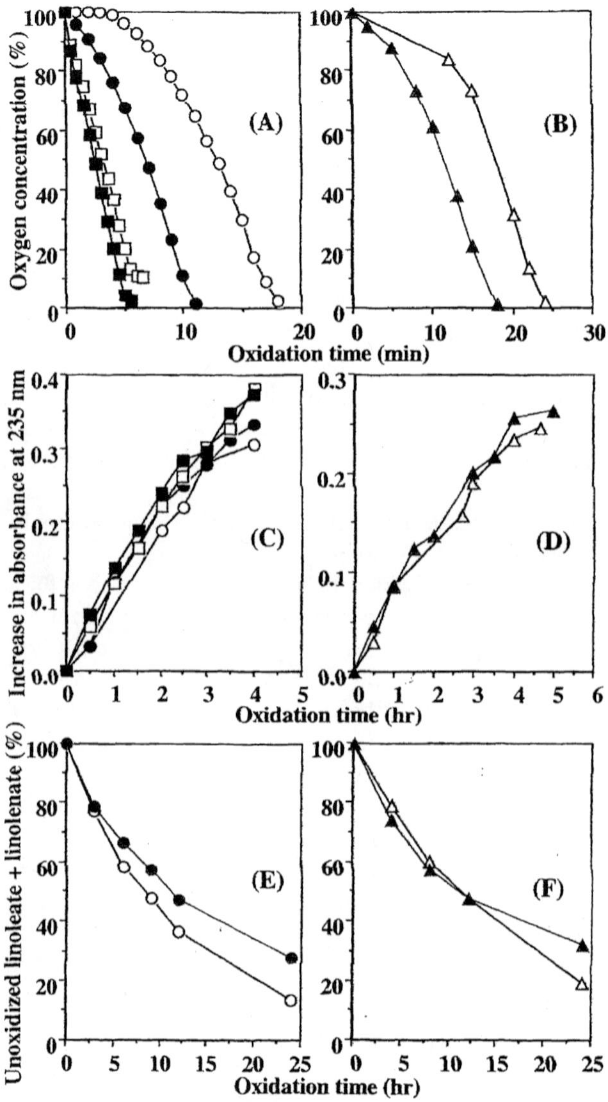

Figure 7. Oxidative stability of soybean phosphatidylcholine in the NaCl solution (open) and in the cathodic solution (solid). Soybean phosophatidylcholine was dispersed as aqueous monomers (square), micelles (circle) or liposomes (triangle). (A and B) Formation of peroxides. (C and D) Decrease in unoxidized linoleate and linolenate. (E and F) Decrease in oxygen concentration.

flavors, much work has been carried out on the effectiveness of many kinds of natural and synthetic antioxidants in various oxidation systems including bulk and aqueous systems (*25*), however, more work is required on the development of effective and new antioxidants. Cathodic solution is expected to be used as a new type of antioxidant that effectively inhibits the aqueous oxidation of lipids and lipid related compounds.

Antioxidants such as α-tocopherol, ascorbic acid and tea catechin can effectively inhibit the oxidation of vegetable oils and development of rancidity in food lipids. However, it has been difficult to protect fish oils containing eicosapentaenoic acid (EPA) and docosahexaenoic acid (DHA) against oxidative deterioration and an effective antioxidant method for fish oils is required. As shown in *Figure 5*, oxidation of ethyl DHA was completely inhibited in the cathodic solution, although it was more easily oxidized in distilled water or in the NaCl solution, therefore, the cathodic solution may be useful as an effective antioxidant for fish oils.

The antioxidant effect of the cathodic solution is due to a number of factors, namely, high hydrogen concentration, radical scavenging effect and alkaline molecules formed in the cathodic solution. However, it has not been clear how the cathodic solution inhibit the lipid peroxidation. Therefore, further investigations are required to elucidate the mechanism for the antioxidant effect of cathodic solution for the practical use of the cathodic solution to foods and other products. Furthermore, the effect of the cathodic solution is also much influenced by the lipid species, and in cases of polar lipids, the cathodic solution acts as prooxidant. This means the limitation of the antioxidant effect of the cathodic solution. More efforts should be made to study the antioxidant effect of the cathodic solution in multi-component aqueous and food emulsion systems.

References

1. Shirahata, S.; Kabayama, S.; Nakano, M.; Miura, T.; Kusumoto, K.; Gotoh, M.; Hayashi, H.; Otsubo, K.; Morisawa, S.; Katakura, Y. *Biochem. Biophys. Res. Commu.* **1997**, *234*, 269.
2. *Lipid Oxidation*; Frankel, E.N., Ed.; The Oily Press, Dundee, Scotland, 1998; p 161.
3. Coupland, J.N.; MaClements, D.J. *Trends Food Sci. & Tech.* **1996**, *7*, 83.
4. Miyashita, K.; Yasuda, M.; Ota, T.; Suzuki, T. *Biosci. Biotechnol. Biochem.* **1999**, *63*, 421.
5. Nara, E.; Kubouchi, H.; Suzuki, T.; Miyashita, K. *J. Oleo Sci.* **2001**, *50* (in press).
6. Nicolaides, N. *Science*, **1974**, *186*, 19.

7. Kohno, Y.; Egawa, Y.; Itoh, S.; Nagaoka, S.; Takahashi, M.; Mukai, K. *Biochim. Biophys. Acta.* **1995**, *1256*, 52.
8. Nara, E.; Kubouchi, H.; Kobayashi, H.; Kotake, M.; Suzuki, T.; Miyashita, K. *J. Oleo Sci.*, **2001**, *50*,575.
9. Barclay, L.R.C.; Ingold, K.U. *J. Am. Chem. Soc.*, **1981**, *103*, 6478.
10. *Cellular Biology and Biochemistry of the Retinoids*; Sporn, M.B.; Roberts, A.B.; Goodman, D.S. Eds.; Raven Press, New York, 1994; p 443.
11. Nagy, L.; Thomazy, V.A.; Shipley, G.L., Fesus, L.; Lamph, W.; Hyeman, R.A., Chandraranta, R.A.S.; Davies, P.J.A. *Mol. Cell Biol.* **1995**, *15*, 3540.
12. Kang, S.; Duell, E.A.; Fisher, G.J.; Datta, S.C.; Wang, Z.-Q., Reddy, A.P.; Tavakkol, A.; Yi, J.Y.; Griffiths, C.E.M.; Elder, J.T.; Voorkeers, J.J. *J. Invest. Dermatol.* **1995**, *105*, 549.
13. Miller, N.J.; Sampson, J.; Candeias, L.P., Bramley, P.M.; Riceevans, C.A. *FEBS Lett.*, **1996**, *384*, 240.
14. Mascio, P.D.; Kaiser, S.; Sies, H. *Arch. Biochem. Biophys.*, **1989**, *274*, 532.
15. Onogi, N.; Okuno, M.; Matsushima-Nishiwaki, R.; Fukutomi, Y.; Moriwaki, H.; Muto, Y.; Koiima, A. *Nutr. Cancer*, **1998**, *32*, 20.
16. Prakash, P.; Jackson, C.L.; Gerber, L.E. *Nutr. Cancer*, **1999**, *34*, 76.
17. Williams, A.W.; Boileau, T.W.-M.; Zhou. J.R.; Clinton, S.K.; Erdman, Jr. J.W. *J. Nutr.*, **2000**, *130*, 728.
18. Kajimoto, G.; Takashima, R.; Murakami, C. *J. Jpn. Oil Chem. Soc.*, **1998**, *47*, 591.
19. Ingold, K.U.; Puddington, I.E. *J. Institute Petroleum*, **1958**, *44*, 168.
20. Weissberger, A.; LuValle, J.E.; Thomas, Jr., D.S. *J. Am. Chem. Soc.*, **1943**, *65*, 1943.
21. Igarashi, O.; Hagino, M.; Inagaki, C. *J. Nutr. Sci. Vitaminol.*, **1973**, *19*, 469.
22. Feldheim, W.; Schulz, H.; Katerberg, R. *Z Lebensm Unters Forsch*, **1984**, *178*, 115.
23. Yohe, G.R.; Hill, D.R.; Dunbar, J.E.; Scheidt, F.M. *J. Am. Chem. Soc.*, **1953**, *75*, 2688.
24. Kawasaki, H. *J. Soc. Chem. Ind. Japan*, **1964**, *67*, 1554.
25. *Lipid Oxidation*; Frankel, E.N., Ed.; The Oily Press, Dundee, Scotland, 1998; p 129.

Chapter 25

Antioxidative Peptides in Porcine Myofibrillar Protein Hydrolysates by Protease Treatment

Ai Saiga and Toshihide Nishimura*

Faculty of Applied Biological Science, Hiroshima University, Hiroshima, Japan

Hydrolysates obtained from porcine myofibrillar proteins by protease treatment (actinase E or papain) exhibited high antioxidative activity in the linolenic acid peroxidation system induced by Fe^{2+}. Antioxidative peptides were isolated from papain hydrolysate by using ion-exchange chromatographies and HPLC. An acidic fraction obtained by chromatography exhibited the higher activity than neutral and basic fractions. Antioxidant peptides in the acidic fraction were isolated on HPLC by ODS column. They possessed the structures, DSGVT, IEAEGE, AEFAES, EELDNALN and VPSIDDQEELM. A peptide, AEFAES showed the highest activity among these peptides.

Lipid peroxidation occurring in food products causes some deterioration in food quality such as rancid flavor, bad taste and shortening of shelf life. The intake of oxidative foods is thought to cause serious diseases such as enlargement of liver (*1*) or necrosis of epithelium tissue. The factors involved in these diseases were lipidperoxidants and low-molecular compounds produced at the latter stage of oxidative reaction (*2*). Furthermore, cancer, coronary heart diseases and Alzheimer's diseases were also reported to be partially responsible for oxidation or free-radical reaction (*3*-*6*). In order to prevent foods from these deterioration and prevent us from serious diseases, it is very important to inhibit lipid peroxidation occurring in food stuffs and living body (*7*). A lipid oxidation is inhibited with antioxidant agents. Artificial antioxidants (BHA, BHT and n-propyl gallate) exhibit strong antioxidant activity toward several oxidation systems. However, as they possess a potential risk in vivo, artificial antioxidants are restricted or prohibited to use in some countries. Therefore, it is required to develop safe antioxidant in vivo occurring in natural resources. Alfa-Tocopherol (*8*), carotenoid from brightly colored vegetables, catechin in tea (*9-10*) and polyphenol compound in red wine (*11*) are well known to be very popular natural antioxidant. These natural antioxidants are almost all derived from plants and non-protein compounds. There is little information on the antioxidant derived from animal foods. Recently, some protein hydrolysates have been reported to exhibit antioxidant activity.

In present study, we investigated antioxidant activity of porcine myofibrillar protein hydrolysates obtained enzymatic treatment in the peroxidation system of linolenic aqueous induced by Fe^{2+}. Furthermore, antioxidant peptides are isolated from its hydrolysate.

Methods

Preparation of myofibrillar protein hydrolysate

Myofibrillar proteins were prepared from fresh pork according to the method reported by Yang *et al* (*12*). One percent actinase E or papain was incubated with myofibrillar proteins in distilled water (pH7.0) at 37°C for 24~48h. After incubation, ethanol was added into the reaction mixture at the final concentration of 80 % in order to stop the enzyme reaction and remove unhydrolyzed proteins. This solution was centrifuged at 2,000×g for 10min. The supernatant was concentrated by evaporation at 45°C.

Amino acid Analysis

A proteolytic hydrolysate of porcine myofibrillar proteins was hydrolyzed in 6 N HCl at 110°C for 24h. Amino acid composition of peptides in the hydrolysate was analyzed with an amino acid analyzer (Shimazu Co, Kyoto Japan).

Peroxidation System

The peroxidation system reported by Chen *et al.* (*13*) was used with a slight modification to measure antioxidative activity. Ten milligrams of linolenic acid in 4 ml of 0.1M K-phosphate buffer (pH7.0) containing 0.5% TrironX-100 (w/v) and 0.05mM $FeCl_2$ (accelerator of oxidation) were sonicated and heated in a water bath at 80°C for 60min. The antioxidant activity was estimated as the inhibition of hydroperoxides and 2-thiobarbituric acid reactive substances (TBARS) production in this peroxidation system.

Measurement of Hydroperoxides and 2-Thiobarbituric Acid Reactive Substances (TBARS)

The hydroperoxides in peroxidation system before and after heating for 60 min were measured according to the method described by Mituda (*14*). That is, 100 μl of reaction mixture were mixed with 4.5 ml of 75% ethanol, 100 μl of 30% ammonium thiocyanate, 200 μl of 0.1 N HCl, and 100 μl of 20mM ferrous chloride in 3.5% HCl. The production of hydroperoxides in this mixture was measured at 500nm.

The 2-thiobarbituric acid reactive substances (TBARS) in peroxidation system before and after heating for 60 min were also measured according to the method described by Tarladgie (*15*). That is, 0.5ml of the solution in peroxidation system was mixed with a thiobarbituric acid solution. This mixture was boiled for 10min and centrifuged at 15,000rpm for 15min. The absorbance of the supernatant at 535nm was measured. The TBARS value before heating was subtracted from that after heating.

Ion exchange column chromatography

Papain hydrolysate (1.4g) was dissolved in 0.05M ammonium acetate solution (pH6.0) and fractionated by cation-exchange chromatography on a Dowex-50W column (2×50 cm) equilibrated with same solvent. After washing unabsorbed peptides, adsorbed peptides were eluted with 0.2M ammonium acetate solution. Adsorbed fractions containing acidic or neutral peptides were concentrated, and further applied to anion-exchange column chromatography on AG1×4 column. The acidic and neutral peptides were applied to this column equilibrated with 0.05M ammonium acetate solution (pH3.5). Adsorbed fractions including acidic peptides were eluted with 1N HCl. These fractions containing acidic peptides were neutralized using 1M NaOH solution and ultrafiltrated to remove salt.

Purification of antioxidative peptides

The antioxidative peptides in the acidic fraction on ion-exchange column chromatography were purified by reversed-phase HPLC on ODS column (VP-318-1251, 4.6×25 mm, Senshu, Japan) using a liner gradient of acetnitrile (0-

30% in 100min) containing 0.1% trifluoroacetic acid at a flow rate of 1.0 mL/min. The eluted peptides were monitored at 220nm.

Mass spectrometry

The molecular masses of purified antioxidative peptides were determined with a LCQ mass spectrometer (Finnigan MAT, San Joes, CA).

Sequence analysis

Amino acid sequence of N-terminal in antioxidant peptides was analyzed with a protein sequencer G1005A (Hewlett-Packard, Palo Alto, CA).

Results and Discussion

Antioxidative activities of the hydrolysates from porcine myofibrillar protein were measured in a linolenic acid oxidation system. The hydrolysates at the concentration of 0.02, 0.2 and 2% exhibited antioxidative activities. All hydrolysates exhibited stronger antioxidative activity, as the concentration was higher in the production of hydroperoxides. On the other hand, the addition of 0.2% hydrolysate suppressed the production of TBARS most strongly, and the antioxidative activity in the addition of 2% hydrolysate was lower than that of 0.2% in the method of TBARS. It is well known that 2-thiobarbituric acid (TBA) reacts with aldehyde compounds including malondialdehyde (MDA) formed by lipid peroxidation. Two percent hydrolysates contained a lot of amino compounds including free amino acids and peptides. Therefore, the production of aldehyde compounds seems to be accelerated by amino-carbonyl reaction between hydrolysate and lipid in lipid peroxidation system including 2% hydrolysate. This might be the reason why the antioxidative activity of 2% hydrolysate was lower than that of 0.2 % hydrolysate in the method of TBARS.

Next, we tried to separate papain hydrolysate into three fractions, such as acidic, neutral and basic fractions, on ion-exchange column chromatography, and characterize the antioxidative peptides. A papain hydrolysate was applied to a cation-exchange column (Dowex 50W). Four peaks containing peptides were detected on this chromatogram. The three unabsorbed fractions including fraction I, II and III contained acidic and neutral peptides, and the adsorbed fraction, fraction IV, contained basic peptides. All four fractions exhibited antioxidative activity in lipid peroxidation system (30-90% inhibition of hydroperoxide production compared with none addition of peptide). Among all fractions, the fraction I including acidic and neutral peptides exhibited the strongest activity. There have already been many reports that peptides consisting of basic amino acid such as His and Lys possess strong antioxidative activity (*16-19*). However, there are few reports that acidic or neutral peptides possessed strong antioxidative activity.

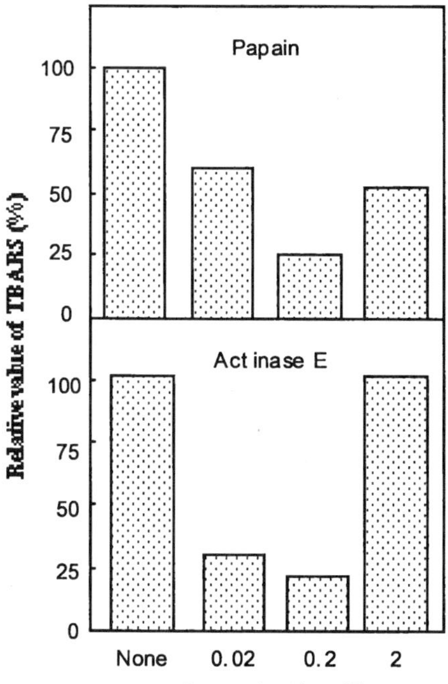

Figure 1. Effects of papain and actinase E hydrolysate concentration on antioxidant activity as shown by relative changes in the 2-thiobarbituric acid reactive substances (TBARS).

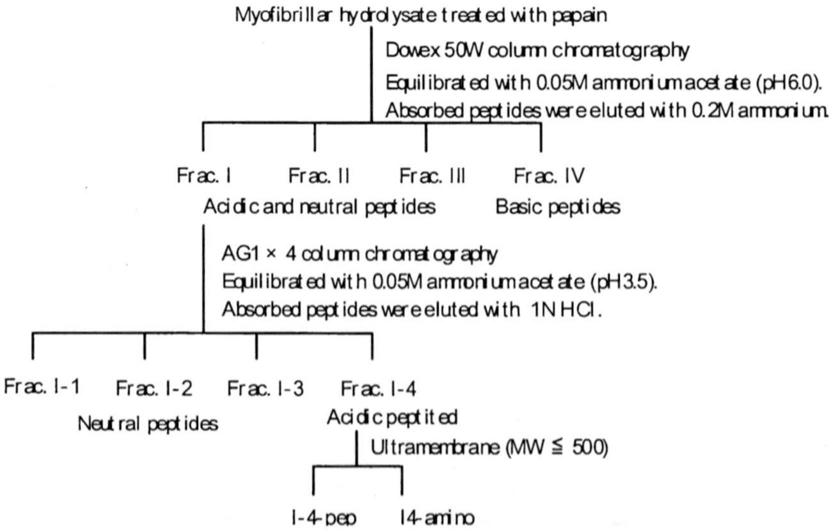

Figure 2. Separation of myofibrillar protein hydrolysate by ion-exchange column chromatography

Next, the fraction I was applied to an anion-exchange column chromatography (AG1×4). Four peaks containing peptides were also detected on this chromatogram. The three unabsorbed fraction including fraction I-1, I-2 and I-3 contained neutral peptides, and the adsorbed fraction, fraction I-4, contained acidic peptides. The yield of acidic peptides was largest among all peptide fractions. This is because major constitute amino acids in porcine myofibrillar proteins are Glu and Asp (14 and 9.5%, respectively). The fraction I-4 was neutralized and then ultrafiltrated with membrane (less than molecular weight 500) to remove salts produced in neutralization. Free amino acids were also removed from the fraction I-4 by ultrafiltration. The filtrate including free amino acids was named the fraction I-4-amino, while the residue by ultrafiltration was named the fraction I-4-peptide.

The antioxidative activity of all fractions (I-1 to I-4) was measured in lipid peroxidation system. The fraction I-4-peptide exhibited the strongest activity. The antioxidative activity of this fraction seems to be caused by the metal chelation of carboxyl group in acidic amino acids such as Glu and Asp, because this fraction contained acidic amino acids. Since carboxyl groups in acidic amino acid are charged to anion (Asp; pKa=3.86, Glu; pKa=4.25) at neutral pH, these groups might bind to metal ion. There are many reasons to suppress lipid peroxidation. A metal chelation is one of the most effective antioxidative actions, because metal irons can attack hydroperoxides directly to produce radical species from oxygen and hydroperoxides. Lipid peroxidations are propagated through this initial reaction (*20,21*). We confirmed that peptides in papain hydrolysate possessed the activity of metal chelation (Data not shown). The metal chelation of peptides in the fraction I-4-peptide seems to lead to inhibit lipid peroxidation.

Antioxidative peptides in the acidic peptide fraction (I-4-peptide) were purified on HPLC by reversed-phase column using a liner gradient (0-30% of acetonitrile including 0.1% TFA). More than 80 peaks were detected. Among them, 26 peaks exhibited antioxidant activity, eight peptides possessing strong antioxidative activity. The N-terminal amino acid sequences of these peptides were clarified and shown in Table 1. They possessed the structures, DSGVT, IEAEGE, AEFAES, EELDNALN and VPSIDDQEELM. A peptide, AEFAES showed the highest activity among these peptides. Acidic amino acids such as Asp or Glu were commonly detected in their sequences. The antioxidative activity was caused by metal chelation, especially metal binding ability of carboxyl residue in acidic amino acid.

Table 1. Sequences of antioxidant peptides

Number	*MW*	*Sequence*
No.4	650.3	Asp-Ser-Gly-Val-Thr
No.33	646.4	Ile-Glu-Ala-Glu-Gly-Glu
No.35-1	N.D	Ala-Glu-Phe-Ala-Glu-Ser
No.35-2	832.5	Asp-Ala-Gln-Glu-Lys-Leu-Glu
No.61	916.9	Glu-Glu-Leu-Asp-Asn-Ala-Leu-Asn
No.81	1275.0	Val-Pro-Ser-Ile-Asp-Asp-Gln-Glu-Glu-Leu-Met
No.82	N.D	Asp-Ser-Ala-Ile-(Asp-Leu-Gly-Asp)

N.D means Not detected.

References

1. Poling, E.; Rice, E. *J. Am. Oil Chem. Soc.* **1962**, *39*, 315.
2. Kanazawa, K.; Kanazawa, E.; Nakane, M. *Lipids* **1985**, 20, 412.
3. Ames, B.N. *Science* **1983**, *221*, 1256-1264.
4 Gey, K.F. *Biochem. Soc. Trans.* **1990**, *18,* 1041-1045.
5. Smith, A.; Perry, G.; Richey, L.; Sayre. M.; Anderson, E.; Beal, F.; Kowel, N. *Nature* **1996**, *382*,120-121.
6. Diaz, N.; Frei, B.; Vita, A.; Keaney, F. *N. Engl. J. Med.* **1997**, *337*, 408-416.
7. Halliwell, B.; Murcia, A.; Chirico, S.; Arumoma, I. *Crit. Rev. Food Sci. Nutr.* **1995**, *35*, 7-20.

8. Liebler, C.; Baker, F.; Kaysen, L. *J. Am.Chem.Soc.* **1990**, *112*, 6995-7000.
9 Amarowicz R.; Shahidi, F. *J. Food Lipids*. **1995**, *2*, 47-56.
10 Huang, W.; Frankel, E.N. *J. Agric Food Chem*. **1997**, *46*, 3033-3038.
11. Urizzi, P.; Monje, C.; Souchard, P.; Abella, A.; Chalas, J.; Lindenbaum, A.; Vergnes, L.; Labidalle. S.; Nepveu, F. *J. Chem. Phys. Chem. Biol.* **1999**, *96*, 110-115.
12. Yang, R.; Okitani, A.; Fujimaki, M. *Agric. Biol. Chem*. **1970**, *34*, 1765-1772.
13. Chen, H.; Muramoto, K.; Yamauchi, F.; Fujimoto, K.; Nokihara, K. *J. Agric. Food Chem*. **1998**, *46*, 49-53.
14. Mituda, H.; Yasumoto, K.; Iwami, K. *Eiyo to Syokuryo (JPN)* **1966**, *19*, 210-214.
15. Tarladgis, B.G.; Watts, B.M.; Younathan, M.T. **1960**, *37*, 44-48.
16. Marcuse, R. *Nature* **1960**, *186*, 886-887.
17. Marcuse, R. *J. Am. Oil Chem. Soc.* **1962**, *39*, 97-103.
18. Karel, M.; Tannenbaum, S.R.; Wallace, D.H.; Maloney, H. *J. Food Sci.* **1966**, *31*, 892-896.
19. Yanmaguchi, N.; Yokoo, Y.; Fujimaki, M. *Nippon Shokuhin Kogyo Gakkaishi* **1971**, *18*, 313-318.
20. Wills, E.D. *Biochim. Biophys. Acta*. **1965**, *98*, 238-251.
21. Yen, G.; Chen, H.; Lee, C. *J. Sci. Food Agric*. **1999**, *79*, 1213-1217.

Fruits and Vegetables

Chapter 26

Structure and Genetic Variation of Cranberry Proanthocyanidins That Inhibit Adherence of Uropathogenic P-Fimbriated *E. coli*

Nicholi Vorsa[1], Amy B. Howell[1], L. Yeap Foo[2], and Yinrong Lu[2]

[1]P. E. Marucci Center, Rutgers, The State University of New Jersey, Chatsworth, NJ 08019
[2]Industrial Research, Gracefield Research Center, P.O. Box 31–310, Lower Hutt, New Zealand

Fruit of the American cranberry (*Vaccinium macrocarpon* Ait.) has long been considered to be beneficial for urinary tract health, and many considered the mechanism of action to be the acidification of urine due to the significant levels of benzoic acid found in the fruit. More recent studies found cranberry juice to have anti-adherence bioactivity against uropathogenic P-fimbriated *E. coli.*, suggesting an alternative mechanism. Proanthocyanidins with A-type linkage were identified to be the component in cranberry fruit responsible for inhibiting adhesion of P-fimbriated *E. coli* to cellular surfaces having disaccharide α-Gal(1→4)β-Gal receptor sequences. Bioactivity was associated with proanthocyanidin polymers, mostly consisting of epicatechin units, having DP 3 to 5 with at least one A-type linkage. Both environmental and genetic variation is observed for overall proanthocyanidin levels in cranberry fruit. Fruit proanthocyanidin levels in cranberry germplasm (collection of domesticated and undomesticated varieties) varied 6-fold. Although significant environmental, e.g. year-to-year, effects are observed, heritability estimates for cranberry fruit proanthocyanidin levels are moderate (h^2 = 0.43), suggesting additive genetic variance exists, and genetic gain for enhanced proanthocyanidin levels is possible.

Introduction

The fruit of the American cranberry (*Vaccinium macrocarpon* Ait.) has been used for the amelioration of urinary tract infections for over 100 years. Women in Cape Cod were known to employ cranberry fruit for dysurea. Many physicians have routinely recommended cranberry juice consumption to patients experiencing urinary tract infections. Women are particularly susceptible to urinary tract infections. An estimated 11 million women in the United States experience a UTI, and many have chronic infections. There is considerable evidence to support the use of cranberries for the prevention of urinary tract infections (*1,2*). Bodel *et al.* (*3*) in 1959 were among the first to report the 'antibacterial action' of cranberry juice, attributing the effect to production of hippuric acid resulting in the acidification of the urine. Subsequent reports supported the use of cranberry juice for urinary tract infection (*4-6*). Reports also suggested the beneficial effect was due to the acidity (*3-7*). However, as experimental techniques improved over the years, the 'acidity theory' was disproved and replaced by a new theory of bacterial anti-adhesion

Sobota (*8*) and Schmidt and Sobota (*9*) were the first to suggest the effect of cranberry juice was due to the inhibition of adherence of uropathogenic bacteria, especially *Escherichia coli,* to uroepithelial cells. Cranberry juice was found to inhibit the adherence of two bacterial phenotypes, type 1 and type P fimbriated *Escherichia coli*, to eucaryotic cells (*10,11*). One hypothesis for the mechanism, is that cranberry juice acts by preventing bacterial adhesion, which presumably facilitates urinary flushing of the causative bacteria, preventing their colonization of the urinary tract (*12*).

Uropathogenic *E. coli* have proteinaceous fibers called fimbriae emanating from the bacterial cell wall which provide a mechanism for adherence to eucaryotic cell surfaces. Fimbriae are heteropolymeric structures composed of protein subunits with adhesins on the fimbrial termini, which have specificity for various carbohydrate receptors on uroepithelial cells (*13*). Fructose, common in most fruits including cranberry, inhibits adherence of *E. coli* phenotypes possessing type 1 or mannose-sensitive fimbrial adhesions (*10*). Another receptor type is based on the recognition of a disaccharide α-Gal (1→4) β-Gal component, and has been shown to be specific for adherence of *E. coli* with P-type (mannose-resistant) fimbriae with PapG adhesin (*14*). The α-Gal (1→4) β-Gal receptor is also found on the surface of uroepithelial cells (*15*). Recently, proanthocyanidins were isolated from cranberries by bioassay-directed fractionation, and identified as the compounds having anti-adherence activity against uropathogenic P-fimbriated *E. coli* (*16*).

As in most crop species, numerous cultivars are available for cultivation and the crop is grown in different areas (environments) across North America, as well on other continents. It is well known that genetic and environmental effects, and phenology play an important role in the biosynthesis of flavonoids, including proanthocyanidins. Quantitative variation for proanthocyanidin content due to genetic factors, e.g. cultivar differences, is significant in a number of species (*17,18*). Numerous varieties from native habitats have been domesticated, as well an increasing number through breeding programs are being developed.

Bioassays

Bioassays enabling bioassay-directed fractionation for anti-adherence activity are available for both type 1 and P-type *E. coli.* Anti-adherence activity for P-type fimbriated *E. coli* is measured through an agglutination assay with cells having glycosphingolipids with α-Gal (1$\rightarrow$ 4) β-Gal receptors or inert materials, e.g., latex beads, whose surface is coated with this disaccharide. The α-Gal (1$\rightarrow$ 4) β-Gal sequence is present on glycosphingolipids of human red blood cells (HRBC), and is analogous to the P blood group antigen (*19*). The anti-adherence tests in these studies measures the amount of agglutination or lack of agglutination of HRBCs (A_1, Rh+) or latex beads coated with a synthetic P receptor analogue (*20*) following incubation with P-fimbriated *E. coli* with cranberry juice or cranberry fruit extracts. P-fimbriated *E. coli* isolated from human patients with urinary tract infections, were cultured under conditions to maintain expression of P fimbriae. Figure 1 exhibits the HRBC agglutination bioassay without and with cranberry juice.

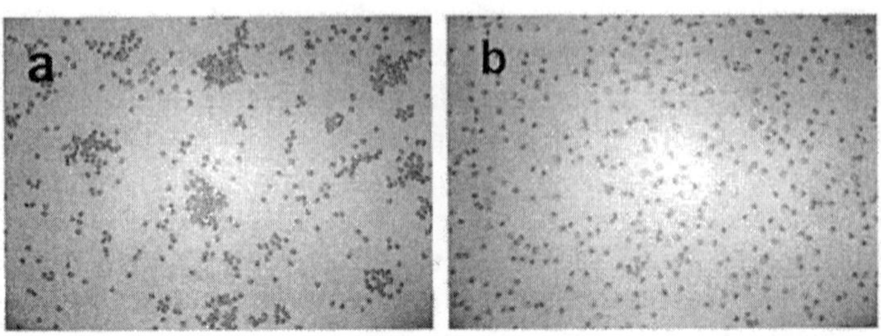

Figure 1 Human red blood cell agglutination bioassay with P fimbriated E. coli, without (a) or with cranberry juice (b).

Extraction and Isolation of Cranberry Proanthocyanidins for Structural Analysis

Proanthocyanidins were extracted from fresh or frozen fruit samples. Fruit were homogenized with acetone and the homogenate filtered and pulp removed. The acetone was evaporated under reduced pressure leaving a residue, which was then diluted with water and defatted by extraction with petroleum ether. The remaining aqueous phase was extracted with ethyl acetate to obtain a red-colored syrup, which was dissolved in ethanol, applied to a Sephadex LH20 column, and washed with ethanol until eluant was clear. The adsorbed proanthocyanidins are eluted from the column with aqueous acetone. The proanthocyanidin fraction isolated from the ethyl acetate extract prevented agglutination activity for P-fimbriated *E. coli* indicating that the fraction had potent bacterial anti-adhesion activity. The anti-adherence activity was evident at concentrations as low as 75 :g/ml. Extraction of higher molecular weight cranberry proanthocyanidins and bioactivity testing of the extracts are described in detail in Foo *et al.* (*12*).

Structure of Cranberry A-type Proanthocyanidins

The ethyl acetate fraction from *V. macrocarpon* fruit exhibits potent anti-adherence activity against P-fimbriated *E. coli.*[12] ^{13}C NMR spectroscopy (Fig. 2) indicated that the ethyl acetate proanthocyanidin fraction contains predominately procyanidin units indicated by the presence of strong peaks at 115-116 ppm and 119.8-121.1 ppm consistent with the C2', C5' and C6' chemical shifts, respectively, of the catechol B-ring. Although the majority of the carbon peaks were found to be consistent with a flavan-3-ol polymeric structure, additional signals were also detected, suggesting that cranberry proanthocyanidins were different from the most commonly found procyanidins. The additional aromatic carbon signals at 151-152 ppm and a quaternary carbon peak at 104.3 ppm in the carbon spectrum, provided evidence of the A-type or double bond interflavanoid linkage (Figure 2).

Although the molecular weight of proanthocyanidins can usually be estimated using relative signal intensity of the C3 signals for the terminating flavanol unit versus the extending flavanol units, the application of this technique is, however, complicated by changes in chemical shifts due to the presence of doubly-bonded procyanidin units. Instead, ES-MS and MALDI-TOF mass spectra of these proanthocyanidins in the ethyl acetate fractions were obtained to estimate molecular weight of the polymers. Both ES-MS and MALDI-TOF spectra exhibited principal ion peaks at *m/z* 1173 and 1464, which

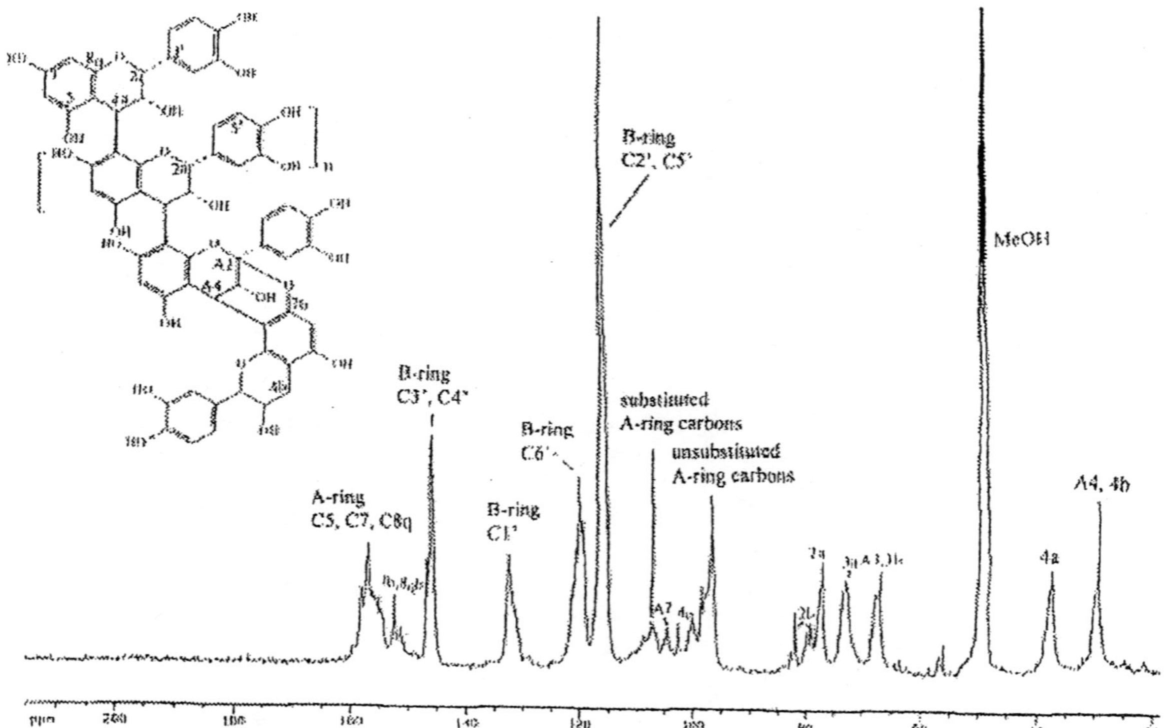

Figure 2. ^{13}C NMR spectrum of cranberry proanthocyanidins showing the presence of A-type linkages (Reproduced with permission from reference 12. Copyright 2000.)

are indicative of procyanidin tetramers and pentamers, respectively, each containing an A-type linkage (*12*). Signals were also observed at *m/z* 1751 and 2038, indicative of procyanidin hexamers and heptamers, respectively, again with each having an A-type linkage. By using MALDI-TOF MS signal intensity as a measure of relative abundance of various oligomers, it was estimated that cranberry procyanidins were made up of 48.6% tetramers, 36.6% pentamers, 11.6% hexamers and 3.1% heptamers.[12] Thus, the ethyl acetate cranberry proanthocyanidin sample consists of predominantly tetramers and pentamers (Figure 3) with 2,3-*cis* stererochemistry linked mostly by C4/C8 interflavanoid linkages and terminated by A2. The terminating A-type linkage is further supported by the isolation of procyanidin A2 which distinctive ^{13}C NMR spectrum showing chemical shifts consistent with a procyanidin dimer but significantly different to those of procyanidin B2 in the higher field region (27-83 ppm) where the chemical shifts of the carbons of the pyran C-ring were located. In particular was the dramatic upfield shift of the C3 and C4 of the upper flavanol unit to 68.5 and 29.7 ppm, respectively, their values being characteristic for those of procyanidin A2 or epicatechin (4β-8, 2β-0-7) epicatechin (*21*,22). Other characteristic features that related to the doubly-linked structure included the transformation of the C2 from a methine carbon in the usual flavan unit to a ketal carbon with the formation of an quarternary carbon 104.7 ppm. As a consequence the resulting substituted oxygenated carbons C7 and C8q of the lower phloroglucinol A-ring involved in the double linkage were shifted upfield to around 152 ppm (*12*).

Employing a technique involving reaction of proanthocyanidins with excess phloroglucinol in the presence of dilute acid, it was established that the C4/C8 interflavonoid bonds were the most common interflavonoid linkages (*12*).

Anti-adherence Bioactivity and Proanthocyanidin Structure

To better understand the structure-activity relationship between proanthocyanidins and inhibition of adherence of P-fimbriated *E. coli*, lower molecular weight cranberry proanthocyanidins were isolated for bioactivity testing (*23*). Column chromatography, alternating between Sephadex LH-20 and MCI Gel CHP 20P, of the ethyl acetate extract of cranberry fruit enabled the separation of epicatechin (**1**) and five proanthocyanidins (**2-6**) (Figure 4), in Foo et al. (*23*).

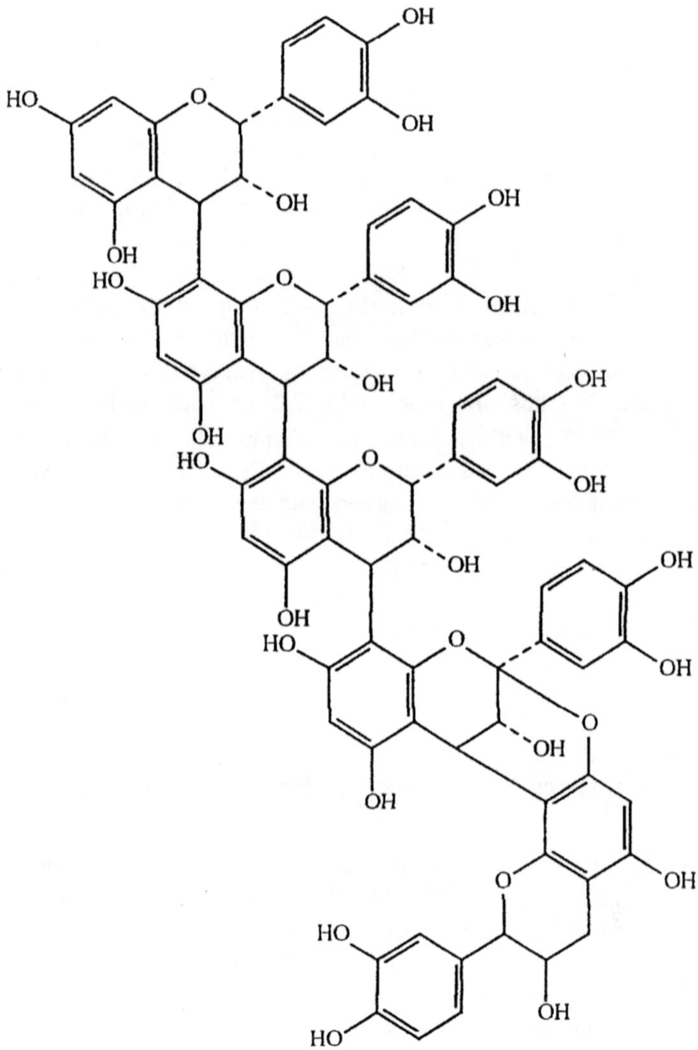

Figure 3. Cranberry A-type procyanidin pentamer.

Table 1 displays the anti-adherence activity of epicatechin and the five proanthocyanidins illustrated in Figure 4. Epicatechin (**1**) and procyanidin B2 (**2**) do not exhibit anti-adherence activity. Procyanidin A2 dimer exhibits relatively weak activity, only apparent at the highest concentration of 2.4 mg/mL. A-type trimers, epicatechin-(4β→6)-epicatechin-(4β→8, 2β→*O*→7)-epicatechin (**4**) and epicatechin-(4β→8, 2β→*O*→7)-epicatechin-(4β→8)-epicatechin (**5**) exhibited the greatest activity, with some anti-adherence activity detected as low as 0.3 mg/mL. A-type trimer epicatechin-(4β→8)-epicatechin-(4β→8, 2β→*O*→7)-epicatechin (**6**) also exhibited relatively high activity, but appeared to be slightly decreased compared to structures (**4**) and (**6**), suggesting that the location of the doubly- bonded units affects bioactivity. All three trimers showed greater bioactivity than the A-type dimer, suggesting a minimum size (MW 863) for bioactivity.

Table I. Ability of compounds 1-6 in Figure 4 to inhibit adherence of uropathogenic P-fimbriated *E. coli* (*23*).

Compound	*Anti-adherence activity (mg/mL)*[a]				
	2.4[b]	*1.2*	*0.6*	*0.3*	*0.15*
1	–	–	–	–	–
2	–	–	–	–	–
3	+	–	–	–	–
4	+	+	+	±	–
5	+	+	+	±	–
6	+	+	±	–	–

[a] Positive anti-adherence activity (+) is measured as the ability of the compounds to suppress agglutimation of both human red blood cells (A_1, Rh+) and latex beads coated with synthetic P receptor analogue following incubation with P-fimbriated E. coli. [b] Dilution of compounds 1-6 in PBS, neutralized with 1N NaOH.

Genetic and Environmental Variation for Fruit Proanthocyanidin Levels in Cranberry: An Analysis of Varieties and Germplasm

Proanthocyanidins from ten cultivars grown in a replicated (Randomized Complete Block Design–RCBD) field trial were quantified from fruit harvested over three dates. The proanthocyanidins were quantified using the standard vanillin/sulphuric acid analysis (*24,25*). Analysis of variance indicated both

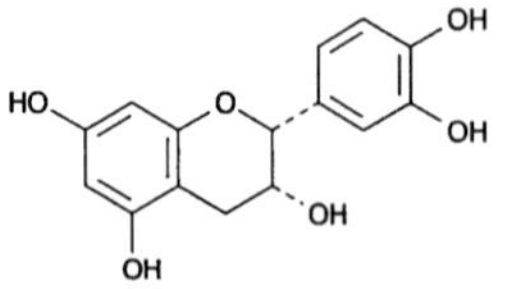

1

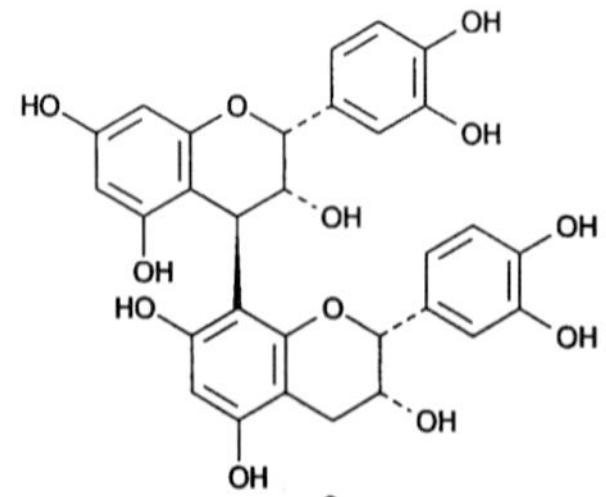

2

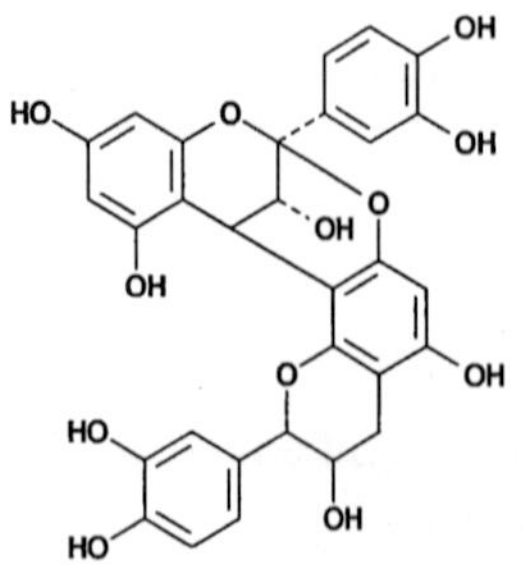

3

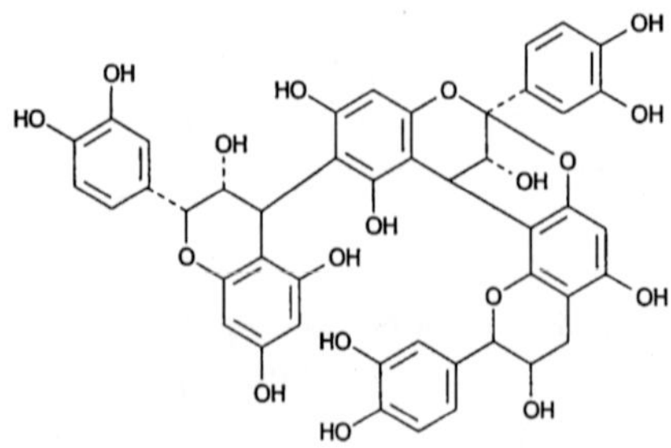

4

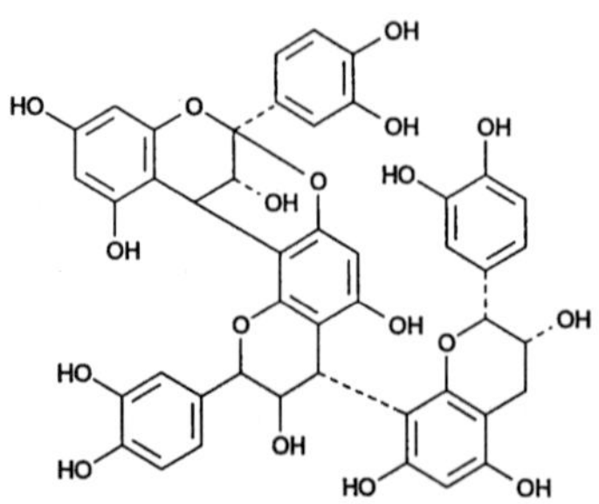

5

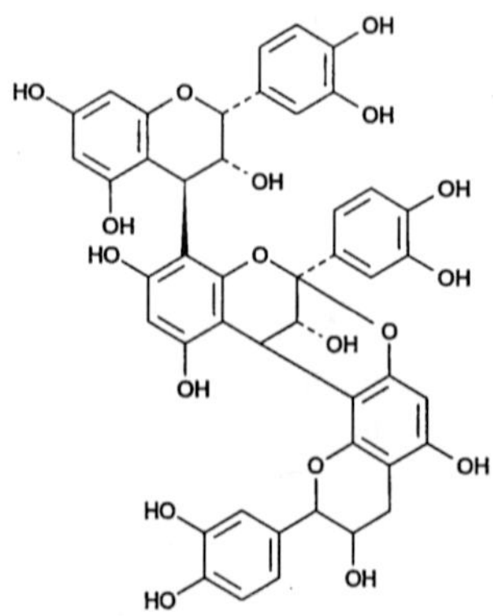

6

Figure 4. Structures of cranberry proanthocyanidins: epicatechin (1), procyanidin B2 or epicatechin-(4β→8)-epicatechin (2), procyanidin A2 or epicatechin-(4β→8, 2β→O→7)-epicatechin (3), and A-type trimers, epicatechin-(4β→6)-epicatechin-(4β→8, 2β→O→7)-epicatechin (4), epicatechin-(4β→8, 2β→O→7)-epicatechin (5), epicatechin-(4β→8)-epicatechin (5), and epicatechin-(4β→8)-epicatechin-(4β→8, 2β→O→7)-epicatechin (6) as from Foo et al. *(23).*

genetic (variety) and harvest date effects were significant (data not shown). Fruit proanthocyandin levels ranged from a low of 4.2 mg/g of fruit for the cultivar 'Ben Lear' to a 11.3 mg/g of fruit for the cultivar 'Early Black' (Figure 5). The most widely grown cultivar 'Stevens' had a mean of 7.8 mg/g fruit which represented intermediate levels of proanthocyanidins.

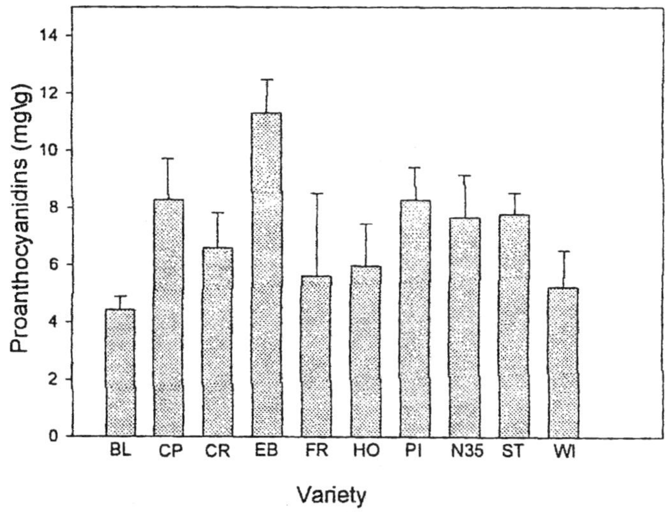

Figure. 5. Mean fruit proanthocyanidin levels in 1996 of ten cranberry cultivars from a replicated field (RCBD – four replicates) trial. Cultivars are 'Ben Lear' (BL), 'Cropper' (CP), Crowley (CR), 'Early Black' (EB), 'Franklin' (FR), 'Howes' (HO), 'Pilgrim' (PI), 'No. 35' (N35), 'Stevens' (ST) and 'Wilcox' (WI).

In 1997, a germplasm collection of over 600 clonal field grown accessions of both domesticated and undomesticated (wild) varieties was evaluated for fruit proanthocyanidin levels from fruit harvested over two harvest dates. The general population distribution of proanthocyanidin content ranged from 5 mg/g fruit to about 35 mg/g fruit, or about six-fold (Fiure. 6). Bog 1 distributions, both cultivated and 'Wild' type, appeared to be slightly higher than the Bog 4 distribution. Two outliers (≥4 units) were apparent in the Bog 1 'Wild' type population. The proanthocyanidin levels of Bog 1 appeared to be somewhat higher than in Bog 4 which may be due to an environmental effect (unpublished data). Bog 1 is essentially a sand base with little or no organic matter, whereas Bog 4 has a 'berryland' soil with about 4 - 5% organic matter and subsequently has higher moisture.

Similar to anthocyanins and overall phenolics, proanthocyanidins were negatively correlated with crop yield and fruit number density for both harvest dates (*26*). Correlation between fruit size (berry weight) and proanthocyanidin

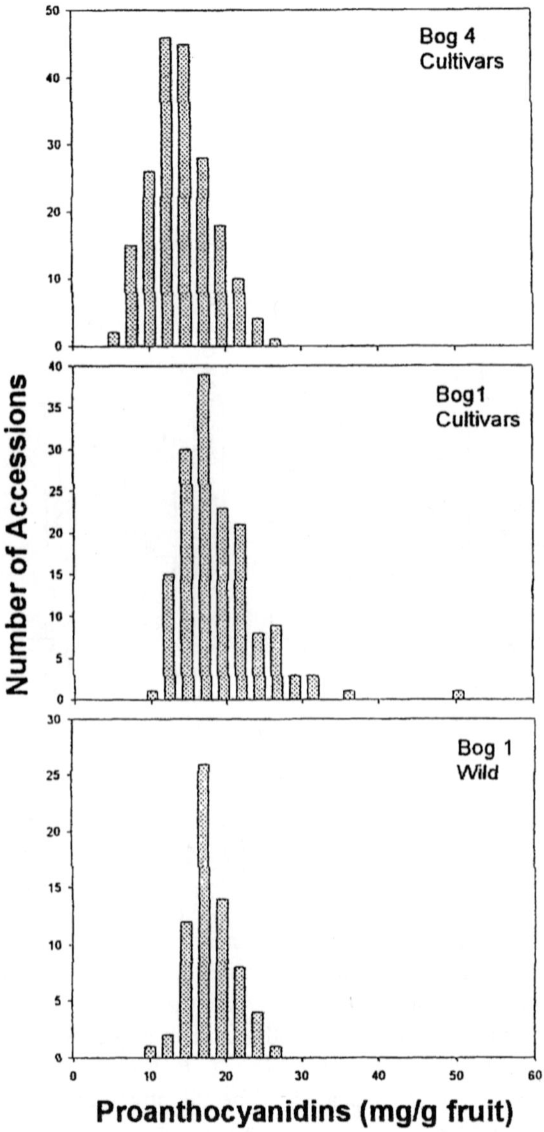

Figure 6. 1997 frequency distributions of variety mean (2 harvest dates) for proanthocyanidin levels of cranberry germplasm. Germplasm includes both cultivated and wild accessions grown in two bogs (Bog 1 and 4). Bog 1 contains both domesticated varieties (cultivars) and clones from the native stands (wild); and Bog 4 contains domesticated varieties.

levels were all negative over both harvest dates suggesting a major portion of proanthocyanidins is located in the fruit epidermis.

However, histological analysis for proanthocyanidins indicated that seeds were also rich in proanthocyanidins. Although these phytochemicals appear to be negatively correlated with yield and components of yield, the correlations are not particularly high, suggesting selection for both yield and phytochemical content should be possible. Fruit anthocyanins, overall phenolics and proanthocyanidins were all positively correlated. A 'partial' correlation (berry weight) analysis was performed to eliminate berry weight as a factor. Proanthocyanidins were not always significantly correlated with anthocyanins and phenolics once correlation to berry weight was eliminated statistically (*26*). Proanthocyanidins were not significantly correlated with anthocyanins and phenolics in the Bog 4 cultivar population, whereas there was a significantly positive correlation of both anthocyanins and phenolics with proanthocyanidins in both the 'Wild' and cultivar populations in Bog 1. Phenolics and anthocyanins were still positively correlated, although *r* values were generally reduced by 5-10%.

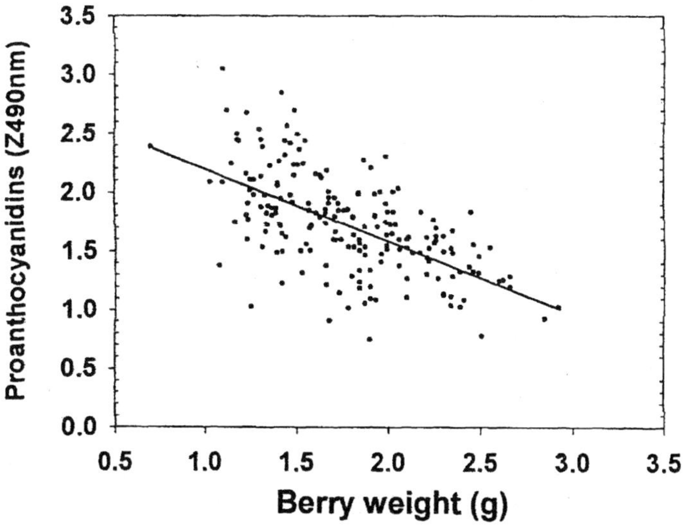

Figure. 7. Relationship between fruit proanthocyanidin content and fruit size (weight) across germplasm accessions.

In a heritability study using parent-offspring regression for the levels of fruit proanthocyanidins, the heritability estimates (h^2) were significantly positive (h^2=0.43), indicating significant additive genetic variance exists for proanthocyandin fruit levels.

The significant variation for proanthocyanidin levels found across cultivars and germplasm suggests genetic enhancement of proanthocyanidin levels is possible in cranberry. Heritability estimates suggest predictable genetic gain is possible. However, the significant negative relationship between fruit size and proanthocyanidin content requires that selection protocols include fruit size as a covariate.

References

1. Avorn, J.; Monane, M.; Gurwitz, J.H.; Glynn, R.J.; Choodnovskiy, I.; Lipsitz, L.A. *JAMA* **1994**, *271*, 751-754.
2. Kontiokari, T.; Sundqvist, K.; Nuutinen, M.; Pokka, T.; Koskela, M.; Uhari, M. *Br. Med. J.* **2001**, *322*, 1571-1573.
3. Bodel, P.T.; Cotran, R.; Kass, E.H. *J. Lab. Clin. Med.* **1959**, *54*, 881-888.
4. Moen, D.V. *Wis. Med. J.* **1962**, *61*, 282-283.
5. Papas, P.N.; Brusch, C.A.; Ceresia, G.C. *Southwest Med.* **1966**, *47*, 17.
6. Sternlieb, P. *New England J. Med.* **1963**, *268*, 57.
7. Kunin, C.M. 1994. *Clin. Infect. Dis.* **1994**, *18*, 1-12.
8. Sobota, A.E. *J. Urol.* **1984**, *131*, 1013-1016.
9. Schmidt, D.R.; Sobota, A.E. *Microbios.* **1988**, *55*, 173-181.
10. Zafriri, D.; Ofek, I.; Adar, R.; Pocino, M.; Sharon, N. *Antimicrob. Agents Chemo.* **1989**, *33*, 92-98.
11. Ofek, I.; Goldhar, J.; Zafriri, D.; Lis, H.; Adar, R.; Sharon, N. *New England J. Med.* **1991**, *324*, 1599.
12. Foo, L.Y.; Lu, Y.; Howell, A.B.; Vorsa, N. *Phytochemistry* **2000**, *54*, 173-181.
13. Beachey, E.H. *J. Infect. Dis.* **1981**, *143*, 325-345.
14. Roberts, J.A.; Marklund, B.; Ilver, D.; Haslam, D.; Kaack, M.B.; Baskin, G.; Louis, M.; Mollby R.; Winberg, J.; Normark, S. *Proc. Natl. Acad. Sci.* **1994**, *91*, 11889-11893.
15. Kallenius, G.; Svenson, S.B.; Mollby, R.; Korhonen, T.; Winberg, J.; Cedergren, B.; Helin, I.; Hultberg, H. *Scand. J. Infect. Dis. Suppl.* **1982**, *33*, 52-60.
16. Howell, A.B.; Vorsa, N.; DerMarderosian, A.; Foo, L.Y. *New England J. Med.* **1998**, *339*, 1085-1086.
17. Yonemori, K.; Matsushima, J. *J. Amer. Soc. Hort. Sci.* **1987**, *112*, 817-821.
18. Bell, A.A.; El-Zik, K.M.; Thaxton, P.M. In *Plant Polyphenols: Synthesis, Properties, Significance*. Eds. R.W. Hemmingway and P.E. Laks. Plenum Press, NY. 1992, pp.517-595.
19. Kallenius, G.; Mollby, R.; Svenson, S.B.; Winberg, J.; Lundblad, A.; Svensson, S.; Cedergren, B. *FEMS Microbiol. Lett.* **1980**, *7*, 297-302.

20. De Man, P.; Cedergren, B.; Enerback, S.; Larsson, A.C.; Leffler, H.; Lundell, A.L.; Nilson, B.; Svanborg-Eden, C. *J. Clin. Microbiol.* **1987**, *25*, 401-406.
21. Nonaka, G.I.; Morimoto, S.; Nishioka, I. *J. Chem. Soc. Perkin Trans. 1*, **1983**, 2139.
22. Balde, A.M.; Pieters, L.A.; Wray, V.; Kolodzies, H.; Vanden Berche, D.A.; Claeys, M.; Vlietrick, A.J. *Phytochemistry* **1991**, *30*, 4129.
23. Foo, L.Y.; Lu, Y.; Howell, A.B.; Vorsa, N. *J. Nat Prod.* **2000**, 63, 1225-1228.
24. Lees G.L. In *Plant Polyphenols: Synthesis, Properties, Significance*. Eds. R.W. Hemmingway and P.E. Laks. Plenum Press, NY. 1992, pp. 915-934.
25. Scalbert A. 1992. In *Plant Polyphenols: Synthesis, Properties, Significance.* Hemmingway, R.W.; Laks, P.E., Eds., Plenum Press, NY. 1992, pp.259-280.
26. Vorsa, N.; Polashock, J.; Howell, A.B.; Cunningham, D.; Roderick, R. *Acta Horticulturae*. 2001, *In press*.

Chapter 27

Fractionation, Antioxidant Activity, and Cytotoxicity of Cranberry Fruit Extracts

Catherine C. Neto, Xiaojun Yan, Brian T. Murphy, Kanayochukwu Azogu, and Gerald B. Hammond

Department of Chemistry and Biochemistry, University of Massachusetts at Dartmouth, North Dartmouth, MA 02747

Cranberries (Vaccinium macrocarpon) are potentially an excellent dietary source of phenolic compounds such as flavonoids, anthocyanins and caffeic acid derivatives which are potent antioxidants. Studies also link a lowered incidence of breast cancer to cranberry juice consumption. In this study, cranberry fruits were fractionated by several methods and tested for radical-scavenging activity in an effort to begin establishing a link between chemical composition and antioxidant activity. The strongest activity was observed in flavonoid-rich extracts. Cytotoxicity assays in several tumor cell lines showed some specificity for HT-29 tumor cells and K562 cells from a methanolic cranberry extract containing several phenolic compounds.

A rapidly growing body of evidence exists for the health benefits of consuming cranberries, an important crop in Southeastern Massachusetts and areas of Wisconsin and New Jersey. Recent studies report that cranberry juice can prevent urinary tract infections (UTIs) and inhibit the growth of several strains of bacteria *(1)*. Researchers have reported that regular consumption of cranberry products inhibits breast cancer development and that cranberry juice prevents oxidation of LDLs, a process involved in the early stages of heart disease *(2)*. Cranberries contain several classes of compounds which can act as antioxidants such as anthocyanins, caffeic acids and flavonoids. However, information about the relative antioxidant activities of specific extracts and components of the cranberry is lacking. The potential anticancer mechanism is still unknown. Information on antioxidant activity of specific extracts and the chemical composition of these extracts may help provide a better understanding of how cranberries and related fruits exert protective effects against cardiovascular disease and some cancers.

In this investigation, an assay-guided fractionation approach was used to identify and evaluate the components of whole cranberries and cranberry parts. The whole cranberries were examined by fractionation into different extracts based on solubility of the components and the relative free-radical-scavenging activity of each cranberry extract as well as the cytotoxicity of cranberry extracts in various tumor cell lines were evaluated. We also have begun to examine the comparative composition of flavonoids and anthocyanins in the various parts of the cranberry. The ultimate goal is to isolate and identify the major antioxidants and anticancer components and to gain a better understanding of how the compounds found in cranberries may provide protection against cardiovascular disease and cancer.

Materials and Methods

Fractionation methods

Two solubility-based methods were used to fractionate whole berries (Stevens variety) harvested by Decas Cranberry, Wareham, MA, in October of 1999.

Method 1 - Sequential solvent extraction of whole berries. One hundred grams of wet weight of frozen whole cranberries were macerated in a blender containing 300 mL of petroleum ether. After vacuum filtration to remove the solvent, the solids were macerated in 200 mL ethyl acetate. After filtration to remove the ethyl acetate, the solid was macerated in 200 mL methanol/2% formic acid. The methanol extracts were removed by filtration. Extracts were dried in vacuo. Yields from 100 g berries were 0.310 g solid from petroleum ether extract, 0.465 g solid from ethyl acetate extract, and 2.137 g solid from methanolic extract. Extracts were assayed for radical-scavenging activity and tumor cell cytotoxicity as described below. Further separation of 0.255 g of dry ethyl acetate extract occurred upon addition of 1:1 methanol/water. Yellow solids (0.120 g) were removed, leaving 0.125 g of a red semisolid material.

Method 2 - Solvent partitioning of crude extract. To prepare the crude cranberry extract, 100 g of frozen whole cranberries were macerated using a blender in methanol/ 2% formic acid (300 mL/100 g berries), vacuum-filtered and washed. The filtrate was lyophilized to produce a dark red semisolid crude extract. The solvent partitioning protocol of Kupchan *(3)* was used to separate components by polarity as follows. Crude extract (8.0 g) was first partitioned between 100 mL water and 200 mL chloroform. The water layer was further partitioned between 100 mL water and 200 mL ethyl acetate to draw some organic-soluble components out of aqueous solution. The chloroform extract was partitioned between 100 mL each of hexane and 90% methanol. Extracts were then dried in vacuo. Extracts were assayed for radical-scavenging activity and tumor cell cytotoxicity as described below. From 100 g berries a typical yield of 8.54 g crude extract was obtained. Partitioning of the crude extract yielded 0.201 g solids from hexane, 0.132 g from methanol, 0.631 g from ethyl acetate and 4.228 g from the aqueous layer.

Method 3 - Physical separation of parts. Cranberries were physically separated by removing the peel and squeezing the juice from the remaining solid. Samples were prepared for HPLC analysis from the peels, solids, juice and the whole berry by extraction with 98:2 methanol/acetic acid. Solutions were passed through Whatman Puradisc 13 mm/0.45 μm filters prior to HPLC analysis. The samples were also analyzed spectrophotometrically for total flavonoid and anthocyanin content using the method of Lees and Francis (4). The data are shown in Table III.

To provide samples for 2,2-Diphenyl-l-picrylhydrazyl radical (DPPH) assay, 500 g (wet weight) of berries were separated into peels, solids and juice. Both the peels and the solids were dried then extracted first with ethyl acetate (300 mL) and then with methanol containing 0.25 % formic acid (300 mL). The juice was extracted with ethyl acetate (400 mL) and the remainder lyophilized as the aqueous extract. Yields are given in Table V.

Antioxidant activity assay

The DPPH assay *(5)* was used to evaluate the free-radical-scavenging capacity of extracts prepared by the methods outlined above, whole berry extract and commercial cranberry juice cocktail (Ocean Spray Inc.). Activity was compared to that of a standard antioxidant (Vitamin E, Aldrich Chemical Co.) measured using the same methods. Varying concentrations of cranberry extracts were mixed with a 60 μM solution of DPPH in methanol. Quenching of the violet DPPH radical was observed as a decrease in absorbance at 515 nm over one hour. EC_{50} values are measured as the sample concentration required to decrease DPPH absorption by 50%. Results are shown in Table I. The DPPH assay was also used to evaluate the extracts of peel, solids and juice; EC_{50} values are reported in Table V.

Cytotoxicity assay

Cytotoxicity of cranberry extracts was evaluated in a variety of tumor cell lines to determine whether cytotoxicity is a likely mechanism of anticancer activity and whether there is any specificity among tumor types. Serial dilutions of each extract were added to the incubating cells (37° C). After 48 h, the live cells remaining were counted. Relative cytotoxicities of each extract are reported based on growth inhibition, as the range of sample concentrations in which GI_{50} occurred (cell count = 50% of control). Cell lines tested were HT-29, H460, ME180, DU145, MCF-7, M-14, K562 and BALB/c3T3. Results are given in Table II.

HPLC analysis

Extracts of peel, solid, juice and whole berry were analyzed for their flavonoid and anthocyanin contents by HPLC. An effective protocol was developed to analyze samples for both flavonoid and anthocyanin content simultaneously using a Waters system consisting of two Waters 515 pumps, a Rheodyne 7725i injector (20 ìL), a Waters 996 photodiode array detector (250 to 600 nm) with Millenium32 operating system and a Waters Nova-Pak ® C18, (3.9× 150 mm) column *(6)*. Solvents used for sample elution were (A) 2% acetic acid and (B) methanol in 2% acetic acid. Elution program was isocratic elution with 100% A from 0 to 10 min, linear gradient to 100% B from 10 to 45 min, finally isocratic elution with 100% B from 45 to 60 min; flow rate 0.8 mL/min.

Anthocyanins were detected at 520 nm; flavonols were detected at 350 nm. The aglycones of flavonol and anthocyanin glycosides in each sample were identified by their spectral characteristics. Compositions are shown in Tables IV and V.

Results

Table I shows the results of a DPPH radical-scavenging assay on each of the whole-cranberry extracts prepared by Methods 1 and 2. For whole cranberries, the highest antioxidant activity was observed in ethyl acetate extracts prepared by both methods, with an IC_{50} value of 0.033 mg/mL for the ethyl acetate extract prepared by Method 2. The ethyl acetate fraction was about twice as effective at radical scavenging as the whole-berry extract (IC_{50} = 0.078 mg/mL). Kinetics of these reactions were slow compared to the standard, Vitamin E; for all cranberry extracts, radical scavenging occurred over a period of approximately one hour as compared to several minutes for vitamin E.

Method 1 was more effective in extracting organic-soluble plant material from berries on a weight basis than Method 2. However, of all extracts prepared, the methanolic fraction obtained from Method 2 showed the most interesting activity against tumor cell lines as is shown in Table II. The GI_{50} for the methanolic fraction was in the range of 31 – 125 μg/mL for HT-29 (colon tumor) cells and 16 – 63 μg/mL for K562 cells (leukemia). These activities were considerably higher than that of the other extracts prepared from whole cranberries. Other tumor cell lines and murine embryonic 3T3 cells were only affected at higher concentrations (most GI_{50} were above 0.250 mg/ml). Initial HPLC analysis of this cytotoxic extract indicates the presence of several phenolic compounds; the identity of these compounds is under investigation.

HPLC analysis of the antioxidant ethyl acetate extract of whole cranberries prepared by Method 1 showed the sample to be composed primarily of flavonoids; in particular, five compounds which were identified mainly as glycosides of quercetin with a small percentage (8%) of myricetin-3-β-$_D$-galactoside. The exact structures of the quercetin glycosides are currently under investigation. Table III indicates the total flavonoid and anthocyanin composition in the whole berry and its parts. Percent composition of flavonoid glycosides in each part of the cranberry is given in Table IV.

The flavonoids occurred mainly as glycosides and there were at least three different glycosides of myricetin and five different glycosides of quercetin in the berry extracts. Much of the flavonoid content of the berries was concentrated in the peel (125 mg/100 g) and solids rather than the juice, which contained only 13.39 mg flavonols/100 g. The peels also contained a higher content of quercetin glycosides and two kaempferol glycosides which did not appear in the juice.

Table I. Comparative antioxidant activities of extracts of whole cranberries measured by a DPPH radical-scavenging assay

Sample origin	EC_{50} *(mg/mL)*[c]
Commercial cranberry juice[a]	0.530
Whole cranberry extract[b]	0.078
Petroleum ether extract, method 1	0.230
Ethyl acetate extract, method 1	0.043
Methanol extract, method 1	0.140
Ethyl acetate extract, method 2	0.033
Methanol extract, method 2	0.140
Aqueous extract, method 2	0.160
Vitamin E (standard)	0.008

[a] Ocean spray cranberry juice cocktail, lyophilized

[b] Prepared as described for method 2

[c] Concentration required to quench 50% of DPPH radical

Table II. Cytotoxicity in tumor cell lines

Sample origin	GI_{50} *(mg/mL)*[a]
Whole cranberry extract[b]	all cell lines: > 0.500
Petroleum ether extract, method 1	all cell lines: 0.125 – 0.500
Ethyl acetate extract, method 1	all cell lines: 0.125 – 0.500
Methanol extract, method 1	all cell lines: 0.500
Aqueous extract, method 2	all cell lines: > 0.500
Ethyl acetate extract, method 2	all cell lines: > 0.500
Methanol extract, method 2	HT-29 cells: 0.031 – 0.125
	K562 cells: 0.016 – 0.063
	all other cell lines: 0.063 – 0.250

[a] Results are reported as the range of sample concentrations in which 50% inhibition of tumor cell growth was observed. Cell lines tested: HT-29, H460, ME180, DU145, MCF-7, M-14, K562 and BALB/c3T3.

[b] Prepared as described for method 2

Table III. Total anthocyanin and flavonoid content in berry and its parts

Sample	*Anthocyanin content (mg/100 g berry)*	*Flavonoid content (mg/100 g berry)*
Whole berry	36.45 ± 3.12	27.89 ± 2.76
Juice	30.17 ± 2.05	13.39 ± 1.23
Peel	101.45 ± 3.86	124.86 ± 4.56
Solid[a]	89.96 ± 5.22	94.77 ± 7.75

[a] Refers to solids remaining after peel is removed

Table IV. Flavonoid composition in cranberry parts

Aglycone[a]	*Retention time (min)*	*% in peel*	*% in solids*	*% in juice*
Myricetin	21.81	8.38	4.55	64.79
Quercetin	23.00	19.83	13.41	---
Quercetin	23.49	---	4.56	17.43
Myricetin	24.40	2.44	7.64	5.10
Quercetin	25.27	4.72	3.48	4.01
Myricetin	26.20	21.08	21.68	3.64
Quercetin	26.20	21.02	0.56	---
Quercetin	29.09	9.10	23.49	---
Kaempferol	30.74	7.66	11.42	2.58
Kaempferol	34.41	5.76	8.22	0.73

[a] Aglycones were determined by uv-visible spectral characteristics

Table V. DPPH-scavenging activity of extracts from peel, solids and juice

Sample	*Mass of extract from 500 g berries*	EC_{50} *in mg/mL*
Peel, ethyl acetate extract	1.225 g	0.055
Peel, methanol extract	5.570 g	0.075
Solids, ethyl acetate extract	0.275 g	0.065
Solids, methanol extract	8.036 g	0.093
Juice, ethyl acetate extract	0.530 g	0.009
Juice, aqueous extract	19.20 g	0.155

Table VI. Anthocyanin composition in cranberry parts

Aglycone[a]	*Retention time (minutes)*	*% in peel*	*% in solids*	*% in juice*
Cyanidin	15.73	24.93	24.95	31.10
Cyanidin	17.24	1.61	---	3.83
Peonidin	17.87	48.21	66.13	49.40
Peonidin	19.01	11.18	8.93	15.67
Petunidin	21.66	6.39	---	---
Petunidin	23.97	7.68	---	---

[a] Aglycones were determined by uv-visible spectral characteristics

The comparative antioxidant activities of extracts from the peels, solids and juice are shown in Table V. Table VI shows the composition of different anthocyanins in cranberry. Cyanidin and peonidin were the principal anthocyanins present in all parts including juice; each existed in two main glycosidic forms. Two glycosides of a third anthocyanin, petunidin, were found only in the peels which accounted for about 14% of the total anthocyanin content in cranberry peels.

Discussion

Among the extracts tested for radical-scavenging efficacy, the greatest antioxidant activity was observed in the ethyl acetate-soluble extracts of whole cranberry which contained primarily quercetin glycosides. The exact glycoside structures are currently under investigation. These results are consistent with the observed strong antioxidant activity of flavonoid compounds in previous studies *(7)*. The DPPH assay shows the increased radical-scavenging power of whole-cranberry extracts over that of the lyophilized commercial juice. This result may perhaps be attributed to the high flavonoid content found in the peel and solids as compared to the juice of the cranberry. For freshly-squeezed juice, excellent radical-scavenging activity was observed in a small ethyl acetate extract but the majority of the water-soluble mass showed a lower activity. Extracts of the peel and solids were moderately active, with the greatest radical-scavenging activity observed in the ethyl-acetate extract of peels (EC_{50} = 0.055 mg/mL). Analysis of solids and juice from berries showed that the highest percentage by weight of both flavonoids and anthocyanins occurred in the peel. The results of both composition analysis and radical-scavenging assays suggest that the high concentration of flavonoids and anthocyanins in the peel and solids of cranberries may help to contribute an additional health benefit for subjects who consume whole cranberries or cranberry products processed in such a way as to derive a higher flavonoid content than juices prepared by current commercial methods. A more detailed investigation of the exact structures of the quercetin glycosides and their comparative antioxidant activities is in progress.

Consumption of cranberry juice has been linked to a decreased proliferation of MDA-MB-435 and MCF-7 breast cancer cells both *in vitro* and *in vivo (8)*. *Vaccinium* fruit extracts also exhibited anticarcinogenic potential in *in vitro* mechanistic screening tests using TPA-induced ornithine decarboxylase activity and quinone reductase induction assay *(9)*. Cytoxicity of cranberry extracts in other tumor cell lines has not been fully reported, nor have the active principles been identified. In assays conducted in this work, most cranberry extracts exhibited low cytotoxicity in tumor cells overall with one exception; a methanol-soluble fraction was found to have increased and selective cytotoxicity against both K562 (leukemia) and HT-29 (colon) tumor cells. Isolation and identification of the major components of this cytotoxic extract is in progress. None of the extracts tested caused DNA mutation in yeast topoisomerase assay (courtesy of D.G.I. Kingston). These data suggest that the cytotoxicity of certain cranberry components may play a role in inhibiting the growth of other cancers besides breast cancer. The cytotoxicity may also be supplemented by the observed antioxidative behavior which may play a role in suppressing tumor initiation.

Further studies will address the structures of the major bioactive components of the antioxidant and cytotoxic cranberry extracts, their compositions in extracts from peel, solids and juice, and their specific molecular and radical targets of activity.

Acknowledgements

We thank Dr. Abraham Vaisberg (Universidad Peruana Cayetano Heredia) for tumor-cell cytotoxicity assays and Dr. David G. I. Kingston and Jeannine Hoch (Virginia Institute of Technology) for DNA mutation assays. We are grateful to David Nolte (Decas Cranberries) for supplying raw materials. This study was supported by a grant from the UMass-Dartmouth Cranberry Agricultural Research Program.

References

1. Foo, L. Y.; Howell, A. B.; Vorsa, N. *Phytochemistry* **2000,** *54*, 173-181.
2. Wilson, T.; Porcari, J.; Harbin, D. *Pharmacol. Lett.* **1998,** *62*, 381-386.
3. Kupchan, S. M.; Dessertine, A. L.; Blaylock, B. T.; Bryan, R. F. *J. Org. Chem.* **1974**, *39*, 2477-2482.
4. Lees, D. H.; Francis, F. J. *J. Food Sci.* **1971**, *36*, 1056-1060.
5. Brand-Williams, W.; Cuvelier, M. E.; Berset, C. Lebensm.-Wiss. U.-Technol. **1995**, *28*, 25-30.
6. Yan, X.; Murphy, B. T.; Hammond, G. B., Vinson, J. A.; Neto, C. C. *J. Agric. Food Chem.* Accepted.
7. Pietta, Pier-Giorgio *J. Nat. Prod.* **2000**, *63*, 1035-1042.
8. Guthrie, N. *FASEB Journal*, **2000**, *14*, Abstract 531.13.
9. Bomser, J.; Madhavi, D. L.; Singletary, K.; Smith, M. A. *Planta Med.* **1996,** *62*, 212-216.

Chapter 28

Conversion of Carotenoids to Retinoids and Other Oxidation Products

Akihiko Nagao and Eiichi Kotake-Nara

National Food Research Institute, Tsukuba, Ibaraki 305–8642, Japan

Dietary provitamin A carotenoids are cleaved to vitamin A at the central double bond by intestinal β-carotene-15,15'-dioxygenase, while eccentric cleavage at random position of conjugated double bonds is proposed for an additional pathway to vitamin A. Pig intestinal homogenate catalyzed exclusively cleavage reaction of the central double bond of β-carotene to produce two molecules of retinal, without any detectable formation of β-apocarotenals. High fat diets enhanced the enzyme activity and the level of cellular retinol binding protein type II in rat intestine. Dietary antioxidants and flavonols with a catechol structure in the B ring inhibited the enzyme activity *in vitro*. Thus, several food components would modulate metabolic conversion of provitamin A in intestinal cells and thereby the level of circulating provitamin A in the body. In contrast, carotenoids can be oxidized at random positions of conjugated double bonds in a non-enzymatic manner. Lycopene was oxidized *in vitro* to *acyclo*-retinal, *acyclo*-retinoic acid, and apolycopenals by autoxidation, and the oxidized lycopene induced apoptosis of HL-60 cells. Oxidation products formed *in vivo* might be involved in biological actions of carotenoids.

Carotenoids are synthesized in microorganisms and plants, and work as antioxidants and antenna pigments in photosynthetic organs. Their oxidative metabolites play important roles as hormones in a wide variety of living organisms. The abscisic acid, which is synthesized through oxidative cleavage of neoxanthin, is a plant hormone related to water stress and senescence (*1*). Trisporic acid synthesized through cleavage of β-carotene in fungi is involved in the formation of zygote. Retinal works as a photo-sensor in vision of animals and retinoic acid regulates gene expression through activation of nuclear hormone receptors in vertebrates. They are synthesized through oxidative cleavage of β-carotene in animals. Thus, oxidative metabolites of carotenoids have been utilized as signal molecules by living organisms. Their formation are mediated and regulated by the enzymes, which catalyze the cleavage of specific double bonds in the respective carotenoids. In mammals, conversion of β-carotene to retinal is mediated by β-carotene-15, 15'-dioxygenase,which catalyzes cleavage reaction at the central double bond of provitamin A carotenoids (*2,3*). Although the dioxygenase plays an essential role for providing animals with vitamin A, the detailed characteristics and regulatory mechanism of the enzyme remain unknown. The enzyme is highly expressed in intestinal epithelium and liver, although the low activity is detected in other peripheral tissues. Thus, the intestinal epithelium is a primary site for conversion of dietary provitamin A carotenoids to vitamin A. Carotenoid absorption to intestinal cells is closely linked to digestion and absorption of dietary fat. The intestinal epithelium is exposed directly to various dietary components, which might influence the dioxygenase activity. The regulatory system of β-carotene dioxygenase in intestinal cells might be considered in this context as well as vitamin A status. In this contribution, effects of dietary fat and antioxidants on the intestinal dioxygenase activity are described.

Carotenoids have excellent quenching activity against singlet oxygen by physical energy transfer, and also have radical-scavenging activity by reaction with oxygen radicals. However, carotenoids are extremely vulnerable to oxidation and thereby work as prooxidants under certain conditions. In addition to the enzymatic cleavage, as described above, a number of compounds are formed from β-carotene by non-enzymatic oxidations, one of which cleaves conjugated double bonds at random positions under oxidative conditions. Retinal and β-apocarotenals are included among the oxidation products (*4*). Therefore, the oxidation products, which might be formed *in vivo* under oxidative conditions, could exert biological actions on human health. This contribution also describes the formation of cleavage products of lycopene, a typical dietary non-provitamin A carotenoid and effects of oxidized carotenoid preparations on proliferation of cancer cells.

Conversion of Provitamin A Carotenoids to Vitamin A

One molecule of β-carotene is converted to two molecules of retinal through the cleavage at central double bond by β-carotene 15,15'-dioxygenase, which was discovered in the mid 1960s by two groups of Goodman and Olson (*2,3*). In the intestinal epithelium, retinal is further reduced to retinol, which is esterified and incorporated into chylomicron as retinyl ester (*5*). This is a central cleavage pathway in conversion of provitamin A carotenoid to vitamin A, and has been confirmed by several groups (*6-8*). In contrast to this symmetrical cleavage, an eccentric cleavage pathway was proposed as an additional pathway of vitamin A formation (*9*). β-Carotene is cleaved by enzyme at random position of conjugated double bonds to retinal, β-apocarotenals, and several short-chain carbonyl compounds. β-Apocarotenals are further cleaved to short-chain compounds or oxidized to retinoic acid through β-oxidation pathway. We have investigated the cleavage reaction with pig intestinal homogenate as the source of enzymes, in order to elucidate the extent to which the eccentric cleavage pathway contributes to vitamin A formation (*10*). The incubation of β-carotene with pig homogenate and subsequent extraction were carefully conducted under the presence of antioxidant to avoid oxidative degradation of β-carotene and retinal, which are extremely susceptible to chemical oxidation. Retinal, which was spontaneously isomerized immediately after formation from β-carotene, was quantified for each geometrical isomer separated by high-performance liquid chromatography on a normal phase column. The low recovery of retinal due to formation of an Schiff base with amino compounds present in tissue homogenate was overcome by formaldehyde treatment prior to extraction. We found more than 94% converson of β-carotene consumed to retinal and no formation of β-apocarotenals. These results clearly indicated that the homogenate of pig intestine converted β-carotene to retinal exclusively by central cleavage. Moreover, in the absence of antioxidant, rat intestinal homogenates was reported to cleave β-carotene randomly to β-apocarotenals (*11*). The results suggested the random cleavage by oxygen radical produced through enzyme reactions. Therefore, the chemical cleavage at random position should be taken into consideration carefully, although it is still uncertain whether the eccentric enzymatic cleavages play significant role in the conversion of β-carotene to vitamin A. Recently, cDNA encoding a carotene dioxygenase, which catalyzed exclusively the asymmetric cleavage at 9', 10' double bond of lycopene as well as β-carotene, was identified from mouse (*12*). In addition to the central cleavage enzyme, the asymmetric cleavage enzyme might work in metabolism of carotenoids in mammals.

Effects of Dietary Fat and Antioxidant on β-Carotene-15,15'-Dioxygenase Activity

β-Carotene-15,15'-dioxygenase was expressed exclusively in the intestinal mucosa and liver, as the brain, kidney and lung exhibited little activity (*13*). The dioxygenase converts dietary β-carotene absorbed into intestinal cells to vitamin A, while in the liver it might attack β-carotene circulated in blood or stored in liver. Therefore, the enzyme would affect the levels of provitamin A carotenoids and vitamin A in the tissues. However, the regulation of β-carotene dioxygenase activity has not been clarified well, although vitamin A status and dietary protein were known to affect the activity (*14-16*). In particular, the intestine is exposed directly to dietary components, which could affect the dioxygenase activity. Several dietary antioxidants were found that remarkably inhibited the enzyme activity *in vitro* (*17*). Flavonoids such as rhamnetin and quercetin with a catechol structure in this ring B inhibited at micromole concentrations. Synthetic antioxidants such as butylhyroxytoluene strongly inhibited the activity at 1 μM. These inhibitory effects were also confirmed in the conversion of β-carotene to retinol by human intestinal Caco-2 cells. These results suggest that some flavonoids, which are ingested with carotenoids, e.g. as green leafy vegetables, might repress the conversion of provitamin A carotenoids to vitamin A. Another factor, which potentially affects the conversion, would be dietary fat, because digestion and absorption of β-carotene are closely related to those of dietary fat. Fat is well known to enhance the absorption of lipophilic vitamins. The dietary fat enhances the formation of mixed micelles composed of bile acid, cholesterol, phospholipids and fat hydrolyzates. Solubilization of carotenoid into mixed micelles is prerequisite to transfer from intestinal tract to the intestinal cells (*18-20*). Moreover, carotenoids and retinyl ester are incorporated into chylomicron rich in triacylglycerol and secreted in the lymph. Dietary unsaturated fat has been reported to enhance the expression of cellular retinol binding protein type II (CRBP-II), which works as carrier protein for retinal and retinol for subsequent metabolism in intestine (*21*). Thus, the effect of dietary fats on the β-carotene dioxygenase activity in rats was investigated (*22*). The rats fed with high fat diets containing 15% of olive oil or soybean oil for 3 weeks showed significantly higher activity of β-carotene dioxygenase in intestinal mucosa than the control rats fed with a low fat diet containing 2.5 % soybean oil (Figure 1). The rats fed with 15% soybean oil showed a higher level of CRBP-II protein in intestinal mucosa than the control rats. The results suggest that the expression of β-carotene dioxygenase is modulated by dietary fat and that the dioxygenase and CRBP-II are closely linked in the conversion of β-carotene. The enhancement of the dioxygenase by dietary fat could be of biological relevance in terms of efficient conversion of β-carotene to vitamin A, when much of β-carotene is absorbed into the intestinal cells. The transcriptional

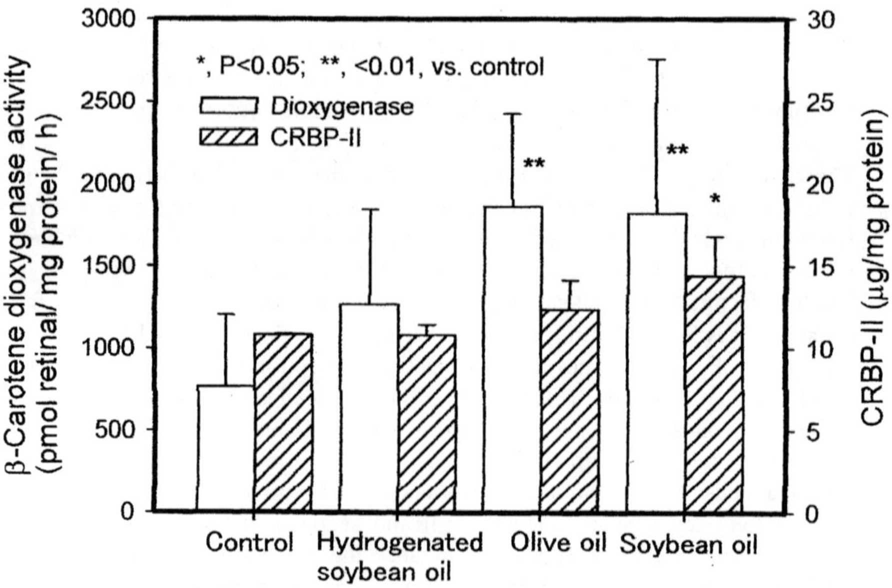

Figure 1. Effects of dietary fats on the levels of β-carotene dioxygenase activity and cellular retinol binding protein type II in rat intestinal mucosa. (Adapted with permission from reference 22. Copyright 1998 The American Society for Nutritional Science)

regulation of CRBP-II by dietary fatty acids has been intensively studied in relation to the peroxisome proliferator-activated receptors (*23*), while it remains unknown whether a similar mechanism for CRBP-II works in regulation of β-carotene dioxygenase. The recent success in the cloning of the dioxygenase (*24,25*) would facilitate the investigation on regulatory mechanism of the dioxygenase at the molecular level.

Non-enzymatic Cleavage of Carotenoids

The oxidation of provitamin A carotenoids to vitamin A is mediated through the specific cleavage at the central double bond by β-carotene dioxygenase. In contrast, non-enzymatic oxidation of carotenoids under *in vitro* oxidative conditions have been reported to produce a number of compounds, which include cleavage products at random positions of conjugated double bonds. 2,6-Cyclolycopene-1,5-diol was reported as an oxidation product of lycopene in human plasma (*26*), and 3-hydroxy-β,ε-carotene-3'-one as a major oxidation product of lutein in human retina (*27*). These oxidation products with a carbon skeleton of carotenoid might be formed *in vivo* by reaction with reactive oxygen species ROS. On the other hand, cleavage products of conjugated double bonds are particularly important, because retinoid-like substances might be formed from diverse carotenoids in addition to provitamin A carotenoids. Retinal and β-apocarotenals were produced under various conditions such as autoxidation in solvent, oxidation with peroxy radical initiators, singlet oxygen, cigarette smoke, and lipoxygenase (*4, 28-33*). A polar oxidation product of β-carotene, 5,8-endoperoxy-2,3-dihydro-β-apocarotene-13-one, which might be formed *in vitro* through cleavage at 13', 14' double bond of β-carotene, was reported to inhibit cell growth and cholesterol synthesis in MCF-7 mammary cancer cells (*34*). Furthermore, 4-oxo-retinoic acid, which was formed as an oxidation product at central double bond of canthaxanthin by incubation in cell culture medium, activated RARβ gene promoter and enhanced gap junctional communications (*35,36*). 3-Hydro-4-oxo-7,8-dihydro-β-ionone and 3-hydroxy-4-oxo-β-ionone were identified as the metabolites of canthaxanthin in rats and astaxanthin in rat hepatocytes, respectively (*37,38*). These two metabolites suggest that the cleavage at the 9', 10' double bond of the respective carotenoids occurs in biological tissues. Moreover, oxidized carotenoid preparations have recently been shown to have adverse effects on biological tissues (*39-43*). These observations strongly suggest that carotenoids are oxidized by reaction with ROS in biological tissues and that some products have potential biological effects, whether beneficial or harmful. Thus, it is worth evaluating the biological effects of oxidation products as well as intact carotenoids.

The cleavage reaction of lycopene, one of typical non-provitamin A carotenoids was investigated (*44*). Lycopene was solubilized in three different media, toluene, Tween 40 aqueous solution, and liposomal suspension, which was used as a model for biological tissues. The lycopene was autoxidized by incubating at 37°C and gave a number of oxidation products with absorption in the UV-VIS region. Among them, a series of carbonyl compounds with different chain length were formed by cleavage of conjugated double bonds of lycopene. Eight cleavage products, namely of 3,7,11-trimethyl-2,4,6,10-dodecatetraen-1-al, 6,10,14-trimethyl-3,5,7,9,13-pentadecapentaen-2-one, *acyclo*-retinal (3,7,11,15,-tetramethyl-2,4,6,8,10,14-hexadecahexaen-1-al), apo-14'-lycopenal, apo-12'-lycopenal, apo-10'-lycopenal, apo-8'-lycopenal, and apo-6'-lycopenal were identified (Figure 2). This result was consistent with the autoxidation of β-carotene in organic solvents (*29,30*). Furthermore, *acyclo*-retinoic acid (3,7,11,15,-tetramethyl-2,4,6,8,10,14-hexadecahexaenoic acid), an acyclic analogue of retinoic acid, was also detected as an oxidation product of lycopene. The incubation of 50 μM lycopene solubilized in liposome for 24 h produced 64 nM *acyclo*-retinal and 1-2 nM *acyclo*-retinoic acid. Although the amount of *acyclo*-retinoic acid formed was far less than that of *acyclo*-retinal in aqueous media, pig liver homogenate showed a remarkable ability to convert *acyclo*-retinal to *acyclo*-retinoic acid. Thus, *acyclo*-retinoic acid is potentially formed from *acyclo*-retinal, when lycopene is oxidized in biological tissues. The results in this study and in previous reports suggest that any carotenoid with long conjugated double bonds is cleaved at random positions by reacting with ROS in biological tissues. Some of the oxidation products and their metabolites might have biological activity, such as retinoids.

Effects of Oxidized Carotenoids on Proliferation of Cancer Cells

Autoxidation of lycopene produced acyclic analogues of retinal and retinoic acid *in vitro*. It is worth evaluating whether the oxidized lycopene preparation works as a retinoid-like substance, in order to elucidate the potential biological effects of oxidized carotenoids. All-*trans*-retinoic acid is known to induce differentiation of human promyelocytic leukemia HL-60 cells to granulocyte. Moreover, lutein (*45*), lycopene (*46*), saffron carotenoids (*47*) and β-carotene (*45, 46, 48*) inhibit the growth of HL-60 cells by inducing differentiation. However, it is still obscure whether the growth inhibition is caused by the intact carotenoids or by their oxidation products. Therefore, the effects of a series of acyclic carotenoids including lycopene and their oxidized preparations on growth and differentiation of HL-60 cells was evaluated (*49*). Oxidation mixture of each carotenoid was prepared by incubating 1 mM carotenoid in toluene at

37°C for 24 h. The carotenoid preparations were incubated at 6 μM as intact carotenoid with HL-60 cells for 5 days, and thereafter the cell growth and differentiation were evaluated. As shown in Figure 3, ζ-carotene and phytofluene significantly inhibited the cell growth to 45.2 and 68.4 % of the control, respectively. Lycopene tended to inhibit cell growth, whereas phytoene and β-carotene did not inhibit the cell growth. ζ-Carotene and phytofluene were unstable in the medium under the culture condition, although they showed a significant growth inhibition against HL-60 cells. On the other hand, β-carotene was stable during incubation in the medium, followed by lycopene. Surprisingly, the oxidation mixture of phytofluene, ζ-carotene, and lycopene more strongly inhibited the growth of HL-60 cells than the respective intact carotenoids. In particular, lycopene drastically increased the inhibitory effect on the cell growth by oxidation prior to supplementation. The oxidation mixture of β-carotene was far less inhibitory than that of lycopene, although the degree of oxidation was at the same level in both preparations. These results suggest that oxidation products formed from specific carotenoids inhibit cell growth rather than intact carotenoids themselves.

Cell cycle-arrest (*50,51*), enhancement of gap junctional communication (*52*) and induction of apoptosis (*53-55*) and differentiation have been reported as possible mechanisms for growth inhibition of cancer cells by carotenoids. The acyclic carotenoid preparations, which inhibited the growth of HL-60 cells, did not induce differentiation in our study, although some carotenoids were reported to induce differentiation in HL-60 cells. Exposure of HL-60 cells to phytofluene, ζ-carotene and oxidation mixture of lycopene at 10 μM for 24 h induced the morphological changes characterized by reduction of cell volume, chromatin condensation, nuclear fragmentation and production of the apoptotic bodies. An apoptotic DNA ladder was observed in HL-60 cells treated with phytofluene, ζ-carotene and oxidation mixture of lycopene at 10 μM for 24 h, but not in those treated with the purified lycopene (data not shown). Thus, phytofluene, ζ-carotene and oxidation mixture of lycopene induced apoptosis in HL-60 cells. These results indicate that acyclic carotenoids and their oxidation products show an apparent growth inhibition by inducing apoptosis.

These carotenoid preparations were also evaluated to examine if they could affect proliferation of human prostate cancer cells. Phytofluene, ζ-carotene, and lycopene significantly reduced the viability of three prostate cancer cells (*56*). Moreover, each oxidation mixture of these carotenoids also reduced the viability as effectively as the intact carotenoids. These results suggest that oxidation products formed from phytofluene, ζ-carotene and lycopene caused reduction of the cell viability of the human prostate cancer cells as well as HL-60 cells. Isolation and identification of oxidation products, which cause apoptosis induction against HL-60 cells, are currently underway. These results strongly

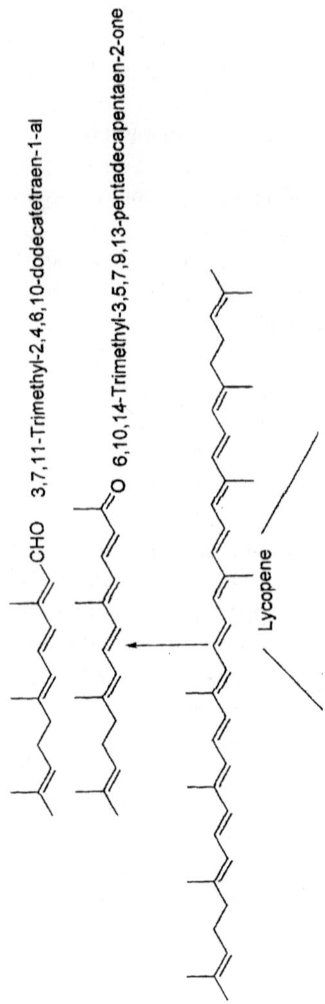
CHO
3,7,11-Trimethyl-2,4,6,10-dodecatetraen-1-al
O
6,10,14-Trimethyl-3,5,7,9,13-pentadecapentaen-2-one
Lycopene

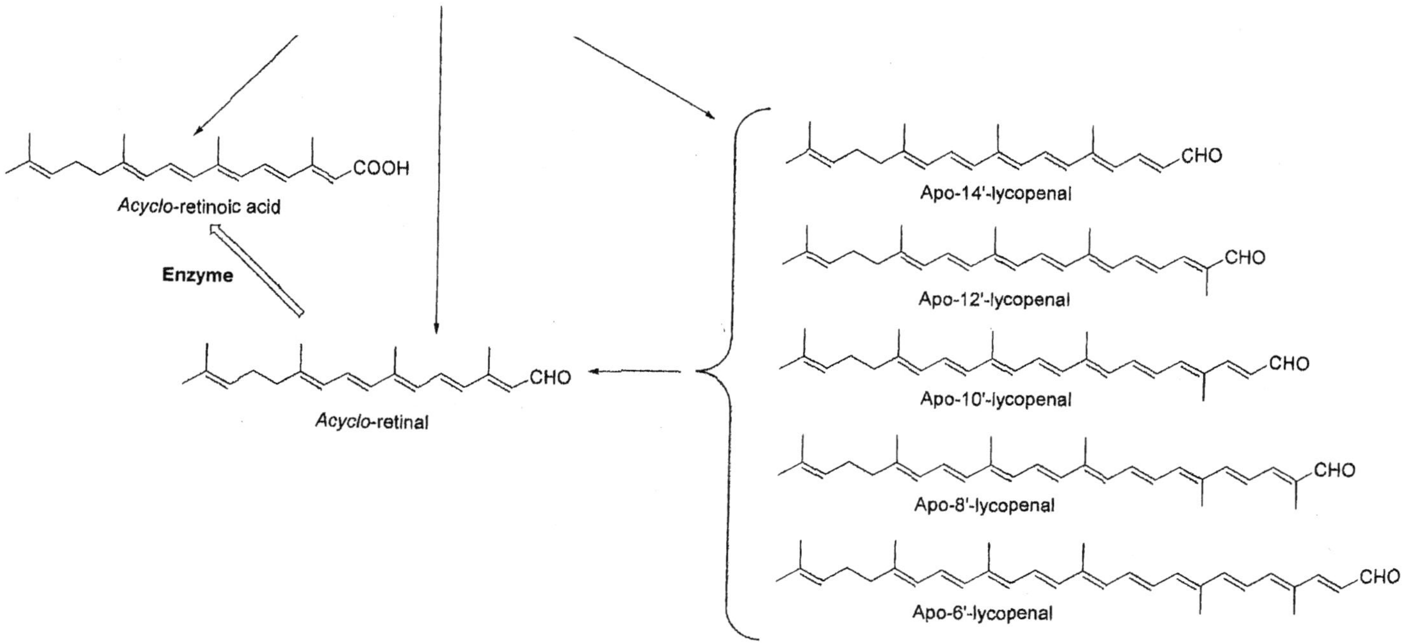

Figure 2. Cleavage products formed from lycopene by autoxidation.

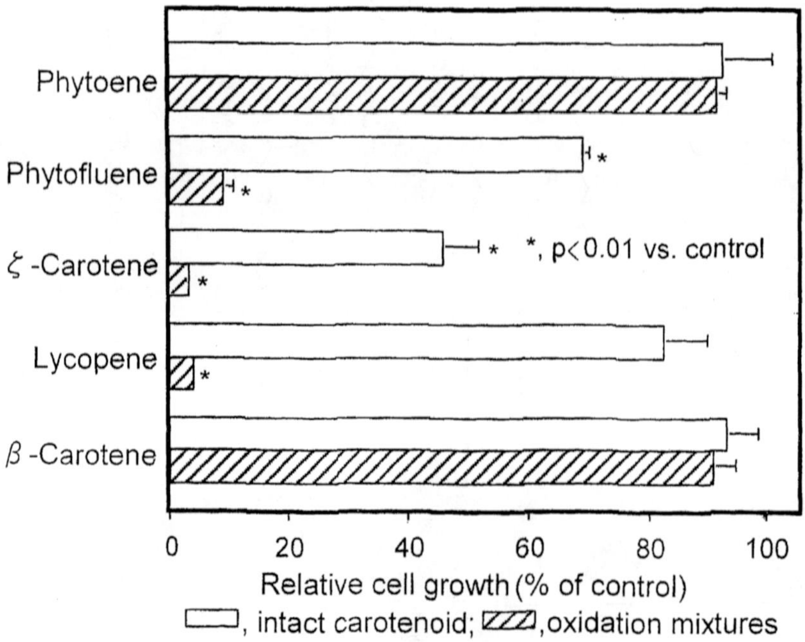

Figure 3. Effects of carotenoid preparations on the growth of HL-60 cells.

suggest that oxidation products as well as intact carotenoids affect proliferation of cancer cells.

Thus, several dietary components were found to affect oxidative metabolism of provitamin A carotenoids. More detailed characterization of regulatory mechanisms is still needed to clarify the bioavailability of provitamin A carotenoids. The non-enzymatic oxidation products of carotenoids have been shown to have the potential to exert biological actions by affecting proliferation of cancer cells. *In vivo* oxidation of carotenoids and its relation to biological actions deserves further studies.

Acknowledgement

This work was supported by the Bio-Renaissance Program of the Ministry of Agriculture, Forestry and Fisheries, Japan and by the PROBRAIN project "Regulation of oxidative stress with phytochemicals from foods" of Bio-oriented Technology Research Advancement Institution.

References

1. Liotenberg, S.; North, H.; Marion-Poll, A. *Plant Physiol. Biochem.* **1999,** *37*, 341-350.
2. Olson, J. A.; Hayaishi, O. *Proc. Natl. Acad. Sci. USA* **1965,** *54*, 1364-1369.
3. Goodman, D. S.; Huang, H. S. *Science* **1965,** *149*, 879-880.
4. Mordi, R.C.; Walton, J.C.; Burton, G.W.; Hughes, L.; Ingold, K.U.; Lindsay, D.A.; Moffatt, D.J. *Tetrahedron* **1993**, *49,* 911-928.
5. Ong, D.E. *J. Nutr.* **1993,** *123*, 351-355.
6. Devery, J.; Milborrow, B.V. *Br. J. Nutr.* **1994,** *72*, 397-414.
7. Lakshman, M.R.; Mychkovsky, I.; Attlesey, M. *Proc. Natl. Acad. Sci. USA* **1989,** *86,* 9124-9128.
8. Nagao, A.; Olson, J. A. *FASEB J.* **1994,** *8,* 968-973.
9. Wang, X. D.; Tang, G. W.; Fox, J. G.; Krinsky, N. I.; Russell, R. M. *Arch. Biochem. Biophys.* **1991,** *285,* 8-16.
10. Nagao, A.; During, A.; Hoshino, C.; Terao, J.; Olson, J. A. *Arch. Biochem. Biophys.* **1996,** *328,* 57-63.
11. Yeum, K. J.; Ferreira, A. L. D.; Smith, D.; Krinsky, N. I.; Russell, R. M. *Free Radic. Biol. Med.* **2000,** *29*, 105-114.

12. Kiefer, C.; Hessel, S.; Lampert, J.M.; Vogt, K.; Lederer, M.O.; Breithaupt, D.E.; von Lintig, J. *J. Biol. Chem.* **2001,** *276,* 14110-14116.
13. During, A.; Nagao, A.; Hoshino, C.; Terao, J. *Anal. Biochem.* **1996,** *241,* 199-205.
14. Grownowska-Senger, A.; Wolf, G. *J. Nutr.* **1970,** *100,* 300-308.
15. Villard, L.; Bates, C. J. *Br. J. Nutr.* **1986,** *56,* 115-122.
16. Vliet, T. van; Vlissingen, M.F. van; Schaik, F. van; Berg, H. van den *J. Nutr.* **1996,** *126,* 499-508.
17. Nagao, A.; Maeda, M.; Lim, B.P.; Kobayashi, H.; Terao, J. *J. Nutr. Biochem.* **2000,** *11*, 348-355.
18. Furr, H. C.; Clark, R. M. *J. Nutr. Biochem.* **1997,** *8,* 364-377.
19. van het Hof, K. H.; West, C. E.; Weststrate, J. A.; Hautvast, J. G. A. J. *J. Nutr.* **2000,** *130*, 503-506.
20. Sugawara, T.; Kushiro, M.; Zhang, H.; Nara, E.; Ono, H.; Nagao, A. *J. Nutr.* **2001**, *in press.*
21. Suruga, K.; Suzuki, R.; Goda, T.; Takase, S. *J. Nutr.* **1995,** *125,* 2039-2044.
22. During, A.; Nagao, A.; Terao, A. *J. Nutr.* **1998,** *128,* 1614-1619.
23. Mochizuki, K.; Suruga, K.; Kitagawa, M.; Takase, S.; Goda, T. *Arch. Biochem. Biophys.* **2001**, *389*, 41-48.
24. von Lintig, J.; Vogt, K. *J. Biol. Chem.* **2000,** *275*, 11915-11920.
25. Wyss, A.; Wirtz, G.; Woggon, W. D.; Brugger, R.; Wyss, M.; Friedlein, A.; Bachmann, H; Hunziker, W. *Biochem. Biophys. Res. Commun.* **2000,** *271*:334-336.
26. Khachik, F.; Spangler, C. J.; Smith, Jr, J. C.; Canfield, L. M.; Steck, A.; Pfander, H. *Anal. Chem.* **1997**, *69*, 1873-1881.
27. Khachik, F; Bernstein, P. S.; Garland, D. L. *Invest. Ophthalmol Vis. Sci.* **1997**, *38*, 1802-1811.
28. Handelman, G. J.; van Kujik, F. J. G. M.; Chatterjee, A.; Krinsky, N. I.; *Free Radical Biol. Med.* **1991**, *10*, 427-437.
29. McClure, T. D.; Liebler, D. C. *Chem. Res. Toxicol.* **1995**, *8*, 128-135
30. Stratton, S. P.; Schaefer, W. H.; Liebler, D. C. *Chem. Res. Toxicol.* **1993**, *6*, 542-547.
31. Baker, D. L.; Krol, E. S.; Jacobsen, N.; Liebler, D. C. *Chem Res. Toxicol.* **1999**, *12*, 535-543.
32. Yeum, K. J.; Lee-Kim, Y. C.; Yoon, S.; Lee, K. Y.; Park, I. S.; Lee, K. S.; Kim, B. S.; Tang, G.; Russell, R. M.; Krinsky, N. I. *Arch. Biochem. Biophys.* **1995**, *321*, 167-174.
33. Wu, Z.; Robinson, D. S.; Hughes, R. K.; Casey, R.; Hardy, D.; West, S. I. *J Agric. Food Chem.* **1999**, *47*, 4899-4906.
34. Hu, X.; White, K. M.; Jacobsen, N. E.; Mangelsdorf, D. J.; Canfield, L. M. *J Nutr. Biochem.* **1998**, *9*, 567-574.

35. Nikawa, T.; Schulz, W. A.; Brink, C. E.; Hanusch, M.; Saag, P.; Stahl, W.; Sies, H. *Arch. Biochem. Biophys.* **1995**, *316*, 665-672.
36. Hanusch, M.; Stahl, W.; Schulz, W. A.; Sies, H. *Arch. Biochem. Biophys.* **1995**, *317*, 423-428.
37. Bausch, J.; Liechti, H.; Oesterhelt, G.; Kistler, A. *Int. Vitam. Nutr. Res.* **1999**, *69*, 268-272.
38. Wolz, E.; Liechti, H.; Notter, B.; Oesterhelt, G.; Kistler, *Drug Metab. Dispos.* **1999**, *27*, 456-462.
39. Gradelet, S.; Astorg, P.; Leclerc, J.; Siess, M. H. *Xenobiotica*, **1996**, *26*, 909-919.
40. Wang, X. D.; Liu, C.; Bronson, R. T.; Smith, D. E.; Krinsky, N. I.; Russell, R. M. *J. Natl. Cancer Inst.* **1999**, *91*, 60-66.
41. Maria, G. S.; Rafael, C.; Gary W. W.; William, A. P. *Free Radic. Biol. Med.* **1999**, *26*, 162-173.
42. Siems, W. G.; Sommerburg, O.; Hurst, J. S.; van Kuijk, F. J. G. M. *Free Radic. Res.* **2000**, *33*, 427-435.
43. Rahman, A.; Parker, R. S. *Nutr. Res.* **2001**, 21, 581-596.
44. Kim, S. J.; Nara, E.; Kobayashi, H.; Terao, J.; Nagao, A. *Lipids* **2001**, *36*, 191-199.
45. Gross, M. D.; Bishop, T. D.; Belcher, J. D.; Jacobs, Jr, D. R. *Nutr. Cancer* **1997**, *27*, 169-173.
46. Amir, H.; Karas, M.; Giat, J.; Danilenko, M.; Levy, R.; Yermiahu, T.; Levy, J.; Sharoni, Y. *Nutr. Cancer* **1999**, *33*, 105-112.
47. Tarantilis, P. A.; Morjani, H.; Polissiou, M.; Manfait, M. *Anticancer Res.* **1994**, *14*, 1913-1918.
48. Biesalski, H. K.; Schäffer, M. Internat. *J. Vit. Nutr. Res.* **1997**, *67*, 357-363.
49. Nara, E.; Hayashi, H.; Kotake, M.; Miyashita, K.; Nagao, A. *Nutr. Cancer* **2001**, *39*, 273-283.
50. Stivara, L.; Savio, M.; Quarta, S.; Scotti, C.; Cazzalini, O.; Rossi, L.; Scovassi, I. A.; Pizzala, R.; Melli, R.; Bianchi, L.; Vannini, V.; Prosperi, E. *Eur. J. Biochem.* **2000**, *267*, 2290-2296.
51. Karas, M.; Amir, H.; Fishman, D.; Danilenko, M.; Segal, S.; Nahum, A.; Koifmann, A.; Giat, Y.; Levy, L.; Sharoni, Y. *Nutr. Cancer* **2000**, *36*, 101-111.
52. Zhang, L. X.; Cooney, R. V.; Bertram, J. S. *Carcinogenesis* **1991**, *12*, 2109-2114.
53. Sumantran, V. N.; Zhang, R.; Lee, D. S.; Wicha, M. S. *Cancer Epidemiol. Biomarkers Prevention* **2000**, *9*, 257-263.
54. Palozza, P.; Maggiano, N.; Calviello, G.; Lanza, P.; Piccioni, E.; Ranelletti, F. O. *Carcinogenesis* **1998**, *19*, 373-376.
55. Muto, Y.; Fujii, J.; Shidoji, Y.; Moriwaki, H.; Kawaguchi, T.; Noda, T. *Am. J. Clin. Nutr.* **1995**, *62*, 1535S-1540S.
56. Kotake-Nara, E.; Kushiro, M.; Zhang, H.; Sugawara, T.; Miyashita, K.; Nagao, A. *J. Nutr.* **2001**, *131*, *in press*.

Chapter 29

Carotenoid and Polyphenol Content of Different Tomato Cultivars and Related Antioxidant Activity

P. G. Pietta[1], P. I. Mauri[1], M. Minoggio[1], C. Gardana[2], I. Iemoli[1], and P. Simonetti[2]

[1]ITB-CNR, V.le F.lli Cervi, 93 20090 Segrate (MI), Italy
[2]Department of Food Science and Microbiology, Via Celoria, 2–20133 Milan, Italy

Different tomato phenotypes were analysed for the content of total polyphenols, selected flavonoids, including flavonols (rutin and a rutin-derivative), flavanones (naringenin and the related chalcone) and carotenoids (lycopene and β-carotene). The identity of these components was based on their chromatographic, ultraviolet and mass spectrometric behavior. All phenotypes were surveyed for their total antioxidant activity (TAA), and correlations betweens TAA values and the content of each group of constituents.

Biological activities of flavonoids and related cinnamic acid derivatives have become well known in recent years. Many studies suggest that these polyphenols have beneficial effects on human health, due to their antioxidant capacity (*1*) and their ability to modulate the activity of different enzymes (*2-4*), interact with specific receptors (*5*), exert vasodilatory effects (*6*) and chelate metal ions such as those of Cu and Fe (*7*).

Based on their daily intake [about 1g (*8, 9*)], which exceeds largely that of other antioxidants (vitamin C, 70-100 mg/day; vitamin E, 7-10 mg/day; β-carotene, 2-3 mg/day), dietary polyphenols may represent an important exogenous defence against the imbalance between prooxidants and antioxidants, that is the oxidative stress.

Indeed, polyphenols play an active role in diminished formation of reactive oxygen species (ROS), since they affect enzymes that catalyse redox reactions, including mitochondrial succinoxidase, NADH-oxidase and enzymes involved in arachidonic acid metabolism (*10*). In addition, the highly oxidizing reactive oxygen species (ROS) are reduced by dietary polyphenols, which in turn are transformed in less aggressive aroxyl radicals (*11*).

Unfortunately, most positive evidence of these activities has been reached using isolated compounds for *in vitro* studies. Thus, it is difficult to extend this evidence to the complex matrix of foods and beverages and *in vivo*.

The occurrence of dietary polyphenols in largely consumed vegetables and their bioavailability need to be known for a proper evaluation of their potential health benefits. In the past years many studies on the uptake and the metabolism of dietary polyphenols have been published, and presently a better information on the absorption and fate of polyphenols from regular food, beverages and supplements is available. By contrast, the polyphenol content of different vegetables consumed in large amounts and with beneficial properties is still poorly defined. This is the case of tomatoes, which represent an important part of the mediterranean diet and are thought to diminish the risk of certain chronic diseases (*12, 13*).

Different factors may influence the polyphenol content of tomatoes, the major being the cultivar followed by climatic conditions and maturity degree. Therefore, it was of interest to evaluate the polyphenol pattern of tomato cultivars selected among those mostly preferred by consumers or processed by food industry.

To this purpose, thirty-one different tomato cultivars were analyzed by spectrophotometric, chromatographic and mass spectrometric methods. Firstly, the content of flavonols (rutin and a rutin-pentoside), flavanones (naringenin and its chalcone), cinnamic acid derivatives (chlorogenic acid, caffeic acid, ferulic acid and a chlorogenic acid analogue), carotenoids (lycopene, β-carotene and lutein) and total polyphenols were determined.

Furthermore, the total antioxidant activity (TAA) of the selected cultivars was assayed, and the obtained TAA values were correlated with the content of tomato components.

Materials and methods

Chemicals

Rutin, naringenin were purchased from Extrasynthese (Genay, France). Ferulic acid, caffeic acid, chlorogenic acid, lycopene, β-Carotene and lutein were purchased from Sigma-Aldrich (Steinheim, Germany). Trolox (6-hydroxy-2,5,7,8-tetramethylchroman-2-carboxylic acid, Aldrich Chemical Co., Gillingham, UK) was used as the antioxidant standard. ABTS [2,2'-azinobis-(3-ethylbenzothiazoline-6-sulfonic acid) diammonium salt] was obtained from Sigma-Aldrich (Dorset-UK). Methanol, acetonitrile and water were HPLC grade from Merck (Darmstadt, Germany).

Extraction of polyphenols fraction from tomatoes

Twenty grams of minced tomatoes were extracted for 3h at 65°C with 200 ml of acetone:water (4:1, v/v). The mixture was filtered and the residue was extracted twice again using the same amount of acetone:water (4:1, v/v). The combined filtrates were evaporated to dryness under vacuum and the residue was dissolved in 10 ml of methanol. The resulting solution was filtered through a 0.22 μm filter and stored at –20°C.

Total polyphenols

The content of total polyphenols was determined by colorimetric assay with Folin-Ciocalteu's phenol reagent, according to Singleton and Rossi (*14*).

Flavonols, flavanones and phenolic acids

The HPLC separation was performed using a Waters 625 LC System (Milford, MA) connected to a Waters model 996 photodiode array detector, equipped with a Rheodyne injector (loop 50 μl) and a Waters Millenium workstation.

The column was a 5 μm X-Terra C_{18} (150x2.1 mm, i.d.) from Waters. The eluents were: (A) 0.1% acetic acid and (B) acetonitrile. Linear gradient was 5% to 35% B in 30 min. Flow-rate was 0.4 ml/min. Acquisition was set at 320 and 350 nm (Spectral acquisition in the range 200-400 nm). Flavonols, flavanones and phenolic acid standards were dissolved in methanol (1 mg/ml) and stored at

0°C. Aliquots of standard solutions in the range of 5-200 μg/ml were injected in HPLC apparatus.

Lycopene and β-carotene

Sample preparation and determination of lycopene and β-carotene was performed according Riso and Porrini (*15*).

Mass spectrometry

Samples were analysed by LCQ_{Deca} ion trap mass spectrometer (Termofinnigan, Milan, Italy) equipped with an electrospray interface (ESI-MS). ESI-MS conditions were optimized by flow injection of rutin standard solution. Analyses were carried out in positive scan mode from m/z 150 to 1000. For MS/MS experiments the collision energy was 30%.

Total antioxidant activity

The TAA of the polyphenol extracts was measured by the ABTS radical cation decolorisation assay, according to Miller and Rice-Evans (*16*).

Results and discussion

Figure 1 shows a typical HPLC cromatogram of a tomato extract. Chlorogenic acid, caffeic acid, ferulic acid, rutin, a chlorogenic acid analogue, naringenin and its chalcone were identified on the basis of their chromatographic and UV characteristics. Concerning peak X, the UV spectrum suggested a rutin-like structure, which was confirmed by comparing its mass spectrum with that of rutin. As indicated by the fragmentation pattern shown in Figure 2, peak X differs from rutin for the presence of a pentose moiety. The nature and the binding site of this pentose is still under investigation, and presently peak X can be assigned as a rutin-pentoside. The content of rutin, its analogue, naringenin and its chalcone in the examined cultivars is shown in Table I. The levels ranged from 0.07 to 2.35 mg/100g for rutin, from 0.03 to 1.38 mg/100g for rutin-pentoside and from 0.04 to 4.90 mg/100g for naringenin and its chalcone. A similar variability was found for the phenolic acids, which were mainly represented by chlorogenic acid ranging from 0.03 to 0.58 mg/100g followed by caffeic acid with a content of up to 0.1 mg/100g (Table II).

Total polyphenols of the examined cultivars were present at higher concentrations (13.15 ± 1.15 mg/100 g, range 4.43 - 25.84 mg/100g), and this may be due to the lack of specificity of the Folin assay.

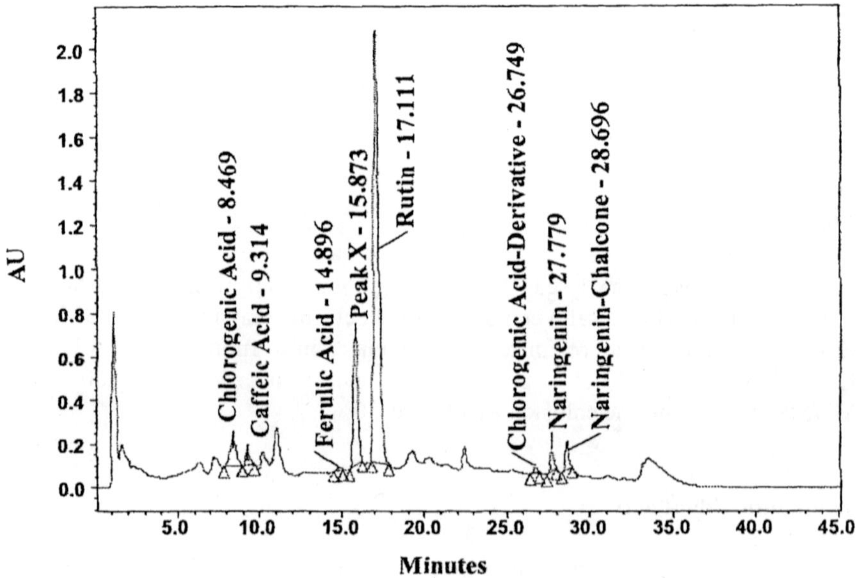

Figure 1. Typical HPLC chromatogram of a tomato extract

Table I. Flavonols and flavanones of selected tomato cultivars (mg/100 g)

	Rutin Pentoside	*Rutin*	*Naringenin + Naringenin Chalcone*
Means ± SE	0.32 ± 0.06	0.74 ± 0.12	0.68 ± 0.16
Range	0.03 – 1.38	0.07 – 2.35	0.04 – 4.90

Table II. Phenolic acids of selected tomato cultivars (mg/100 g)

	Chlorogenic acid	*Caffeic acid*	*Ferulic acid*	*Chlorogenic acid analogue*
Means ± SE	0.20 ± 0.03	0.03 ± 0.01	0.01 ± 0.01	0.02 ± 0.01
Range	0.03 – 0.58	0.00 – 0.10	0.00 – 0.01	0.00 – 0.07

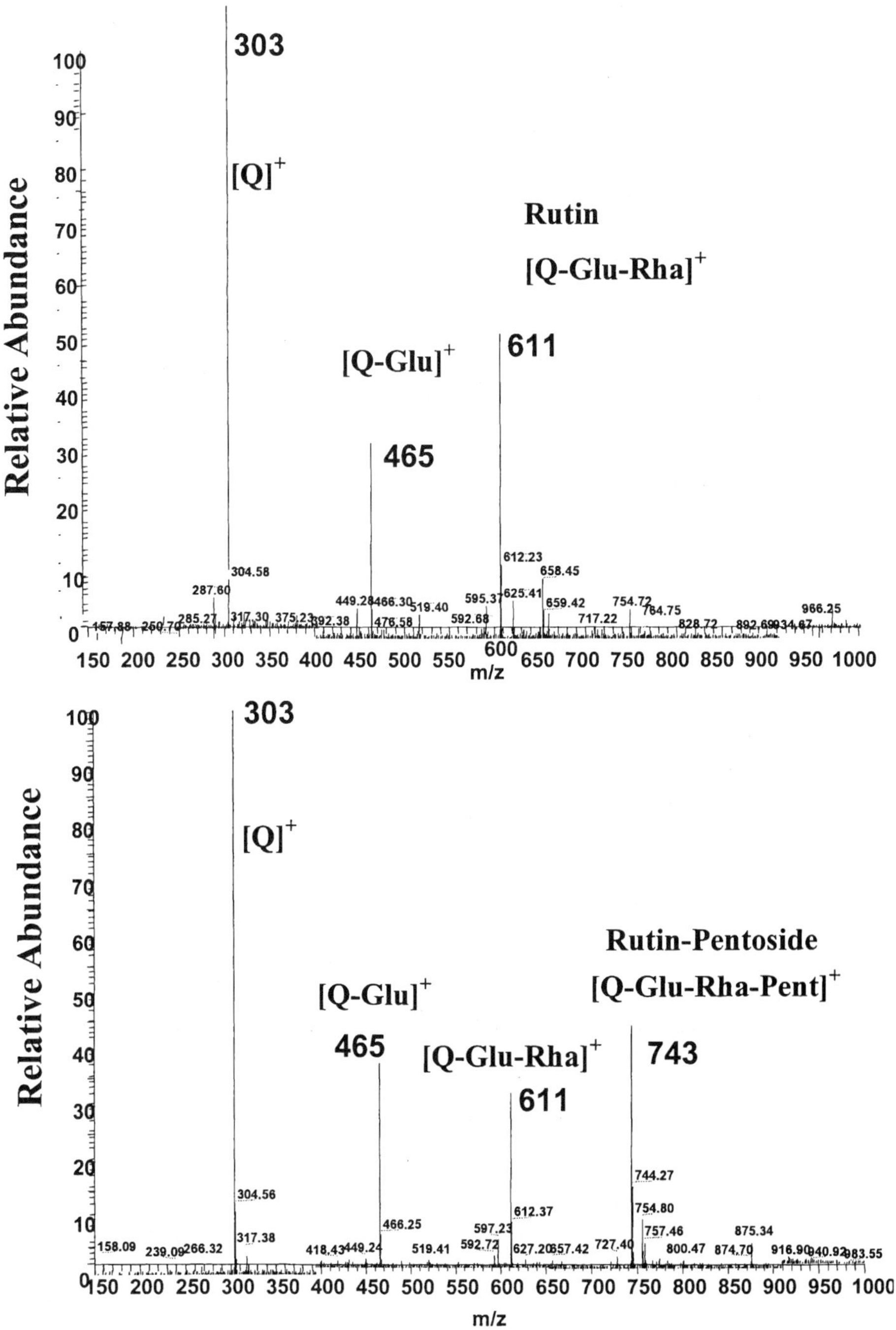

Figure 2. MS/MS of rutin (top) and rutin-pentoside (bottom)

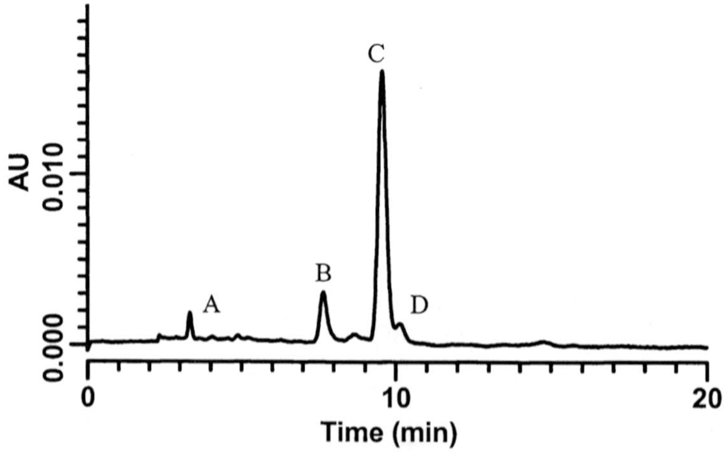

Figure 3. Carotenoids of tomato extract. A = lutein, B = β-carotene, C = trans-lycopene, D = cis-lycopene

Figure 3 shows a typical HPLC of lycopene, β-carotene and lutein in the selected samples.

As for the other components, the contents of lycopene (concentration from 0 to 17 mg/100g) and β-carotene (from 0.12 to 13.54 mg/100g) were scattered over a large range (Table III).

Table III. Carotenoids of selected tomato cultivars (mg/100 g)

	lycopene	*β-carotene*
Means ± SE	5.38 ± 0.90	1.18 ± 0.40
Range	0.00 – 17.00	0.12 – 13.54

Each tomato extract was analysed for its TAA (Table IV), and the obtained values were in good correlation with the total polyphenol content (Figure 4).

When considering the contribution of each polyphenol sub-class to TAA, an acceptable correlation was obtained for phenolic acids ($R^2 = 0.7796$). No correlation between TAA values and flavonols and flavanones was found.

Table IV. Total antioxidant activity of selected tomato cultivars (mmol/ g)

	TAA
Means ± SE	1.30 ± 0.10
Range	0.60 – 2.30

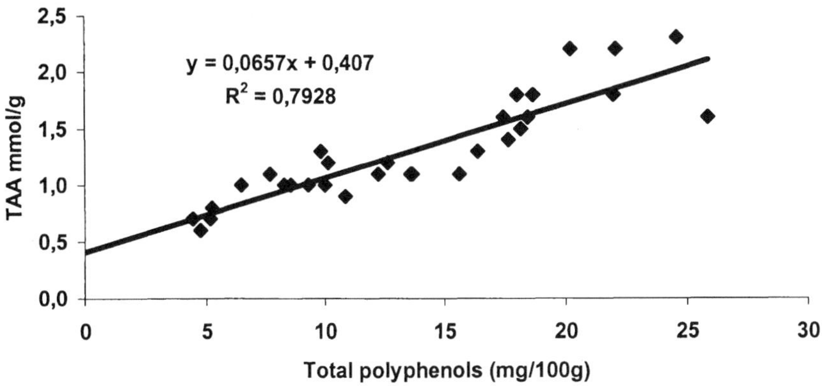

Figure 4: Correlation between TAA and total polyphenols

These results are not surprising, since components present in the polyphenolic extracts at levels higher than those of phenolic acids, rutin/rutin-pentoside and naringenin/naringenin chalcone are responsible for the total antioxidant activity.

Concerning a possible relationship between the content of lycopene and that of polyphenols, it can be assumed that cultivars with low lycopene content have higher concentrations of rutin/rutin-pentoside and naringenin/naringenin chalcone (Figure 5).

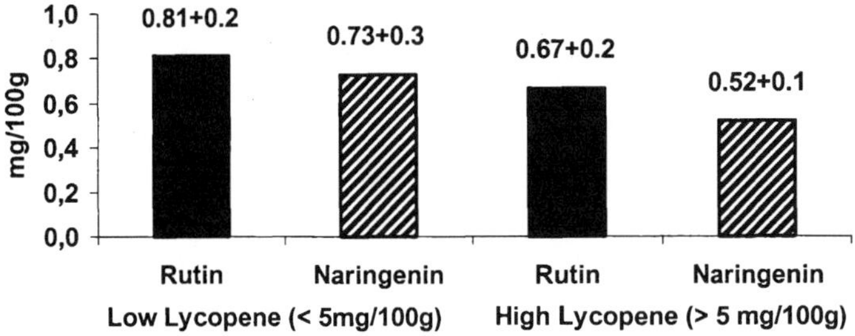

Figure 5. Flavonols and flavanones in tomato cultivars with low and high lycopene content

However, in the case of a cultivar producing almost exclusively high levels of lycopene, the trend observed for most cultivars is reversed, in the sense that also rutin/rutin-pentoside and naringenin/naringenin chalcone levels are high. By contrast, another cultivar synthetising mainly β-carotene was poor in both rutin/rutin-pentoside and naringenin/naringenin chalcone.

Conclusions

Based on the results, it may be concluded that total antioxidant activity (TAA) of the examined tomato cultivars is mainly correlated to the content of total polyphenols, and this reinforces the need for further studies on the chemical identity of all phenolics present in tomatoes (as well as in other common vegetables).

Acknowledgements

The authors acknowledge the contribution of Enrico Rosti to this work. COPOM is acknowledged for its support.

References

1. Pietta, P.G. *J. Nat. Prod.* **2000**, *63,* 1035-1042.
2. Kameoka, S.; Leavitt, P.; Chang, C.; Kuo, S.M. *Cancer Letters* **1999**, *146,* 161-167.
3. Huang, Y.T.; Hwang, J.J.; Lee, P.P.; Ke, F.C.; Huang, J.H.; Huang, C.J;. Kandaswami, C.; Middleton, E.; Lee, M.T. *Br. J. Pharm.* **1999**, *128,* 999-1010.
4. Kavutcu, M.; Melzig, M.F. *Pharmazie.* **1999**, *54*, 457-459.
5. Liang, YuChih.; Chen, YenChou.; Lin, YuLi.; Lin-Shiau, ShoeiYn.; Ho ChiTang.; Lin, JenKun. *Carcinogenesis.* **1999**, *20,* 733-736.
6. Ko, F.N.; Huang, T.F.; Teng, C.M. *Biochimica et Biophysica Acta - General Subjects.* **1991**, *1115,* 69-74.

7. Cook, N.C.; Samman, S. *Nutr. Biochem.* **1996**, *7,* 66-76.
8. Pietta, P.G. and Simonetti, P. *Biochem. Mol Biol. Int.* **1998**, *44,* 1069-1074.
9. Kuhnau, J. *World Rev. Nutr.Diet.* **1976**, *24,* 117-191.
10. Middleton, E.J.R. and Kandaswami, C. *The flavonoids: advances in research since 1986.* Harborne, J.B. Ed.; Chapman and Hall: London, 1993, p 619-652.
11. Jovanovic, S.V.; Steenken, S.; Simic, M.G.; Hara, Y. *Flavonoids in health and disease;* Rice-Evans, C.A.; Packer, L. Eds.; Dekker: New York, 1997; p 137-161.
12. Agarwal, S.; Rao, A.V. *Drug Metabolism & Drug Interactions.* **2000**, *17,* 189-210.
13. Agarwal, S.; Rao, AV. *CMAJ.* **2000**, *163,* 739-744.
14. Singleton, V.L.; Rossi, J.A. *Am. J. Enol. Vitic.* **1965**, *16,* 144-158.
15. Riso, P.; Porrini, M. *Internat. J. Vit. Nutr. Res.* **1997** *67,* 47-54.
16. Miller, N.J. and Rice-Evans, C.A. *Free Rad. Res.* **1997** *26,* 195-199.

Chapter 30

Garlic Chemistry: Chemical and Biological Properties of Sulfur-Containing Compounds Derived from Garlic

Yukihiro Kodera, Hiromichi Matsuura, Hiromichi Sumiyoshi, and Shin-ichiro Sumi

Healthcare Research Institute, Wakunaga Pharmaceutical Company, Ltd., 1624, Shimokotachi, Koda-cho, Takata-gun, Hiroshima 739–1195, Japan

Garlic (*Allium sativum* L.) is rich in biologically active organosulfur compounds. Although intact garlic cloves contain a limited number of organosulfur compounds, such as alliin, methiin and γ-glutamyl-S-alk(en)yl-cysteines, processing initiates a cascade of chemical transformation reactions. Allicin is one of the well-known transformation compound, however, it is highly unstable and reactive, and quickly decomposes into other organosulfur compounds including alk(en)ly-polysulfides, ajoenes and vinyldithiins. Thus, allicin is a transient compound and likely only its transformation compounds contribute to the health benefits of garlic. Recently, biological activities of water-soluble organosulfur compounds derived from garlic, such as S-allyl-L-cysteine and S-allylmercapto-L-cysteine, have become the center of attention because they are stable, odorless and safe. Studies on structure-activity relationships have revealed that the S-allyl group plays an important role in the pharmacological activities of organosulfur compounds derived from garlic. Further, consumption of garlic shows feasibility to prevent cancer and affect immunomodulation or enhancement of the immune systems.

For thousand of years, people have used garlic for medicinal purposes because they were aware of the existance of its biologically active constituents from their own experience. One may ask in what form(s) the garlic yielded such benefits. Various processing methods have been noted in the historical remedies using garlic for treatment and healing (*1-4*). It is generally believed that the biological activities of garlic are derived from organosulfur compounds, however, intact constituents in raw garlic do not have strong biological activities. There is a legend called "***Four Thieves' Vinegar***" that states that the lives of four condemned criminals were saved from terrible plague in Marseilles by drinking a concoction consisting of macerated garlic in wine, and this legend is still in circulation today (*5*). Macerated preparation do not contain the allicin which has strong antimicrobial activity (*3,4*), but it might be possible that there were other beneficial compounds derived from garlic in that ***Vinegar***. Processing activates constituents in garlic preparations through enzymatic and/or chemical reactions and composition of generated compound varies greatly depending on the processing method employed.

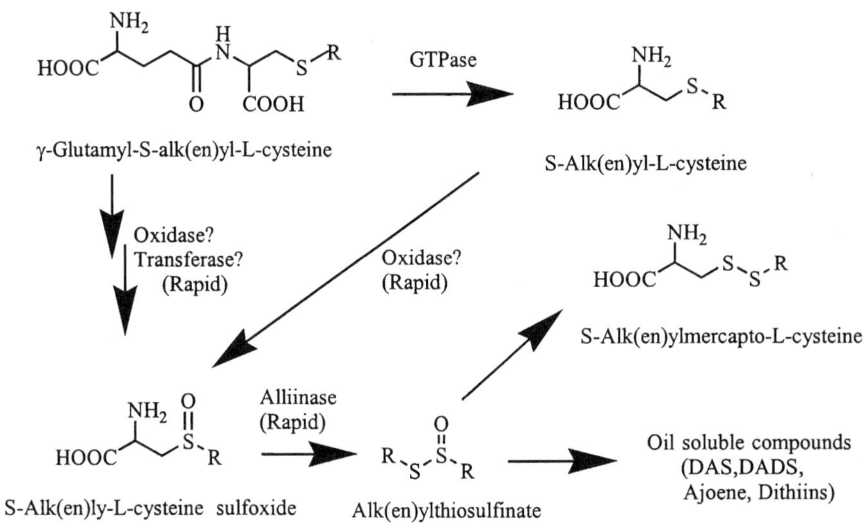

Figure 1. Key reaction pathway in transformation reaction of sulfur containing compound derived from garlic

Additionally, processing methods greatly effect biological activities of resulting preparations. In this chapter, the effect of processing on chemical constituents and biological activities of garlic preparation will be discussed and potential benefits of various processing methods be elucidated.

Processing

Intact garlic contains sulfur constituent such as S-alk(en)yl-L-cysteine sulfoxides and γ-glutamyl-S-alk(en)yl-L-cysteines. These constituents in garlic dramatically change to other compounds by processing (Figure 1). Processing involves various reactions and these reactions greatly affect constituents in each preparation (Table 1) (*3,4*). In the garlic cells, S-alk(en)yl-L-cysteine sulfoxide (for example, alliin) stably exists as the end product which is produced from S-alk(en)yl-L-cysteine and/or γ-glutamyl-S-alk(en)yl-L-cysteines by hypothetical oxidase and/or transferase (Figure 1). However, once garlic is processed, C-S lyase, such as alliinase, stored in vacuoles produces alk(en)ylthiosulfinates (for example, allicin) which are highly reactive. Produced

Table I. Content of Organosulfur Containing Compounds in Intact Garlic and Garlic Preparations

	Raw Garlic	FD[a)] Garlic	Garlic Oil	Oil[b)] Macerate	Soaking (AGE)[c)]	Heating[d)]
Alliin	5.4-14.5	>1	ND	ND	0.01>	>1
Allicin	ND	ND	ND	ND	ND	ND
Allicin-Release[e)]	>2	>1	ND	ND	ND	ND
Dithiin	ND	ND	ND	0.6-0.7	ND	ND
Ajoene	ND	ND	ND	0.02-0.12	0.01	ND
Allylpoly-Sulfide	ND	ND	>1	0.06-0.22	0.01-0.05	0.01>
γ-GSAC	1.9-8.2	>1	ND	ND	0.2-1	>1
SAC	Trace	Trace	ND	ND	>1	0.01>
SAMC	ND	ND	ND	ND	0.01-0.05	ND

NOTE: *a)* Freeze dried garlic. *b)* Clear oil isolated from maceration or grinding of garlic cloves in vegetable oil. *c)* Sliced garlic was soaked with alcohol containing water for more than 10 months at room temperature. *d)* Whole raw garlic was boiled for one hour. e) Amount of allicin produced after homogenating or mixing with water. γ-GSAC ; γ-glutamyl-S-allyl-L-cysteine, SAC ; S-allyl-L-cysteine, SAMC ; S-allylmercapto-L-cysteine, ND ; Not detected. Units are mg/g-materials.

alk(en)ylthiosulfinates then transform to various compounds through non-enzymatic chemical cascade reactions. Thus, alk(en)ylthiosulfinates are important transient compounds that generate various organosulfur compounds via chemical transformations (genaration of oil soluble compounds, see Figure 1) (*6*).

On the other hand, enzymatic reaction was related to production of S-alk(en)yl-L-cysteines form γ-glutamyl-S-alk(en)yl cysteines, such as production of S-allyl-L-cysteine (SAC), in processing. GTPase activity during aging of garlic, which is one of soaking in an aqueous-alcoholic solution, was examined and it was observed that its activity was retained even after 300 days with a resultant increase in SAC content (Figure 2) (*7*). There is more evidence that GTPase relate to SAC production. When cysteine was added to the soaking mixture, the amount of SAC produced was dramatically increased as compared with no addition of L-cysteine (Figure 3). The assumed reaction mechanism is that added cysteine became a glutamin acceptor on transformation of SAC and SAC was released by GTPase, as shown in Figure 4. Processing under around room temperature, such as soaking, generates various compounds because both chemical and enzymatic reactions are able to work at same time, however, enzymatic reactions, such as reaction of GTPase, are inhibited at high temperatures (i.e. distillation or heating). Therefore, the number of compounds in preparation produced under high temperature treatment are fewer than those produced under low temperture treatment (Table I).

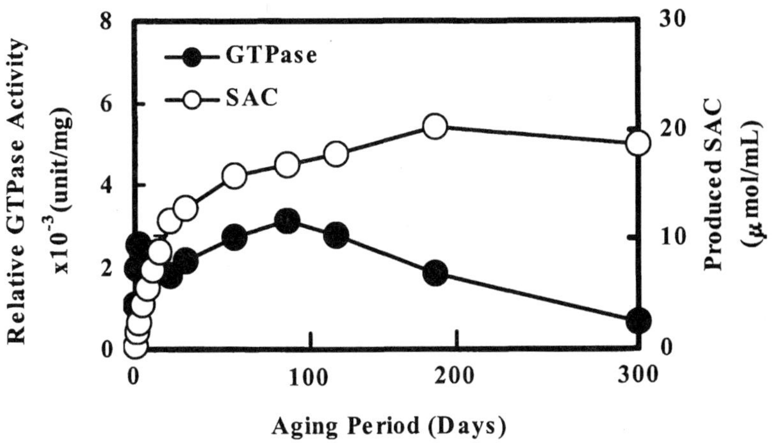

Figure 2. The content of S-allyl-L-cysteiene and GTPase activity during aging process.

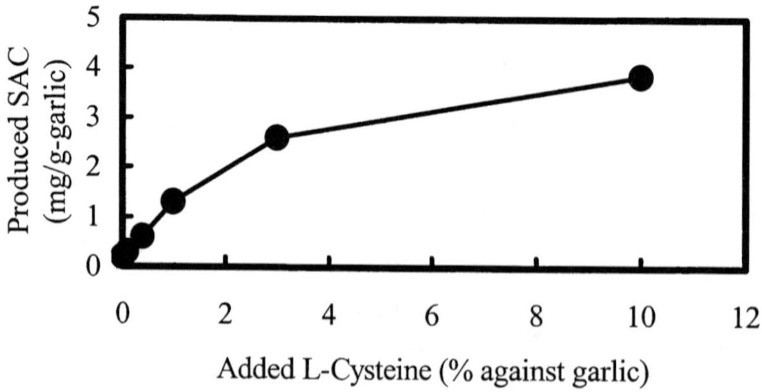

Figure 3. Effect of L-cysteine addition for S-allyl-L-cysteine (SAC) production. The preparation was incubated at 37°C for 7 days after addition of L-cysteine.

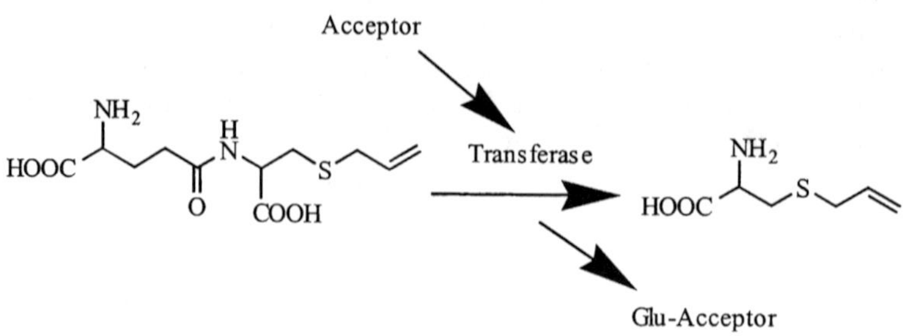

Figure 4. Hypothetical mechanism of S-allyl-L-cysteine production with addition of L-cysteine.

Processing affects not only the cascade reactions of sulfur containing compounds, but also other constituents, such as saponins, amino acids and carbohydrates, among others. For example, proto-eruboside-B, one of intact saponins in raw garlic, transforms to eruboside-B during the extraction process. Eruboside-B inhibits tumor promotion activity but intact compound, proto-eruboside-B, does not (*8,9*). Recently, several kind of strong and unique antioxidants, Nα-(1-deoxy-D-fructos-1-yl)-L-arginine (*10*) and 1,2,3,4-tetrahydro-β-carbolines, were isolated from aged garlic extract (AGE). These antioxidants did not exist in raw garlic, but increased upon soaking, and their antioxidant activity was stronger than ascoribic acid in H_2O_2 scavenging assay system. Additionally, processing change the potency of biological activity of garlic. Two research groups investigated the improvement of peripheral blood circulation by garlic preparations, independently (*11,12*). They observed that the effectiveness of AGE and potency of AGE was greater than raw garlic or heat-treated garlic on both rats and human. Considering the above findings, processing is obviously necessary for taking advantage of the beneficial biological activity of garlic.

Pharmacokinetic Behavior and Metabolism

To evaluate biological activities of herbs or chemicals for human health promotion, it is also important to assess chemistry, pharmacokinetic behavior and metabolism of action of these mateirals. To find interaction or metabolism of sulfur-containing compounds with biological materials, some representative compounds derived from garlic, such as allicin, diallyldisulfide (DADS), ajoene, vinyldithiins, were incubated with blood and allylmercaptan was detected (*13*). Additionally, DADS, one representative compound in garlic oil, was also detected along with allylmercaptan in our follow-up reinvestigations. A perfusion experiment of DADS in isolated rat livers yielded allylmercaptan as the metabolite (*14*). Pushpendran *et al.(15)* found that sulfates were recovered as main metabolite in the mouse liver cytosol fraction in their pharmacokinetic study using radioactive DADS. Therefore, it is suggested DADS was first reduced to allylmercaptan which was then oxidized to sulfate by hepatic oxidases. Vinyldithiins, representative compounds in oil macerate, were quickly absorbed (T_{max}:15min, rat) and metabolic rate between 1,2-dithiin and 1,3-dithiin was very different in peroral administration. A part of both administrated vinyldithiins remained in the kidney and fat tissue even 24 hours after administration, but metabolites were not identified (*16*). Metabolites and metabolic pathway of vinyldithiins is still unknown. There are no clear reports which have studied the absorption and detection of allicin, but not transformation compounds, in a living body, though more than half a century has passed since allicin was discovered. When allicin was added to whole blood, allicin completely disappeared in whole blood within a few minutes and allylmercaptan and DADS were identified (*6,13,17*). In addition, it has been shown that hemoglobin in the blood rapidly and irreversibly changes to methemoglobin through interaction with allicin. High reactivity is one chemical property of allicin, thus, detection of allicin and its mechanism of action in living body is difficult to elucidate.

Table II. LD_{50} Values of S-Allyl-L-cysteine in Rat and Mice

Route	Sex	LD_{50} values(g/kg)[a] Mice	Rat
p.o.	Male	8.89	10.94
	Female	9.39	9.50
i.p.	Male	6.91	3.34
	Female	3.65	3.34

NOTE : *a)* LD_{50} values were calculated by Probit method.

On the other hand, alliin, a hydrophilic compound in the intact garlic and the precursor of allicin, was investigated along with its pharmacokinetic behavior including allicin production in *in vivo* (*4,6,14,17*). T_{max} of this compound was 10 min and its bioavailability was 16.5%. In addition, no evidences was found of allicin production in living bodies. S-Allyl-L-cysteine, produced during the soaking of garlic in aqueous alcohol, was investigated in detail. This compound was quickly absorbed and excreted slowly in both experimental animals and humans. Bioavailability of SAC was very high, in mice – 100%, in dog – 87%. N-Acetyl-S-allyl-L-cysteine was identified as the metabolite of this compound in rats urine after administration of SAC (*6*) and also human urine after consumption of garlic (*18*). Toxicity of this compound was very weak and its

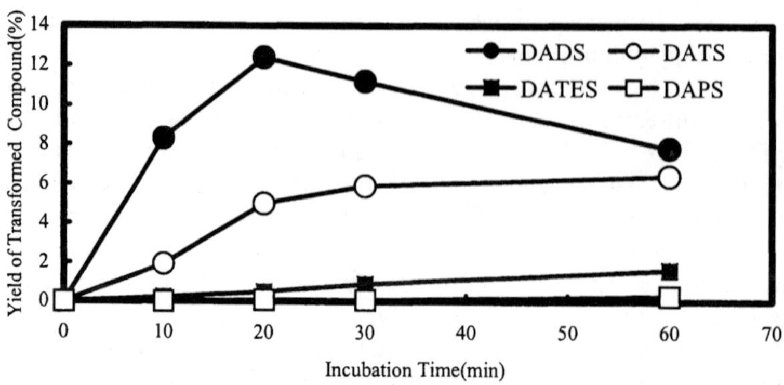

Figure 5. Biotransformation of S-allylmercapto-L-cysteine (SAMC) in rat liver homogenate. DADS, diallyldisulfide; DATS, diallyltrisulfide; DATES, diallyltetrasulfide; and DAPS, diallylpentasulfide.

LD_{50} was >8.8g/kg on *p.o.* and >3.3g/kg on *i.p.* in mice and rat, respectively (Table II), and subacute toxicity test revealed non-toxic dose for rats with as much as 250mg/kg. LD_{50} values of this compound were almost the same as for essential amino acids such as Ile (6.81g/kg), Leu(6.54g/kg), Phe(5.28g/kg) and Met(4.31g/kg) in rat by *i.p.* administration (*19*).

Another hydrophilic compound, S-allylmercapto-L-cysteine (SAMC), showed a unique metabolite profile in which allylpolysulfides (S=2~5) gradually increased after incubation of SAMC with rat liver homogenete (Figure 5) (*6*). Allylpolysulfides have been reported to have protective effects on lipid peroxidation in a rat liver microsome. SAMC has been shown to have antioxidative activity *in vitro* and hepatoprotective effect both *in vitro* and *in vivo*. Therefore, these results suggest that SAMC might be responsible for some of biological activity of garlic through biotransformation.

Considering these findings, metabolic passway shown in Figure 6 suggests that the allyl-$(S)_n$- group containig compounds (n>1) might be first reduced to allylmercaptan and then either oxidized to SO_4^{2-} by hepatic oxidases or reversibley transformed to allylpolysulfides (*15*). These reactions may occur concurrently.

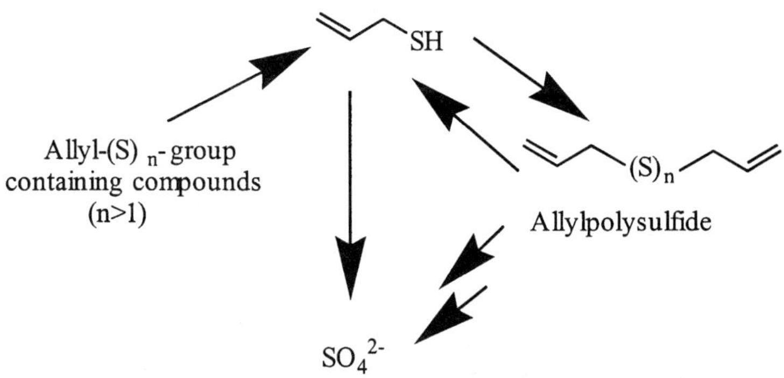

Figure 6. Hypothetical metabolic passway of allyl - $(S)_n$- group containing compounds derived from garlic.

Important Structure

It is obvious that sulfur containing compounds derived from garlic are responsible, at least in part, for biological activity of garlic. However, there is little knowledge of specific chemical structures responsible for biological compounds containing S-allyl group were effective. In addition, they revealed the necessity of allyl group being attached to the sulfur atom for manifestation of neurotrophic activity. These findings strongly indicated that the structure of S-allyl group plays important roles in biological activity of sulfur containing compounds derived from garlic.

activity although numerous garlic compounds have been investigated for biological activities. Considering the cascade reaction of sulfur containing compounds following processing and transformation in living bodies, the S-allyl group might be the key structure responsible for biological activity of garlic and for generation of new compounds. To evaluate the importance of S-allyl group, investigations were conducted to reveal the relationships between chemical structure and biological activities.

Inhibition of platelet aggregation was investigated using garlic compounds containing methyl and allyl moieties, and compounds containing the allyl moiety were found to be more active than those containing the methyl moiety (*20*). Hatono *et al.(21)* investigated structure-activity relationship of garlic chemicals and chemopreventive activity using the rat aberrant crypt assay. Figure 7 shows re-evaluation of their results with regard to carbon number, sulfur number, unsaturated bonds and their position. Some relationships were observed among these factors. First, crypt number decreased by increasing of carbon numbers on thioalkyl and thioalkenyl compounds. Second, the crypt number increased by increasing of carbon numbers on alkyl disulfide compounds, and other findings indicated that S-allyl group had the highest potency for colon cancer prevention and was safer than the other groups. Moriguchi *et al. (22)* investigated the importance of the S-allyl group on the survival of neurons using analogues or derivatives of S-allyl-L-cysteine and γ-glutamyl-S-alk(en)yl cysteines. Only

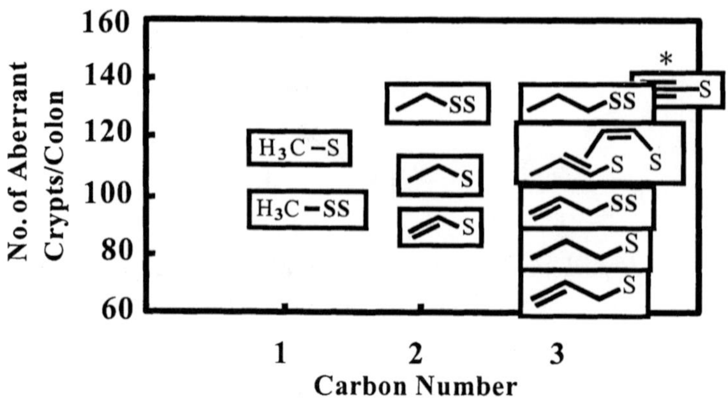

*Figure 7. The relationships between carbon number, sulfur number, unsaturated bond of alk(en)ylsulfides and number of aberrant crypts. Position of each boxes with chemical structure indicates the score of aberrant crypt assay. * ; the score of S-propargyl was almost the same as for propyldisulfide.*

Potency of Cancer Prevention

National Cancer Institute (NCI) has considered numerous natural products for their cancer preventive activity; garlic was given the most crucial position in the NCI experimental foods program (*23*). Recently, several epidemiological or intervention studies for cancer prevention have been reported or are on-going. These reports show that garlic consumption has a tendency to prevent cancer(*24-28*). For example consumption of 28g-garlic/week (about half to one bulb of garlic) is associated with cancer protective effects against stomach and colorectal cancers (*28*).

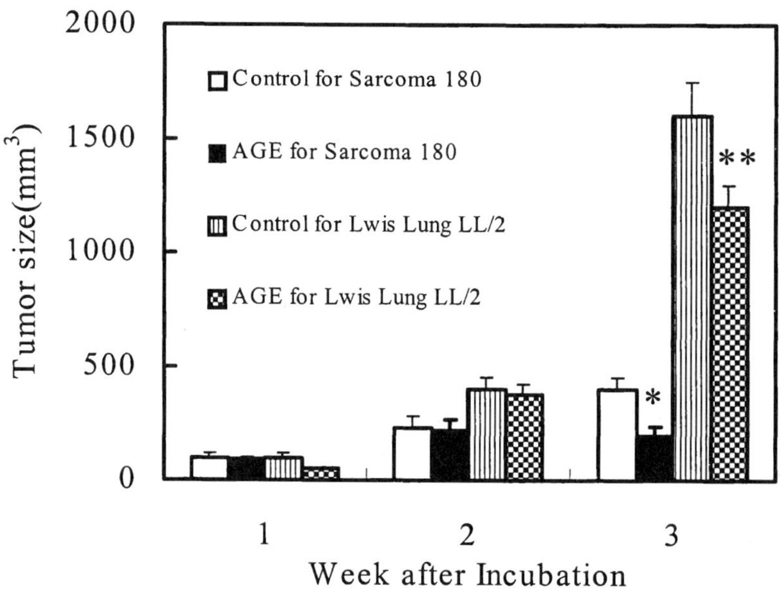

*Figure 8. Anti-tumor activities of aged garlic extract. Astarisks denote significant difference from control : * ; p<0.05 on experiment of Salcoma 180, ** ; p<0.05 on experiment of Lwis Lung LL/2.*

It is well known that there are three steps in the onset of cancer, namely initiation, promotion and progression. Many garlic compounds generated by processing have been reported to be effective for prevention of the onset of cancer through antioxidation mechanism (SAC and allylpolysulfides), antimutagenesis (ajoene and SAC), and apoptosis (ajoene and SAMC), among others (*3,4*). Recently, some researchers have come up with an interest prevention mechanisms related to the immune system. Enhancement of the immune system is not only effective for cancer prevention but also for prevention of other diseases. Kyo *et al. (29)* examined the antitumor activities and immunomodulation of aged garlic extract responsible for the inhibition of tumor growth and stimulation of natural killer (NK) activities. As seen in Figure 8, the size of implanted cancer cell in the AGE-treated group was obviously much smaller than the control group, and NK activity was significantly increased by AGE treatment. Another group observed that garlic extract stimulates the secretion of lymphokines, such as IL-1 and IL-2 (*30*). Therefore, these results indicate that garlic augments cancer prevention through immunomodulation or enhancement of the immune system.

Conclusions

Processing plays very important roles in chemical and biological transformation of garlic constituents and processing has the potential to induce beneficial pharmaceutical activities. Organosulfur compounds derived from garlic were quickly absorbed and metabolites identified contained S-allyl moiety. The S-allyl moiety in organosulfur compounds plays important roles in chemical and biological transformations and biological activity. Further, garlic shows promise for cancer prevention.

Acknowledgements

We greatly thank Miss Brenda Lynn Petesch, M.S., Nutritionist, Supervisor, Research and Development, Wakunaga of America Co., Ltd., for suggestion for our present report.

References

1. Blackwood, J.; Fulder,S. *Garlic, Nature's Original Remedy;* Javelin Books: U.K., 1986.
2. Wilen, J.; Wilen, L. *Garlic: Nature's super healer;* Prentice Hall, Englewood Cliffs, NJ, 1997.
3. Koch, H.P.; Lawson, L.D. *Garlic: The Science and Therapeutic Application of Allium sativum L. and Related Species;* Williams & Wilkins: Baltimore, ML,1996, pp37-52.
4. *Garlic Science (Ninniku no kagaku, Japanese);* Saitoh, H., Eds, Asakura Shoten, Tokyo, 2000, pp107
5. Block, E. *Sci. Am.* **1985,** 252(3), 114-119
6. Kodera,Y. In *Nutraceuticals: Designer Foods III Garlic, Soy and Licorice*; Lachance, P.A., Eds.; Food and Nutrition Press, Inc., Trumbull, CT, 1997; p95.
7. Matsuo, H.; Ogasawara, K.; Yoshida, J.; Sasaoka, T.; Ryu. K. This investigation was performed in Healthcare Institute, Wakunaga Pharm. Co., Ltd., 2000, *Unpublished data.*

8. Matsuura, H.;Ushiroguchi, T.; Itakura. Y.;Hayashi, N.; Fuwa,T, *Chem. Pharm. Bull.,* **1989,** 36, 3659-3663.
9. Matsuura H. In *Nutraceuticals: Designer Foods III Garlic, Soy and Licorice*; Lachance, P.A., Eds.; Food and Nutrition Press, Inc., Trumbull, CT, 1997; p55.
10. Ryu, K.; Ide, N.; Matsuura,H.; Itakura, Y. *J. Nutr. Supplements*, **2001**,131(3S), 972S-976S
11. Okuhara, T. *Jpn. Pharmacol. Ther.* **1994**, 22(8), 335-341.
12. Ushijima, M.; Sumioka, I.; Kakimoto, M.; Yokoyama, K.; Uda, N.; Matsuura, H.; Kyo, E.; Suzuki, A.; Kasuga, S.; Itakura, I.; Brenda, L.P.; Amagase, H. *Phytothrapy Res.* **1997**, 11, 226-230.
13. Lawson, L.D.; Wang, S.J. *Planta Med.* **1993**, 59, A688
14. Egen-Schwind, C.; Eckard, R.; Kemper, F.H. *Planta Med.* **1992**, 58,301-305.
15. Pushpendran, C.K.; Devasagayam, T.P.A.; Chintalwar, G.J.; Banerji, A.; Eapen, J. *Experimentia,* **1980**, 36, 1000-1001.
16. Egen-Schwind, C.; Eckard, R.; Jekat, F.W.; Winterhoff, H. *Planta Med.* **1992**, 58, 8-13.
17. Freeman, F.; Kodera,Y. *J.Agr. Food Chem.* **1995,** 43, 2332-2338
18. Nandke, J.; Spiteller, G. J. Chromatog. **1987,** 421, 1-8
19. Gullino.P.; Winitz, M.; Birnbaum, S.M.; Otey, M.C.; Cornfield, J.; Greenstein, J.P. *Arch. Biochem. Biophys.* **1955**, 58. 253-257
20. Lawson, L.D.; Ransom, D.K.; Hughes, B.G. *Throm. Res.* **1992**, 65, 141-156.
21. Hatono,S.; Wargovich, M.J. In *Nutraceuticals: Designer Foods III Garlic, Soy and Licorice*; Lachance, P.A., Eds.; Food and Nutrition Press, Inc., Trumbull, CT, 1997; p139
22. Moriguchi, T.; Matsuura, H.; Kodera, Y.; Itakura, Y.; Katsuki, H.; Saitoh, H.; Nishiyama, N. *Neurochem. Res.*, **1997**, 22,1449-1452.
23. Caragay, A. B. *Food Technol.*, **1992**, 4, 65-68.
24. You, W.C.; Blot, W.J.; Chang, Y.S.; Ershow, A.; Young, Z.T.; An, Q.; Henderson, B.E.; Fraumeni Jr.J.F.; Wang,T.G., *J. National Cancer Int.* **1989,** 81(2), 162-164.
25. Buiatti, E.; Palli, D.; Decarli, A.; Avellini, C.; Bianchi, S.; Biserni, R.; Cipriani, F.; Cocco, P.; Giacosa, A.; Marubini, E.; Puntoni, R.; Vindigni, C.; Fraumeni Jr., J.; Blot, W. *Int. J. Cancer,* **1989**, 44, 611-616.
26. Steinmetz, K.A.; Kushi, L.H.; Bostick, R.M.; Folsom, A.R.; Potter, J.D. *Am. J. Epidemiol.* **1994,** 139(1), 1-15.
27. Dorant, E.; van den Brandt, P.A.; Goldbohm, R.A. *Cancer Res.* **1994**, 54, 6148-6153.
28. Fleischauer, A.T.; Poole, C.; Arab, L. *Am. J. Clin. Nutr.* **2000**, 72(4), 1047-1052.
29. Kyo, E.; Uda, N.; Suzuki, A.; Kashimoto, N.; Ushijima, M.; Kasuga,S.; Itakura, *Phyomed.*, **1998,** 5(4), 259-267.
30. Burger, R.A.; Warren, R.P.; Lawson, L.D. *Int. J. Pharmacog.* **1993**, 31(3), 169-174.

Chapter 31

Isothiocyanates as Inducers of Phase II Drug-Metabolizing Enzyme: Involvement of Cellular Redox Alteration

Yoshimasa Nakamura

Laboratory of Food and Biodynamics, Graduate School of Bioagricultural Sciences, Nagoya University, Nagoya 464–8601, Japan

A simple system for the rapid measurement of glutathione *S*-transferase placental form (GSTP1) that detoxifies polycyclic aromatic hydrocarbons using the cultured rat liver epithelial cell line, RL34 was recently developed. During the course of our studies, benzyl isothiocyanate (BITC) was isolated from papaya as a strong inducer of GST activity. BITC induced the depletion of glutathione and the generation of reactive oxygen species (ROS) in the cells. The structure-activity relationship of isothiocyanates also indicated that the ROS producing activities closely correlated with their GST inducing potencies. Moreover, the GSTP1 enhancer I (GPEI)-containing region was found to be essential for the induction of GSTP1 gene by BITC. These data suggest the involvement of redox regulation in the induction of GSTP1 by BITC.

Several lines of evidence indicate that phase II enzymes such as NAD(P)H:(quinone-acceptor) oxidoreductase (NQO1) and glutathione *S*-transferase (GST) play a role in the cellular detoxification of genotoxic and carcinogenic chemicals. Recently, two transgenic rodent studies clearly demonstrated that Class π GST (GSTP1), one of the GST isozymes, can profoundly alter the susceptibility to chemical carcinogenesis in mouse skin (*1*) and rat liver (*2*). The Class π rat and human GST isozymes have been shown to be highly efficient in the glutathione (GSH) conjugation of carcinogenic benz[*a*]pyrene derivatives (*3,4*), and widespread environmental pollutants in cigarette smoke and automobile exhaust. Thus, the induction of GSTP1 is regarded as one of the important determinants in the cancer chemoprotection potential of food stuffs or phytochemicals.

Talalay and his colleagues have identified many kinds of inducers of NQO1 activity using murine hepatoma cell lines (*5-7*). Some of them have proven to induce not only NQO1 activity but also GST activity *in vivo* (*6,7*). An antioxidant/electrophile response element (ARE/EpRE; consensus sequence TGACNNNGC) or the related element, regulating both its basal and inducible expression, was mostly found in the 5'-flanking region of the genes of phase II enzymes and may be recognized by a similar series of transcriptional factors (*8*). Thus, an inducer of NQO1 is regarded as a common inducer of phase II enzymes. However, in the case of GSTP1, few intensive studies on inducers in food stuff and their molecular mechanisms have been described. Therefore, we have briefly screened malignant and nonmalignant rat liver cell lines for their sensitivity to GST activity induced by *t*-butylhydroquinone, a well-known phase II inducer (*5,9*). Because normal rat liver epithelial RL34 cells exhibited the greatest enhancement of GST induction in response to *t*-butylhydroquinone treatment, this cell line was utilized for the chemical studies such as the screening and identification of novel type of inducers.

Benzyl isothiocyanate as a GST inducer

Common fruits in Japan were preliminary screened as sources of GST inducers using RL34 cells (*9*), because epidemiological studies have suggested that the intake of fresh fruits reduces cancer risk, particularly for the lung, stomach and pancreas (*10*). The GST-induction potency of EtOAc extracts of a total of 25 samples (part tested; fruit, peel or seed) from 19 fruits were examined. Papaya and avocado fruits exhibited a significant enhancement of GST activity even at a concentration of 25 μg/ml. Thus, the activity-guiding separation of a principal inducer from papaya was performed. The spectroscopic data of the isolated compound were completely identical to those of benzyl isothiocyanate (BITC), that has already been isolated from papaya (*11*) and cruciferous vegetables including cabbage (*12*), and the GST inducing ability in rodents (*13*).

Isothiocyanates (ITCs) are organosulfur compounds that occur as glucosinolates in a variety of cruciferous vegetables such as *Brussica* species (Fig. 1). ITCs have been shown to protect chemical carcinogenesis in experimental animals. In mice, BITC blocked the neoplastic effects of diethylnitrosamine or benz[*a*]pyrene on the lung and forestomach (*14-16*), and a variety of phenylalkyl ITCs reduced the pulmonary carcinogenesis of the tobacco-derived nitrosamine (*17*). The anticarcinogenic effects of ITCs may be related to their capacity to induce phase II enzymes including GSTs,

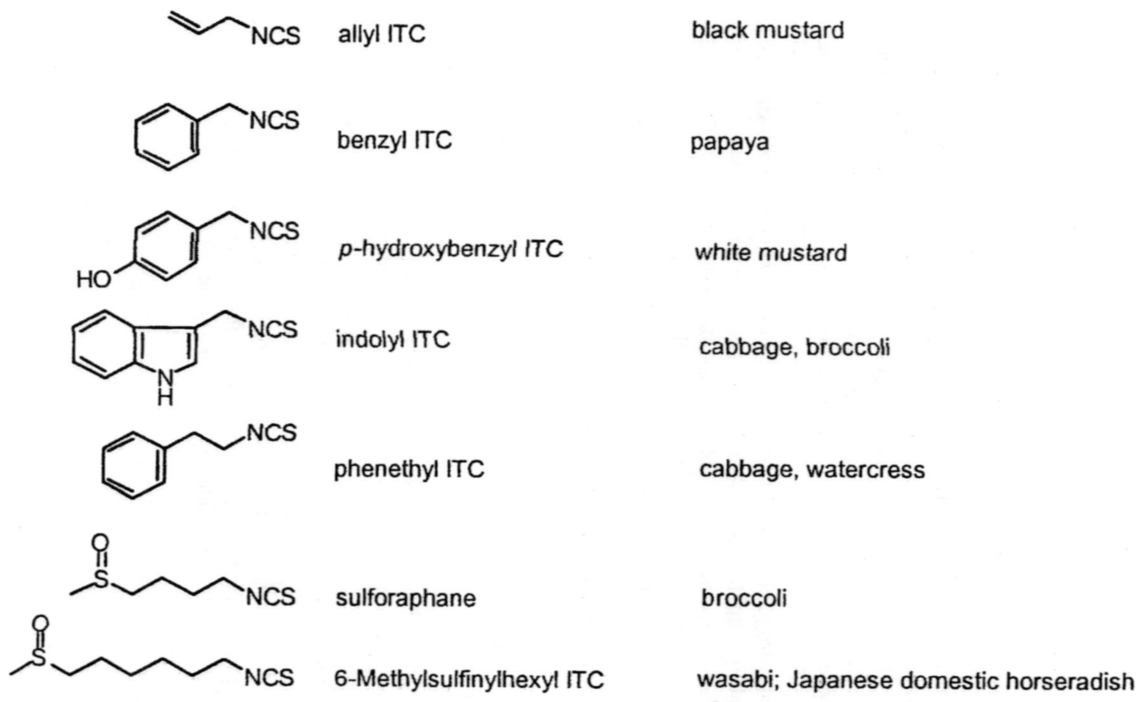

Figure 1. Structures and sources of the representative isothiocyanates.

which are involved in the metabolism of carcinogens. ITCs indeed induce phase II enzymes in rat liver (*18*). BITC is a monofunctional inducer, which induces phase II enzymes but not phase I enzymes, in cultured liver cells (*6*), as confirmed in a recent study (*9*).

Structure-activity relationship of isothiocyanates

Since there are few systematic studies on ITC-induced GST activity or GSTP1 protein elevation, the cells were exposed to a variety of ITCs to examine the effect of ITCs including BITC on the GST activity. The structure-activity relationship of ITCs is summarized in Fig. 2. The ability of the GST induction increased with lengthening of the carbon chain in aliphatic ITCs (C1~6), likely to increase in cellular uptake. Arylalkyl ITCs including BITC and phenethyl ITC showed the most potent inducing ability of the GST activity. Introduction of an electron donating to α-carbon (R-$\underline{C}X_1X_2$-NCS) significantly enhanced the GST activity compared with methyl ITC. The ITC group (-NCS) is essential to express GST activity induction since the corresponding derivatives of BITC, such as thiocarbamate, isocyanate, and thiocyanate, showed no inducing ability. Some of the isocyanates favor reacting with nucleophiles, such as nucleic acids (*19*) and proteins (*20*), and are regarded as mutagens (*21*). From the aspect of a biomolecular-chemical interaction, it is interesting that mutagenic isocyanates lack the GST inducibility, though there is only a small (one atom) difference between isocyanates and ITCs (oxygen atom versus sulfur atom). An analysis by a simple linear regression clearly demonstrated a significant correlation ($P < 0.01$, $r = 0.913$) between the GST activity and GSTP1 protein induction. These results indicated that the induction of GST activity in RL34 cells resulted, at least in part, from the enhanced expression of GSTP1.

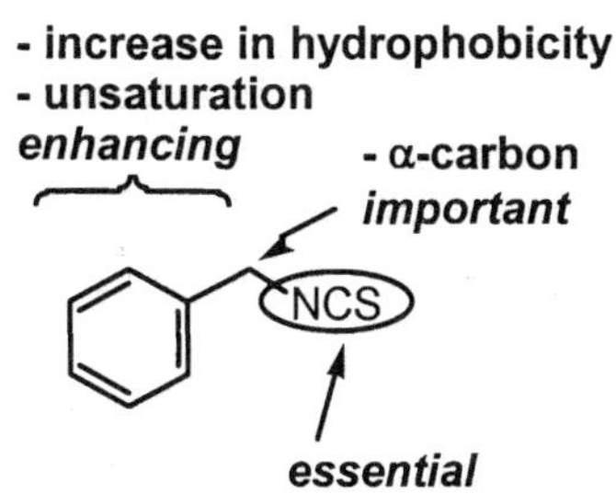

Figure 2. Deduced important structural factors of BITC for GST induction.

Talalay *et al.* (*7*) have speculated that the presence of a proton atom at α-carbon is required for the induction activity. On the other hand, this study revealed for the first time that *p*-nitrophenyl ITC, having no α-proton, exhibited a significant enhancement in the GST activity and GSTP1 protein level. As for the phenyl ITC derivatives, the reactivity of ITC with nucleophiles increases with decreasing density of π-electrons on the carbon atom of the -NCS group by substitution of an electron-withdrawing group at the *para*-position, explainable by Hammett equation theory (*22*). However, as mentioned above, some of isocyanates favor reacting with nucleophiles but lack GST induction potential. Therefore, it is not sufficient to explain that the GST inducibility of the phenyl ITC derivatives is only correlated with their electrophilicity.

Involvement of redox alteration in GST induction by BITC

Recent findings indicate that the GSTA1 gene expression is related to intracellular oxidative stress presumably mediated by hydroxyl radical or the pro-oxidative potential of GSTA1 inducers (*23,24*). It is increasingly recognized that an adequate extent of oxidative stress stimulates a variety of signal transduction pathways under circumstances that do not result in cell death. In a recent study, the treatment of RL34 cells with the major end product of oxidized fatty acid metabolism results in GSTP1 induction (*25*) and shows a quick cellular GSH depletion, generation of intracellular ROS and activation of stress signaling pathways (*26*). We recently observed that BITC-induced enhancement of GST activity was blocked by the antioxidant GSH and enhanced by the thiol blocker diethyl maleate (DEM). These results suggest that the initial signal for GST induction is likely to be transduced to a plausible cytosolic sensor(s) or receptor(s). Talalay and Zhang (*27*) have recently manifested the possibility that cytosolic GSH, as a target of direct alkylation with ITCs, plays a negative regulating role in the phase II induction based on the result that depletion of GSH by buthuonine sulfoximine (BSO) increased the inducer potencies of several ITCs (*27*). We indeed observed that the treatment of BITC, but not inactive phenyl ITC, for 15 min resulted in depletion of the cellular GSH level (Fig. 3). However, downregulation of the cytosolic GSH is unlikely to be an initial signal for GST induction, since BSO, reducing the cytosolic GSH level, showed no GST inducing potency.

The treatment of BITC quickly and significantly enhanced the intracellular ROS production in RL34 cells detected by a fluorescence probe H_2DCF-DA, as demonstrated recently for the first time (Fig. 4). The experiments using the membrane-impermeable catalase and superoxide dismutase also suggested that BITC-induced ROS generation might occur within the cells (*28*). In the structure-activity relationship study of ITCs, the ROS producing activities correlated closely with their GST inducing potencies. The oxidative stress inducible effect of BITC was blocked by the pretreatment of an antioxidant such as GSH or quercetin. The treatment of

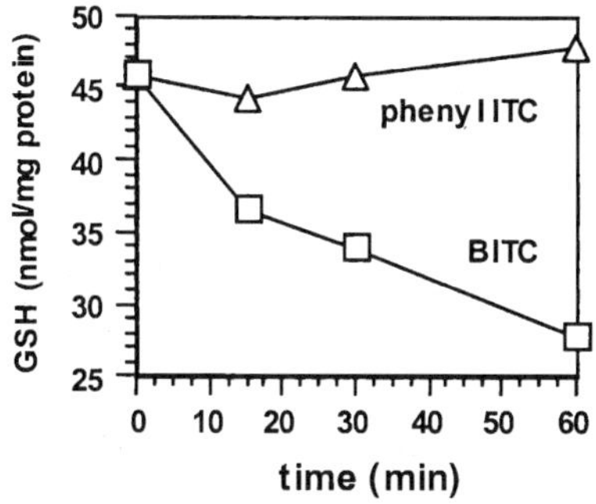

Figure 3. BITC-induced intracellular GSH depletion. The cells were treated with 25 μM BITC (open square) or phenyl ITC (open triangle) for different time intervals. Intracellular GSH levels were coloremetrically measured using commercial kit GSH-400 (BIOXYTECH).

BSO, only in part, mimicked the elevation of cellular oxidative stress. It has been reported that BSO mainly depleted the cytosolic GSH content by blocking the GSH synthesis and GSH reductase but does not appreciably affect the mitochondrial GSH pools (*29*). On the other hand, the pretreatment of DEM, which blocks intracellular thiol groups including mitochondrial GSH (*30*), solely produced ROS and enhanced BITC-induced oxidative stress. Moreover, the pretreatment of diphenylene iodonium (DPI), acting not only as a NAD(P)H oxidase inhibitor (*31*) but also as an inhibitor of mitochondrial reactive oxygen species production (*32*), resulted in a significant decrease in the BITC-induced ROS accumulation (Fig. 4). BITC is likely to enhance the accumulation of 2,7-dichlorofluorescein (DCF) produced by the basal oxidative metabolism (*28*). These results, taken together, strongly suggested that ROS detected in the cells exposed to BITC may originate from the mitochondria, one of the major ROS producing organelles. More recently we observed that BITC modified the mitochondrial function including respiration and that most of the ROS produced by the BITC treatment were hydrogen peroxide derived from the dismutation of superoxide (unpublished results).

GPEI is a BITC response element

Recently, the mechanism of transcriptional regulation of GSTP1 has been revealed by a number of studies. The GSTP1 gene expression is dominantly regulated by the GSTP1 enhancer I (GPEI), a ARE/EpRE of GSTP1, containing a palindromic dyad of the 12-*O*-tetradecanoylphorbol-13-acetate responsible element (TRE)-like sequence (*33*). Our recent study

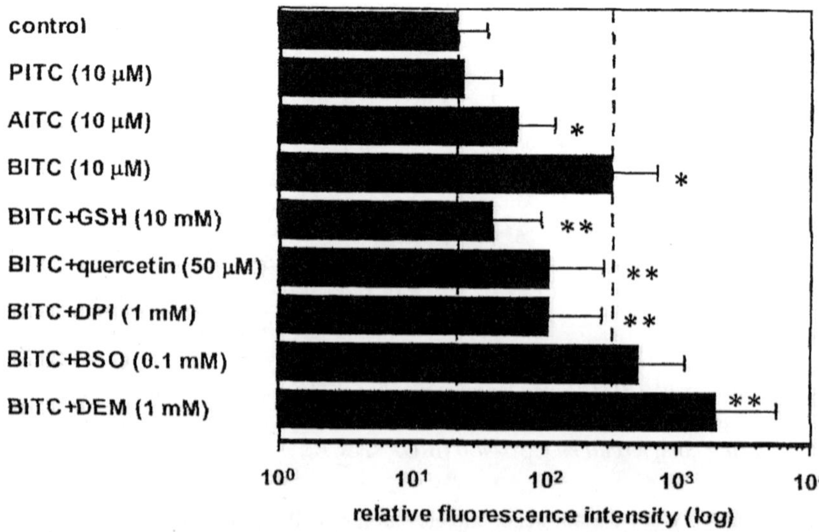

Figure 4. Effects of a variety of agents on intracellular ROS accumulation. The DCF fluorescence of more than 10,000 cells was monitored on a flowcytometer.

revealed for the first time that GPEI is an essential cis-element required for the activation of the GSTP1 gene by redox alteration by BITC or DEM in the experiment using a chloramphenicol acetyltransferase assay (*28*). The GSTP1 gene is thus activated by some trans-activator(s) since TRE is known to be a specific binding site of AP-1 or related transcriptional factors. ITCs-induced oxidative stress is reported to be involved in the ITCs-induced activation of JNK (*34*), which phosphorylates transcriptional factors, such as c-Jun, ATF-2, and Elk-1, and strongly augments their transcriptional activity (*35-38*). Identification of the factor(s) that bind GPEI and activate the GSTP1 gene expression are required for further understanding of the regulation of GSTP1 induction by BITC. In addition, it is noteworthy that π-class GST isozyme is closely related with regulation of JNK signaling (*39*). It is within the range of possibility that the primary target of BITC or BITC-induced ROS is GSTP1 itself, whose modification may result in direct stimulation of the JNK signaling pathway. The observation that the GST activity was inhibited by the incubation with BITC for 30 min (*28*) also supports this hypothesis.

Venugopal and Jaiswal (*40*) have reported that the transcription factor Nrf2 positively regulates the antioxidant response element-mediated (ARE-mediated) expression of Phase II detoxification enzyme genes. Itoh *et al.* (*41*) have also shown by gene-targeted disruption in mice that Nrf2 is a general regulator of the Phase II enzyme genes in response to electrophiles and ROS. More recently, the general regulatory mechanism underlying the electrophile counterattack response has been demonstrated in which electrophilic agents alter the interaction of Nrf2 with its repressor protein (Keap1), thereby liberating Nrf2 activity from repression by Keap1, culminating in the induction of the Phase II enzyme genes and antioxidative stress protein genes via ARE/EpREs (*42*). Keap 1 contains 25 cysteine residues, 9 of which are expected to have highly reactive sulfhydryl groups (*43*). Because most of the inducers are redox-active, the Keap1-Nrf2 complex is a plausible candidate for the cytoplasmic sensor system that recognizes inducers including BITC. More recently, our group found that a sulforaphane analogue potently activates the Nrf2-dependent GST induction pathway (submitted for publication), thus supporting this speculation. Further studies of factors interacting with GPEI and other functional *cis*-acting elements should be required for elucidation of the specific expression of the gene in association with the possible chemoprotective response of BITC.

Conclusion

The Redox alteration by intracellular ROS is likely to mediate the BITC-induced GSTP1 gene expression because 1) a short time (1 h) exposure to BITC was sufficient to evoke the elevation of GST activity (*28*), 2) DEM enhanced BITC-induced ROS production and accelerated both basal and BITC-induced GST activity and GSTP1 gene expression, while the antioxidant GSH inhibited them (*9,28*). Many researchers have thus far confirmed that phase II enzymes play an important role in the cellular detoxification of polycyclic aromatic hydrocarbons. In tumors, however, the same enzymes promote spreading of cancer cells by inactivation of cytoplastic drugs or other agents used to control and eliminate the malignant cells. Chemopreventive agents during the initiation period, most of which induce phase II enzymes, do not necessarily exert beneficial effects in the post initiation phase (*44,45*). Thus, the exact chempreventive potential of the phase II enzyme inducers in multistage carcinogenesis is controversial. As mentioned above, the profound relationship between GSTP1 and stress signaling pathways (*39*) indicated that GSTP1 is one of the most important

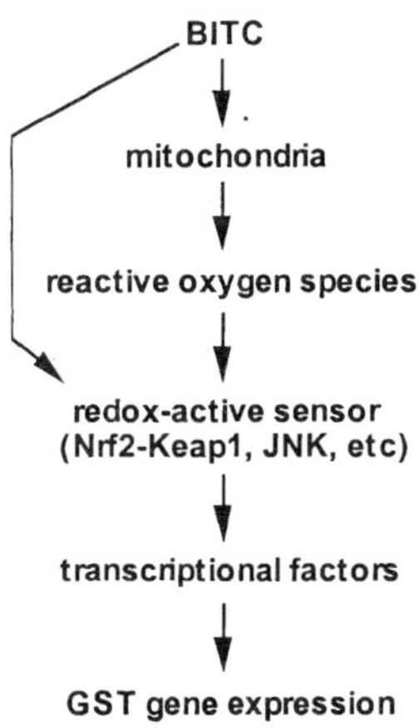

Scheme. A proposed mechanism for the BITC-induced GSTP1 expression

components that could influence key cellular functions including growth, apoptosis, and transformation. Since the cancer preventive or promoting potential, threshold, and the target organ of ITCs have to be distinguished in detail, further mechanistic studies on intracellular oxidative stress and the following events induced by ITCs are essential to provide supporting information. As mentioned above, phenylethyl ITC has been reported to be a bifunctional inducer upregulating both phase I and II enzymes in rat liver (*46*), while BITC was a monofunctional inducer, which induces phase II enzyme but not phase I enzyme, in cultured liver cells (*6*). This suggested one possibility that the metabolism of phase II inducer may play some roles in the induction of phase I enzymes. To understand the mechanism or nature of chemoprevention mediated by inducers, all the biological activities including apoptosis induction (*47*) of the probable phase II enzyme-inducing compounds and their metabolites also have to be demonstrated.

Acknowledgment

The author thanks Profs. K. Uchida, T. Osawa (Nagoya University), H. Ohigashi (Kyoto University), A. Murakami (Kinki University), and Y. Morimitsu (Ochanomizu University) for their kind collaborations and valuable discussions. This work was supported by a grant-in-aid for Encouragement of Young Scientists (No. 13760102) from the Japanese Society for the Promotion of Science and by Program for Promotion of Basic Research Activities for Innovation Biosciences.

References

1. Henderson, C. J.; Smith, A. G.; Ure, J.; Brown, K.; Bacon, E. J.; Wolf, C. R. *Proc. Natl. Acad. Sci. USA* **1998**, *95*, 5275-5280.
2. Nakae, D.; Denda, A.; Kobayashi, Y.; Akai, H.; Kishida, H.; Tsujiuchi, T.; Konishi, Y.; Suzuki, T.; Muramatsu, M. *Jpn. J. Cancer Res.* **1998**, *89*, 1118-1125.
3. Robertson, I. G. C.; Guthenberg, C.; Mannervik, B.; Jernström, B. *Cancer Res.* **1986**, *46*, 2220-2224.
4. Robertson, I. G. C.; Jensson, H.; Mannervik, B.; Jernström, B. *Carcinogenesis* **1986**, *7*, 295-299.
5. De Long, M. J.; Prochaska, H. J.; Talalay, P. *Proc. Natl. Acad. Sci. USA* **1986**, *83*, 787-791.
6. Prochaska, H. J.; Talalay, P. *Cancer Res.* **1988**, *48*, 4776-4782.
7. Talalay, P.; De Long, M. J.; Prochaska, H. J. *Proc. Natl. Acad. Sci. USA* **1988**, *85*, 8261-8265.
8. Primiano, T.; Sutter, T. R.; Kensler, T. W. *Comp. Biochem. Physiol.* **1998**, *118B*, 487-497.
9. Nakamura, Y.; Morimitsu, Y.; Uzu, T.; Ohigashi, H.; Murakami, A.; Naito, Y.; Nakagawa, Y.; Osawa, T.; Uchida, K. *Cancer Lett.* **2000**, *157*, 193-200.

10. World Cancer Research Fund. In *Food, Nutrition and the Prevention of Cancer: A Global Perspective.* The American Institute for Cancer Research, Washington DC, 1997.
11. Flath, R. A.; Forrey, R. R. *J. Agric. Food Chem.* **1977**, *25*, 103-109.
12. Huang, M.-T.; Ferraro, T.; Ho, C.-T. In *Food Phytochemicals for Cancer Prevention I, ACS symposium series 546;* Editors, M.-T. Huang, T. Osawa, C.-T. Ho and R.T. Rosen. American Chemical Society, Washington, DC, 1994; pp. 2-16.
13. Sparnin, V. L.; Venegas, P. L.; Wattenberg, L. W. *J. Natl. Cancer Inst.* **1982**, *68*, 493-496.
14. Wattenberg, L. W. *Carcinogenesis* **1987**, *8*, 1971-1973.
15. Hecht, S. S. *J. Cell. Biochem.* **1995**, *22 (Suppl.)*, 195-209.
16. Sparnins, V. L.; Wattenberg, L. W. *J. Natl. Cancer Inst.* **1981**, *66*, 769-772.
17. Stoner, G. D.; Morrissey, D. T.; Heur, Y. H.; Daniel, E. M.; Galati, A. J.; Wagner, S. A. *Cancer Res.* **1991**, *51*, 2063-2068.
18. Vos, R. M. E.; Snoek, M. C.; van Berkel, W. J. H.; Mueller, F.; van Bladeren, P. J. *Biochem. Pharm.* **1988**, *37*, 1077-1082,.
19. Medesto, R. R.; Pesce, A. J. *Biochim. Biophys. Acta* **1973**, *295*, 283-295.
20. Segal, A.; Solomon, J. J.; Li, F. *Chem.-Biol. Interact.* **1989**, *69*, 359-372.
21. Caspary, W. J.; Myhr, B. *Mutat. Res.* **1986**, *174*, 285-293.
22. Podhradsky, D.; Drobnica, L.; Kristian, P. *Experientia* **1978**, *35*, 154-155.
23. Pinkus, R.; Weiner, L. M.; Daniel, V. Biochemistry **1995**, *34*, 81-88.
24. Pinkus, R.; Weiner, L. M.; Daniel, V. *J. Biol. Chem.* **1996**, *271*, 13422-13429.
25. Fukuda, A.; Nakamura, Y.; Ohigashi, H.; Osawa, T.; Uchida, K. *Biochem. Biophys. Res. Commun.* **1997**, *236*, 505-509.
26. Uchida, K.; Shiraishi, M.; Naito, Y.; Torii, Y.; Nakamura, Y.; Osawa, T. *J. Biol. Chem.* **1999**, *274*, 2234-2242.
27. Zhang, Y.; Talalay, P. *Cancer Res.* **1998**, *58*, 4632-4639.
28. Nakamura, Y.; Ohigashi, H.; Masuda, S.; Murakami, A.; Morimitsu, Y.; Kawamoto, Y.; Osawa, T.; Imagawa, M.; Uchida, K. *Cancer Res.* **2000**, *60*, 219-225.
29. Reed. D. J. *Ann. Rev. Pharmcol. Toxicol.* **1990**, *30*, 603-631.
30. Shrieve, D. C.; Bump, E. A.; Rice, G. C. *J. Biol. Chem.* **1988**, *263*, 14107-14114.
31. Cross, A. R.; Jones, O. T. G. *Biochem. J.* **1986**, *237*, 111-116.
32. Li, Y.; Trush, M. A. *Biochem. Biophys. Res. Commun.* **1998**, *253*, 295-299.
33. Sakai, M.; Okuda, A.; Muramatsu, M. *Proc. Natl. Acad. Sci. USA* **1988**, *85*, 9456-9460.
34. Chen, Y.-R.; Wang, W.; Kong, A.-N. T.; Tan, T.-H. *J. Biol. Chem.* **1998**, *273*, 1769-1775.
35. Livingstone, C.; Patel, G.; Jones, N. *EMBO J.* **1995**, *14*, 1785-1797.

36. Gupta, S.; Campbell, D.; Derijard, B.; Davis, R. J. *Science* **1995**, *267*, 389-393.
37. Cavigelli, M.; Dolfi, F.; Claret, F.-X.; Karin, M. *EMBO J.* **1995**, *14*, 5957-5964.
38. Whitmarsh, A. J.; Shore, P.; Sharrocks, A. D.; Davis, R. J. *Science* **1995**, *269*, 403-407.
39. Adler, V.; Yin, Z.; Fuchs, S. Y.; Benezra, M.; Rosario, L.; Tew, K. D.; Pincus, M. R.; Sardana, M.; Henderson, C. J.; Wolf, C. R.; Davis, R. J.; Ronai, Z. *EMBO J.* **1999**, *18*, 1321-1334.
40. Venugopal, R.; Jaiswal, A. K. *Proc. Natl. Acad. Sci. USA* **1996**, *10*, 14960-14965.
41. Itoh, K.; Chiba, T.; Takahashi, S.; Ishii, T.; Igarashi, K.; Katoh, Y.; Oyake, T.; Hayashi, N.; Satoh, K.; Hatayama, I.; Yamamoto, M.; Nabeshima, Y. *Biochem. Biophys. Res. Commun.* **1997**, *236*, 313-322.
42. Itoh, K.; Ishii, T.; Wakabayashi, N.; Yamamoto, M. *Free Radic. Res.* **1999**, *31*, 319-324.
43. Itoh, K.; Wakabayashi, N.; Katoh, Y.; Ishii, T.; Igarashi, K.; Engel, J. D.; Yamamoto, M. *Genes Dev.* **1999**, *13*, 76-86.
44. Ogawa, K.; Futakuchi, M.; Hirose, M.; Boonyaphiphat, P.; Mizoguchi, Y.; Miki, T.; Shirai, T. *Int. J. Cancer* **1998**, *76*, 851-856.
45. Hirose, M.; Yamaguchi, T.; Kimoto, N.; Ogawa, K.; Futakuchi, M.; Sano, M.; Shirai, T. *Int. J. Cancer* **1998**, *77*, 773-777.
46. Manson, M. M.; Ball, H. W. L.; Barrett, M. C.; Clark, H. L.; Judah, D. J.; Williamson, G.; Neal, G. E. *Carcinogenesis* **1997**, *18*, 1729-1738.
47. Nakamura, Y.; Kawakami, M.; Yoshihiro, A.; Miyoshi, N.; Ohigashi, H.; Kawai, K.; Osawa, T.; Uchida, K. *J. Biol. Chem.* **2002**, *277*, 8492-8499.

Chapter 32

Separation and Bioactivity of Diarylheptanoids from Lesser Galangal *(Alpinia officinarum)*

Zhihua Liu[1,2], M. Mohamed Rafi[2], Nanqun Zhu[2], Kenjiro Ryu[1,3], Shengmin Sang[2], Chi-Tang Ho[1,2], and Robert T. Rosen[1,2]

[1]Center for Advanced Food Technology and [2]Department of Food Science, Cook College, Rutgers, The State University of New Jersey, 63 Dudley Road, New Brunswick, NJ 08901–8520
[3]Healthcare Research Institute, Wakunaga Pharmaceutical Company, Ltd., 1624, Shimokotachi, Koda-cho, Takata-gun, Hiroshima 739–1195, Japan

Diarylheptanoids from the rhizomes of *Alpinia officinarum* were isolated by column chromatography and HPLC. Normal phase column chromatography followed by semi-preparative reversed-phase HPLC was used to isolate five diarylheptanoids, which were identified as 5-hydroxy-7-(4″-hydroxy-3″-methoxyphenyl)-1-phenyl-3-heptanone (**AO-1**), 5-methoxy-7-(4″-hydroxy-3″-methoxyphenyl)-1-phenyl-3-heptanone (**AO-2**), 7-(4″-hydroxyphenyl)-1-phenylhept-4-en-3-one (**AO-3**), 7-(4″-hydroxy-3″-methoxyphenyl)-1-phenyl-hept-4-en-3-one (**AO-4**), 1,7-diphenylhept-4-en-3-one (**AO-5**). This paper discusses the separation and isolation of these compounds and their biological as well as antioxidant activity.

Lesser Galangal is native to the island of Hainan, in the southern part of China. The most commonly used part is its rhizome, which has a pungent, spicy taste and aromatic odor. In Asia, the root has long been used as a spice or flavoring. Lesser galangal has a long history of traditional medicinal use in China due to its significant therapeutic properties for the spleen and stomach (*1*).

Its usage includes reducing flatulence, control of vomiting and facilitating digestion. It also has reputation as a remedy for chronic gastritis.

Of the many compounds identified in lesser galangal, flavonoids and diarylheptanoids are among the most important. A variety of flavonols and diarylheptanoids were isolated from this plant and found to display antioxidative activity as demonstrated by an anti-lipid peroxidation assay (*2*). *In vitro* and *in vivo* studies indicated that the flavonoid galangin had antioxidative and free radical scavenging activities and was able to modulate enzyme activities and suppress the genotoxicity of chemicals, making it a promising candidate for cancer chemoprevention (*3*). Recently using bioassay-guided fractionation, several flavonoids and diarylheptanoids were isolated from the plant and characterized as COX-2 inhibitor (*4*). Yakuchinone A, a diarylheptanoid obtained from lesser galangal, was determined to be a very potent inhibitor against prostaglandin synthase (*5*).

Apoptosis, also known as programmed cell death, plays a very important role in many normal biological processes. For instance, failure to properly execute apoptosis may lead to various disease states such as cancer (*6*), and a variety of anticancer drugs which kill cancer cells inducing apoptosis have been well documented (*7*). Screening of herbal extracts for bioactive compounds that could effectively induce apoptosis may provide some promising candidates for cancer chemoprevention. Solvent extracts of various plants were screened with respect to induce apoptosis and it was found that methanol extract of *Alpinia officinarum* was one of the most potent. Until now, no work has been done comparing the bioactivity of the diarylheptanoids in lesser galangal. Therefore our research objective was to isolate and study the compounds that accounted for this activity.

A variety of diarylheptanoids present in *Alpinia officinarum* were determined to display antioxidative activity demonstrated by an anti-lipid peroxidation assay (*2*). The DPPH assay has been extensively used to test the free radical scavenging ability of various chemicals (*8,9*) and therefore we used the DPPH method to explore five isolated compounds capacity to act as free radical scavengers.

Materials and Methods

General Procedures

^{1}H NMR and ^{13}C NMR spectra were recorded on a VXR-200 instrument. Mass spectra were obtained by using direct probe electron ionization (EI) and by atmospheric pressure chemical ionization (APCI) in the negative-ion mode.

Direct probe EI-MS was performed on a Finnigan MAT 8230 high-resolution mass spectrometer (San Jose, CA). APCI MS analysis was carried out on a Micromass Platform II system (Micromass Co., MA) equipped with a Digital DECPc XL 560 computer for analysis of data. The ion source temperature was set at 150 °C and the probe temperature was set at 450 °C. The sample cone voltage was 10 V and the corona discharge was 3.2 kV. HPLC analysis was performed on a Varian 5500 Liquid Chromatograph pump coupled to a Varian 9065 Polychrom diode array detector (Sugar Land, TX). Semi-preparative fractionation of mixture was done on an ABI Spectroflow 400 HPLC pump coupled to an ABI Spectroflow 183 Programmable Absorbance Detector (Ramsey, NJ). Column chromatography was carried out on silica gel (32-60Å, particle size) using a glass chromatography column purchase from Kontes (Vineland, NJ). Formic acid (FA), methanol, 1-butanol, ethyl acetate, hexanes, water and acetonitrile, were purchased from Fisher Scientific (Springfield, NJ). All solvents used for extraction and chromatographic analysis were of HPLC grade. Mixture of solvents for HPLC were degassed using a sonic cleaner purchased from Fisher Scientific. The UV absorbance was measured using a spectrophotometer (Milton Roy, Model 301).

Plant Material and Cell Line

The rhizomes of *Alpinia officinarum* were purchased from Nuherbs Co. (Oakland, CA). Du-145 prostate tumor cells were obtained from the American Type Culture Collection (ATCC). Cells were maintained at 37°C in an atmosphere of 5% CO_2 and grown in Roswell Park Memorial Institute (RPMI) media 1640 (GIBCO/BRL) with 10% fetal bovine serum and with 5% penicillin and streptomycin. Cells ere routinely checked and found to be free of contamination by mycoplasma.

Extraction and Isolation Procedures

The powdered roots of *Alpinia officinarum* were extracted with methanol and concentrated under vacuum using rotary evaporation. The dried residue was then partitioned with hexanes, ethyl acetate and 1-butanol successively. The three extracts were subjected to bioassays. It was determined that the ethyl acetate extract was the most potent fraction which induced apoptosis in Du-145 cancer cell lines.

The dried ethyl acetate extract was then chromatographed on a normal phase silica gel column (2.5 × 30 cm) to perform bioassay-directed fractionation. The extract was first dissolved in methanol and loaded onto the column packing material. The prepared extract was then placed on top of the column and elution was performed using a solvent mixture of chloroform/methanol with an increasing amount of methanol (30:1, 20:1, 10:1, 5:1, 0:100; each 1000 mL). Successive fractions were collected and tested for biological activity. The fraction eluted with 30:1 chloroform/methanol was found to be most active. This fraction was then rechromatographed on a semipreparative Zorbax Rx-C18 reversed phase HPLC column (9.4 mm × 240 mm, 5 μm) purchased from MacMod Analytical (Chadds Ford, PA). Compounds were eluted by an isocratic solvent system: 55% A, water with 0.05% formic acid (FA); 45% B, ACN (v/v) at a flow rate of 4 mL/min. The wavelength monitored was 205 nm. Successive fractions (1-3) were collected and sent for biological testing again. It was found that all three fractions were able to induce apoptosis.

The 30:1 chloroform/methanol extract was then rechromatographed on a normal phase silica gel column and eluted with hexanes/chloroform 20:80, 10:90, 0:100 successively to get the above three fractions. Fraction 3 was a pure compound. Final separation of pure compounds from fractions 1 and 2 were obtained using semipreparative HPLC on a Zorbax Rx-C18 reversed phase column. Isocratic solvent systems were used for the two fractions: fraction 1, 50:50 (Water with 0.05%FA: ACN), v/v; fraction 2, 55:45, (water with 0.05% FA: ACN), v/v.

Quantification of Diarylheptanoids in *Alpinia officinarum*

At least five different concentrations were prepared for each purified diarylheptanoid, i.e. AO-1 to AO-5, and then each sample in term of a specific concentration was chromatographed using an analytical reversed phase HPLC column. The calibration curve for each compound was obtained by plotting concentration versus UV absorbance. The ethyl acetate extract of lesser galangal was then subjected to the same HPLC program and the concentration of each diarylheptanoid in the ethyl acetate extract was obtained from the calibration curve. The concentrations of the five diarylheptanoids in the rhizomes of *Alpinia officinarum* were determined by comparing the amount of each compound to that of plant material (dry basis) used in this study.

Cytotoxicity Assessed by Cell Viability Assay

Cellular growth in the presence or absence of experimental agents was determined using the modified method as previously described MTT – microculture tetrazolium assay (*10*). Briefly, rapidly growing cells were harvested, counted, and inoculated at the appropriate concentrations (100 μL volume) into 96-well micro-titer plates using a multichannel pipet. After 24 hours, AO-1 to AO-5 were applied in different concentrations to triplicate culture wells, and cultures were incubated for 72 hours at 37 °C. MTT (Sigma, St. Louis, MO) was prepared at 2 mg/mL in Phosphate buffered saline (PBS) and 50 μL were added to microculture wells. After 4 hour incubation at 37 °C, 250 μL were removed from each well, and 150 μL of 100 % DMSO were added to solubilize the MTT-formazan product. After thorough mixing with a mechanical plate mixer, absorbence was measured at 570 nm using a Dynatech microplate reader. Treatment of prostate tumor cell line Du-145 with the various diarylheptanoids resulted in IC_{50} values (drug concentration in a 50% inhibition of growth). This assay is based on the reduction of MTT tetrazolium salt to a formazan product by the metabolic activity of live cells and which was measured in a multiwell scanning spectrophotometer. Cell line growth and growth inhibition were expressed in terms of mean absorbance units and following the subtraction of mean background absorbance.

Measurement of Radical-Scavenging Activity by DPPH

This method was adapted from that of Brand-Williams, *et al.* (*8*). At least seven different concentrations were prepared for each purified compound. 25 μL pure compound solution and 975 μL DPPH solution (63.4 μM) were mixed together and left in the dark for 30 min. Each sample was triplicated and the values were averaged. The absorbance of the samples was measured at 515 nm against methanol solution without DPPH as the blank reference. The absorbance was measured every 30 min until the reaction reached a plateau. The reaction kinetics were then plotted using the above data and the percentage of $DPPH^{\bullet}$ remaining at the steady state was obtained. IC_{50} values were determined by extrapolation from linear regression analysis.

Results and Discussion

Our previous screening work showed that the methanol extract of *Alpinia officinarum* exhibited potent activity in the apoptosis assay. Then the column chromatography indicated that 30:1 chloroform/methanol fraction was the most active one in the bioassay. This fraction was then analyzed by reverse phase HPLC and its corresponding HPLC chromatogram at 205 nm is presented in Figure 1. The 30:1 fraction was further subfractionated into three fractions and subjected to the bioassay again. It was shown that all three were active and the second fraction was the most potent.

Fraction 1 obtained from column chromatography was subjected to reverse phase HPLC and three peaks were collected. Peak 2 and 3 were identified to be flavonoids and had no activity at all. Peak 1 showed biological activity to some level and tentatively designated as AO-1. EI mass chromatogram of AO-1

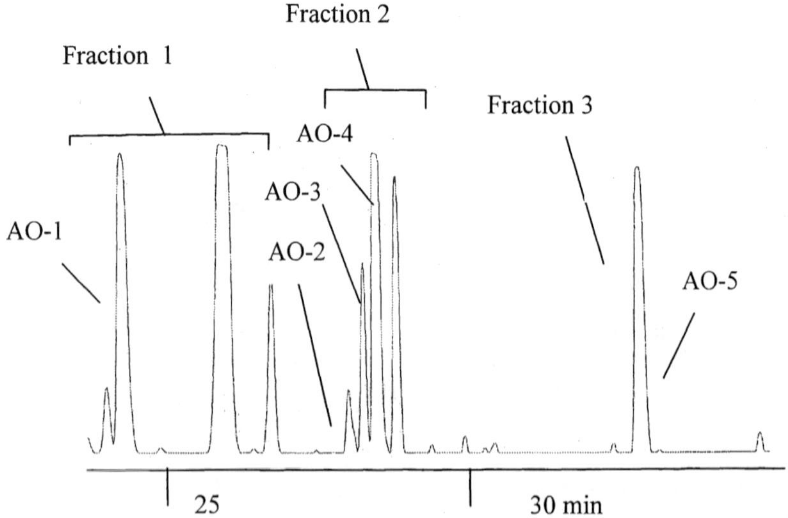

Figure 1. *Reversed phase HPLC chromatogram of Alpinia officinarum 30:1 chloroform/methanol fraction at 205 nm using a Discovery C18 reversed phase HPLC column (250 mm × 4.6 mm, 5 µm).*

exhibited three major peaks with m/z 310 $[M-H_2O]^{+\bullet}$, 180 $[C_6H_3(OH)(OMe)CH_2CH_2CHO]^{+\bullet}$, 148 $[C_6H_3CH_2CH_2COCH_3]^{+\bullet}$.

Fraction 2 contained three main peaks and each compound displayed some activity. These were designated as AO-2, AO-3 and AO-4. The EI mass spectrum of AO-2 exhibited peaks at m/z 342 $[M]^{+\bullet}$, 310 $[M-CH_3OH]^{+\bullet}$, 205 $[C_6H_3(OH)(OMe)CH_2CH_2CHCHCO]^+$, 137 $[CH_2C_6H_3(OH)(OMe)]^+$, 105 $[C_8H_9]^+$ and 91 $[C_7H_7]^+$, which along with the NMR data, indicated the presence of a 4-hydroxy-3-methoxyphenyl and a phenyl moiety as well as the position of the ketone and aliphatic methoxy group. The EI mass spectrum of AO-3 showed ion at m/z 280 $[M]^{+\bullet}$, 133 $[C_9H_9O]^+$, 107 $[C_7H_7O]^+$, 91 $[C_7H_7]^{+\bullet}$ and with the NMR data, indicated the presence of 4-hydroxyphenyl and a phenyl moiety as well as the position of the ketone and a α,β-unsaturated ketone grouping. The EI mass spectrum of AO-4 had ion at 310 $[M]^{+\bullet}$, 205 $[C_6H_3(OH)(OMe)CH_2CH_2CHCHCO]^+$, 137 $[CH_2C_6H_3(OH)(OMe)]^+$, 105 $[C_8H_9]^+$, 91 $[C_7H_7]^+$, which suggested the same substitution on the benzene ring as sample AO-2. The data also showed the same position of the double bond as well as the ketone group like AO-3. Fraction 3 obtained from column chromatography was a pure compound and exhibited a molecular ion at m/z 264 $[M]^{+\bullet}$ as well as a characteristic fragment ion peak at m/z 159 $[C_6H_4CH_2CH_2COCHCH_2]^+$, which indicated the position of the ketone group. On the basis of MS and NMR spectra, AO-1 to AO-5 were identified to be all diarylheptanoid compounds and determined to be 5-hydroxy-7- (4″-hydroxy-3″-methoxyphenyl)-1-phenyl-3-heptanone, 5-methoxy-7-(4″-hydroxy-3″-methoxy-phenyl)-1-phenyl-3-heptanone, 7-(4″-hydroxyphenyl)-1-phenylhept-4-en-3-one, 7-(4″-hydroxy-3″-methoxyphenyl)-1-penylhept-4-en-3-one and 1,7-diphenyl-hept-4-en-3-one successively. Structures of these five compounds are shown in Figure 2. The concentration of AO-1 to AO-5 in the powdered roots of *Alpinia officinarum* were approximately 134 μg/g, 40 μg/g, 74 μg/g, 168 μg/g, 138 μg/g respectively.

In order to identify the active compounds contributing to the biological activity, the IC_{50} values for the above five diarylheptanoids were obtained and summarized in Table 1. AO-1 and AO-2 with IC_{50} 100 and 88 μM were significantly less active than AO-3, AO-4 and AO-5. The IC_{50} values for AO-3 to AO-5 were 20 μM, 12.5 μM and 32 μM, respectively. Among the five diarylheptanoids, AO-4 showed the most potent activity followed by AO-3 and AO-5. Regarding their structures and the $IC_{50,}$ the importance of α,β-unsaturated ketone grouping is evident from the fact that substituting the double bond on the carbon seven moiety (AO-4) with hydroxy (AO-1) or methoxy (AO-2) groups decreases the biological activity significantly. It also could be seen from the Figure 2 and Table 1 that substitution at the *para* position (AO-5) with a hydroxyl group (AO-3) on the B benzene ring enhances the ability to induce apoptosis. Furthermore, substitution at the *meta* position (AO-3) with a methoxy group (AO-4) further enhances the bioactivity. Therefore, substitution on the B benzene ring with different functional groups as well as the presence of α,β-unsaturated ketone grouping may significantly affect biological activity.

Table I. Effects of Diarylheptanoids on Inducing Apoptosis in Du-145 Cancer Cell Line

Compound	*IC_{50} (μM)*
AO-1	100
AO-2	88
AO-3	20
AO-4	12.5
AO-5	32

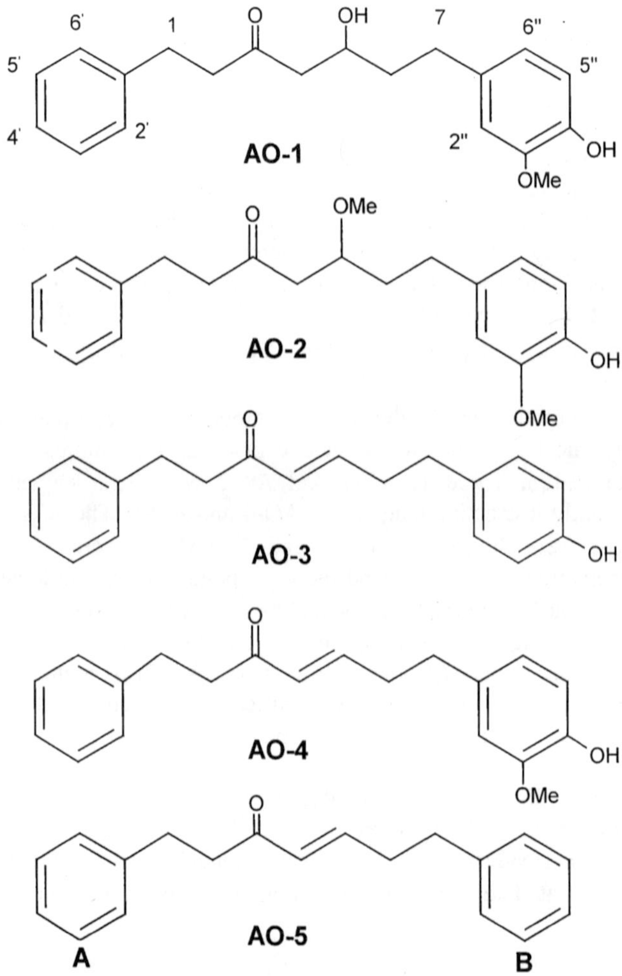

Figure 2. *Structures of diarylheptanoids isolated from Alpinia officinarum. AO-1 (5-hydroxy-7-(4"-hydroxy-3"-methoxyphenyl)- 1-phenyl-3-heptanone), AO-2(5-methoxy-7-(4"-hydroxy-3"-methoxyphenyl)-1-phenyl-3-heptanone), AO-3 (7-(4"-hydroxyphenyl)-1-phenylhept-4-en-3-one), AO-4 (7-(4"-hydroxy-3"-methoxyphenyl)- 1-phenylhept-4-en-3-one), AO-5 (1,7-diphenylhept-4-en-3-one).*

DPPH, 2,2-Diphenyl-1-picrylhydrazyl ($DPPH^{\bullet}$), is a stable radical in methanol solution. In its radical form, $DPPH^{\bullet}$ absorbs at 515 nm, but the absorption ceases upon reduction by an antioxidant (AH) or a radical species ($R^{\bullet}$) (*8*). The concentration of tested chemicals needed to decrease the initial $DPPH^{\bullet}$ concentration by 50% (IC_{50}) is a parameter widely used to measure the antioxidant potential (*11, 12*). The lower the $IC_{50,}$ the higher the free radical scavenging power. The IC_{50} of the above five diarylheptanoids were shown in Table 2. It could be seen from the table that AO-3 and AO-5 almost have no antioxidant power with their IC_{50} larger than 1000 μm. The introduction of a methoxy group to AO-3's *ortho* position on the right benzene ring leads to a significant increase of antioxidant activity (AO-4). This agrees with the Burton *et al.* and Cuvelier *et al.* 's reports that the *ortho* substitution with an electron donor such as methoxy, methyl etc., increases the antioxidant activity of phenols by enhancing the stability of phenoxyl radical through inductive effect (*13,14*). The substitution on the right benzene ring of AO-1, AO-2 and AO-4 are the same and their structures' difference comes from the substitution of hydroxy (AO-1) and methoxy (AO-2) to the α,β-unsaturated ketone group (AO-4). Their IC_{50} are close to each other showing that the presence of the α,β-unsaturated ketone group is not an important factor for the antioxidant activity. However, the introduction of a methoxy group to the *ortho* position of the phenol ring results in the significant increase of free radical scavenging activity.

Table II. IC_{50} of Diarylheptanoids in Scavenging DPPH Free Radicals

Compound	*IC_{50} (μM)*
AO-1	11.44
AO-2	12.71
AO-3	More than 1000
AO-4	13.7
AO-5	More than 5000

Structure Determination of Isolated Compounds

(AO-1) 5-Hydroxy-7-(4"-hydorxy-3"methoxyphenyl)-1-phenyl-3-heptanone; MW=328: APCI, m/z 327 [M-H^- ion]; EI-MS: 310(12), 205(6), 137(100), 122(10), 105(6), 91(14), 77(7); UV λ_{max} nm: 279.2; ^{1}H NMR δ 1.64-1.88 (2H, m, H-6), δ 2.48-2.94 (8H, m, H-1, 2, 4, 7), δ 3.84 (3H, s, 3″-OCH_3), δ 4.22 (1H, m, H-5), δ 6.64 (1H, dd, J=8 Hz, J=2 Hz, H-6″), δ 6.72 (1H, d, J=8 Hz, H-5″), δ 6.78 (1H, d, J=2 Hz, H-2″), δ7.12-7.34 (5H, m, H2′-H6′); ^{3}CNMR δ 28.6 (C-1), δ 30.4 (C-7), δ 38.5 (C-6), δ 44.8 (C-2), δ 47.5 (C-4), δ 54.4 (3″-OCH_3), δ 69.7 (C-5), δ 111.2 (C-2″), δ 114.2 (C-5″), δ 119.8 (C-6″), δ 125.6 (C-4′), δ 128.4 (C-2′, 6′), δ128.5 (C-3′, 5′), δ 132.9 (C-1″), δ 140.4 (C-1′), δ 143.8 (C-4″), δ 146.9 (C-3″), δ 209.6 (C-3). (*15,16*)

(AO-2) 5-Methoxy-7-(4″-hydroxy-3″-methoxyphenyl)-1-phenyl-3-heptanone; MW=342: APCI, m/z 341 [M-H^- ion]; EI-MS: 342(30), 310(36), 205(8), 177(17), 163(30), 137(100), 105(70), 91(68); UV λ_{max} nm: 231, 279.9; ^{1}H NMR δ 1.6-1.8 (2H, m, H-6), δ 2.4-2.9 (8H, m, H-1, 2, 4, 7), δ 3.28 (3H, s, 5-OCH_3), δ 3.67 (1H, m, H-5), δ 3.84 (3H, s, 3″-OCH_3), δ 6.60 (1H, dd, J=8 Hz, J=2 Hz, H-6″), δ 6.72 (1H, d, J=8 Hz, H-5″), δ 6.76 (1H, d, J=2 Hz, H-2″), δ 7.1-7.3 (5H, m, H2′-6′); ^{13}CNMR δ 29.6 (C-1), δ 30.9 (C-7), δ 36.0 (C-6), δ 45.0 (C-2), δ 47.5 (C-4), δ 54.4 (3″-OCH_3), δ 56.2 (5-OCH_3), δ 76.0 (C-5), δ 111.2 (C-2″), δ 114.2 (C-5″), δ 119.8 (C-6″), δ 126.2 (C-4′), δ128.4 (C-2′, 6′), δ 128.5 (C-3′, 5′), δ 132.8 (C-1″), δ 140.6 (C-1′), δ 143.6 (C-4″), δ 146.9 (C-3″), δ 209.1 (C-3). (*16,17*)

(AO-3) 7-(4″-hydroxyphenyl)-1-phenyl-hept-4-en-3-one; MW=280: APCI, m/z 279; EI-MS: 280(12), 174(5), 159(14), 133(5), 107(100), 105(8), 91(16), 77(10); UV λ_{max} nm: 224, 278; ^{1}H NMR δ 2.48 (2H, q, J=7.3 Hz, H-6), δ 2.69 (2H, t, J=7.3 Hz, H-7), δ 2.88 (4H, s, H-1, 2), δ 6.10 (1H, d, J=16.2 Hz, H-4), δ 6.71 (2H, d, J= 8.4 Hz, H-3″, 5″), δ 6.92 (1H, double t, J=16 Hz, 6 Hz, H-5), δ 7.02 (2H, d, J=8.4 Hz, H-2″, 6″), δ 7.12-7.33 (5H, H2′-6′); ^{13}C NMR δ 30.4 (C-1), δ33.6 (C-7), δ 34.7 (C-6), δ 41.4 (C-2), δ 115.2 (C-3″, 5″), δ 126.1 (C-4′), δ 128.4 (C-2′, 6′), δ 128.5 (C-3′, 5′), δ 129.4 (C-2″, 6″), δ 130.7 (C-4), δ 132.0 (C-1″), δ 140.5 (C-1′), δ 147.3 (C-5), δ 154.7 (C-4″), δ 200.4 (C-3). (*16,18,19*)

(AO-4) 7-(4″-hydroxy-3″-methoxyphenyl)-1-phenyl-hept-4-en-3-one; MW=310: APCI, m/z 309 [M-H^- ion]; EI-MS: 310(18), 205(16), 162(10), 150(4), 138(14), 137(100), 105(7), 91(11); UV λ_{max} nm: 224.9, 279.7; ^{1}H NMR δ 2.51 (2H, q, J=7.3 Hz, H-6), δ 2.72 (2H, t, J=7.3 Hz, H-7), δ 2.88 (4H, s, H-1, 2), δ 3.82 (3H, s, 3″-OCH_3), δ 6.10 (1H, d, J=16 Hz, H-4), δ 6.64 (1H, dd, J=8, J=2 Hz, H-6″), δ 6.72 (1H, d, J=8 Hz, H-5″), δ 6.92 (1H, double t, J=16, J=6 Hz, H-5), δ 7.10-7.32 (5H, m, H2′-6′); ^{13}C NMR δ 29.9 (C-1), δ 33.5 (C-7), δ 34.2 (C-6), δ 41.4 (C-2), δ 54.4 (3″-OCH_3), δ 111.2 (C-2″), δ 114.4 (C-5″), δ 119.9 (C-6″), δ 126.1 (C-4′), δ 128.4 (C-2′, 6′), δ 128.5 (C-3′, 5′), δ 129.9 (C-4), δ 132.4 (C-1″), δ 141.2 (C-1′), δ 143.9 (C-4″), δ 146.5 (C-3″), δ 146.9 (C-5), δ 200.4 (C-3). (*16,19,20*)

(AO-5) 1,7-diphenylhept-4-en-3-one; MW=264: APCI, m/z 263 [M-H^- ion]; EI-MS: 264(26), 172(8), 159(72), 131(11), 105(11), 91(100), 77(8), 65(14); UV λ_{max} nm: 226.6; ^{1}H NMR δ 2.54 (2H, q, J=7.3 Hz, H-6), δ 2.78 (2H, t, H-7), δ 2.87 (4H, s, H-1, 2), δ 6.10 (1H, d, J=16.0 Hz, H-4), δ 6.80 (1H, double t, J=16 Hz, J=6 Hz, H-5), δ 7.10-7.32 (10H, m, H2′-6′, 2″-6″); ^{13}C NMR δ 30.2 (C-1), δ 34.2 (C-7), δ 34.4 (C-6), δ 41.4 (C-2), δ 125.2 (C-4″), δ 125.4 (C-4′), δ 128.4 (C-2′, 2″, 6′, 6″), δ 128.6 (C-3′, 3″, 5′, 5″), δ 130.7 (C-4), δ 140.3 (C-1″), δ 141.2 (C-1′), δ 146.4 (C-5), δ 199.3 (C-3). (*19,20*)

Conclusion

Column chromatography and HPLC has led to the isolation of five diarylheptanoids from the roots of *Alpinia officinarum*. Bioassays of them showed that AO-4 was the most potent in inducing apoptosis in the Du-145 cancer cell line. The results indicated that the presence of a α,β-unsaturated ketone grouping may significantly affect bioactivity. In addition, DPPH data showed that AO-1, AO-2, AO-4 could act as very good free radical scavengers.

Acknowledgments

CAFT is an initiative of the NJ commission of Science and Research. This is New Jersey Agricultural Experiment Station publication # D99101-02-01. The work was supported by the New Jersey Commission on Cancer Research, NCI CA 80654, Cap Cure, and CA 77135 and the New Jersey Commission of Science and Research.

References

1. World Health Organization (ED.), *Medicinal Plants in China,* WHO Regional Publications, **1989**, 21.
2. Shen, J.; Zhang, H.; Xu, B.; Pan, J. *Tianran Chanwu Yanjiu Yu Kaifa.* **1998**, *10*, 33-36.
3. Ray, P. G.; Majumdar, S. K. *Indian Journal of Experimental Biology.* **1976**, *14*, 712-714.
4. Heo, M. Y.; Sohn, S. J.; Au, W.W. *Mutation Research.* **2001**, *488*, 135-150.
5. Kang, S. S.; Kim, J. S.; Son, K. H.; Kim, H. P. *Saengyak Hakhoechi.* **2000**, *31*, 57-62.
6. Kiuchi, F.; Iwakami, S.; Shibuya, M.; Hanaoka, F. *Chem. Pharm. Bull.* **1992**, *40*, 387-391.
7. Reed, J. C. *Curr. Opin. Oncol.* **1995**, *7*, 541-546.
8. Brand-Williams, W.; Cuvelier, M. E.; Berset, C. *Lebensm. Wiss. Technol.* **1995**, *28*, 25-30.

9. Dinis, T. C.; Maderia, V. M., Almeida, L. M. *Arch. Biochem. Biophys.* **1994**, *315*, 161-169.
10. Scudiero, D. A.; Shoemaker, R. H.; Paull, K. D. *Cancer Res.* **1988**, *48*, 4827-4833.
11. Kanner, J.; Frankel, E.; German, B.; Kinsella, J. E. *J. Agric. Food Chem.* **1994**, *42*, 64-69.
12. Vinson, J. A.; Dabbagh, Y. A.; Serry, M. M. *J. Agric. Food Chem.* **1995**, *43*, 2800-2802.
13. Burton, G. W.; Doba, T.; Gabe, E. J.; Hughes, L. *J. Am. Chem. Soc.* **1985**, *107*, 7053-7065.
14. Cuvelier, M. E.; Richard, H.; Berset, C. *Biosci. Biotech. Biochem.* **1996**, *56*, 324-325.
15. Inoue, Takehisa; Shinbori, T.; Fujioka, M. *Yakugaku Zasshi.* **1978**, *9*, 1255-1257.
16. Kikuzaki, H.; Kobayashi, M.; Nakatani, N. *Phytochemistry.* **1991**, *11*, 3647-3651.
17. Kiuchi, F.; Shibuya, M.; Sankawa, U. *Chem. Pharm. Bull.* **1982**, *30*, 2279-2282.
18. Itokawa, H.; Morita, H.; Midorikawa, I. *Chem. Pharm. Bull.* **1985**, *33*, 4889-4893.
19. Endo, K.; Kanno, E.; Oshima, Y. *Phytochemistry* **1990**, *29*, 797-799.
20. Itokawa, h.; Morita, M.; Mihashi, S. *Chem. Pharm. Bull.* **1981**, *29*, 2383-2385.

Chapter 33

Inhibition of Carcinogenesis by Tea Aqueous Non-Dialyzates Fractionated from Crude Tea Extracts

Yoshiyuki Nakamura[1], Mamoru Isemura[2], Sumio Hayakawa[2], Kouichi Saeki[2], Yu Koyama[2], Takashi Kimura[2], Masanori Kuroyanagi[3], Tadataka Noro[2], Kyoji Yoshino[4], and Toshihiro Tsuneyoshi[5]

[1]School of Pharmaceutical Sciences and [2]Graduate University of Food and Environmental Sciences, University of Shizuoka, Shizuoka 422–8526, Japan
[3]Hiroshima Prefectural University, Syobara, Hiroshima 727–0023, Japan
[4]Numazu College of Technology, Numazu, Shizuoka 410–8501, Japan
[5]Shizuoka Institute of Science and Technology, Fukuroi, Shizuoka 437–8555, Japan

High molecular weight tea fractions TNDs (tea non-dialysates) were found to induce apoptosis in mouse JB6 cells, human leukemia U937 cells, stomach cancer MKN-45 cells, and colon cancer WiDr cells. Black tea non-dialysate caused the decrease in the expression of mRNAs for caspase 1 and TNF-α and the increase in mRNA expression for several cell surface proteins related to apoptosis in U937 cells. Peroral administration of green tea non-dialyzate (0.05 % in water) resulted in the decrease in the polyp number in the stomach and colon of *APC* knockout mice and the increase in the apoptosis index in the small tumors. These data suggest that drinking of tea is beneficial for prevention of cancer of the digestive tract on the basis of apoptosis-inducing activities of its constituents.

Many animal studies have shown that tea and tea components have anti-cancer activities (1, 2). Green tea and black tea catechin compounds such as epigallocatechin gallate (EGCG) and theaflavin have been investigated most intensively to reveal molecular basis for their anti-tumor activities (3-8). However, tea infusion contains many compounds other than catechins and we have been interested in water-soluble high molecular weight fractions of tea extracts.

We have previously reported that the green tea non-dialyzate (GTND), a green tea high molecular weight fraction, could inhibit carcinogenesis induced by chemical carcinogen, *N*-ethyl-*N*'-nitro-*N*-nitrosoguanidine in the mouse duodenum. For example, the 0.05 % GTND-treated group had a half of the number of tumors compared with the untreated control group (9).

This contribution describes the results of further studies on the anti-tumor activities of high molecular weight tea fractions TNDs (tea non-dialysates), with special reference to its apoptosis-inducing activity.

Preparation of TNDs

Leaves of green tea, black tea, Oolong tea or Pu-erh tea were extracted with hot water. The extracts were then extracted with chloroform, ethyl acetate and butanol, and the residual aqueous layer was dialyzed exhaustively against water and non-dialyzable fractions were freeze-dried and used as TNDs. The yields were 0.42, 2.01, 1.78, and 4.52% for green tea GTND, black tea BTND, Oolong tea OTND, and Pu-erh tea PTND, respectively (10). These high molecular weight fractions are considered to be a complex mixture of tannins and contain several monosaccharides such as glucose and galactose and polyphenols. As polyphenolic compounds, kaempherol, quercetin, gallic acid, and catechins were identified (10).

Anti-tumor Promotion Activity of TNDs

Murine JB6 cells cannot grow in soft agar. However, after treatment with 12-*O*-tetradecanoylphorbol-13-acetate they can grow in soft agar. When BTND was added to this system, the number of the colonies was reduced dose-dependently. The reduction of the colony number was concentration-dependent and 30 μg/ml of BTND inhibited colony formation almost completely (10). Other TNDs also inhibited neoplastic transformation induced by TPA in a concentration-dependent manner.

Apoptosis-inducing Activity of TNDs

It was noticed that BTND and EGCG induce apoptosis in the transformant of JB6 cells. These transformant cells were prepared by the treatment of JB6 cells with *N*-ethyl-*N*'-nitro-*N*-nitrosoguanidine. Apoptotic cells were detected as fluorescent cells by the terminal deoxynucleotidyl transferase-mediated dUTP-biotin nick end labeling (TUNEL) method (Figure 1). With BTND at 80 μg/ml, 12% of the cell population underwent apoptosis, while no apparent apoptosis was observed for the untreated cells. Other TNDs also induced apoptosis, but the effects were weaker than BTND. JB6 cells before transformation did not show any apoptotic feature under these conditions. Thus, the effects of BTND and EGCG on mouse tumor cells appear to be stronger than those on the normal counterpart.

TNDs and EGCG were also found to inhibit cell proliferation by inducing apoptosis in human leukemia U937 cells, human stomach cancer MKN45 cells, and human colon cancer WiDr cells (11).

Effects on Expression of Apoptosis-related mRNAs

It is generally accepted that immediate-early response oncogenes are activated in the course of apoptosis (12,13). The reverse transcription-polymerase chain reaction (RT-PCR) method detected the increase in the levels of these oncogenes, particularly in c-*fos*, by treatment with EGCG or BTND (Figure 2).

The expression of mRNAs related to apoptosis was also examined using RT-PCR with primer sets for several proteins, called Multiplex supplied by Maxim Biotech, Inc. (South San Francisco, CA; Figure 3). EGCG did not affect so much the expression of mRNAs for these, while BTND caused drastic changes of these mRNA levels. The mRNAs for ICE or caspase 1 and TNF-α were greatly reduced, but there was no change in bcl-2 (Figure 3, a and b).

There were also several other changes. The m-RNA for caspase 8 (Flice) was increased and mRNAs for cell-membrane-associated proteins, Fas, Fas-ligand, Fadd and Tradd were also increased (Figure 3, c and d). However the mechanism of apoptosis induction by TNDs has not yet been elucidated. The data, however, suggest that the apoptosis induction mechanism of BTND is different from that of EGCG.

Carcinogenesis in *APC* Knockout Mice

The APC1309 knockout mice with a mutated adenomatous polyposis coli gene were generously supplied by the Japanese Foundation for Cancer Research, Cell Biology Department, Cancer Institute, Tokyo, Japan. By 15-weeks of age, they developed polyps of about 30 in average in the gastrointestinal tract. The oral administration of EGCG (0.05% w/v in water) or GTND (0.05% w/v in water) was started at 4 weeks of age. Table I shows the number of tumors larger than 0.5 mm in size in each gastrointestinal segment of APC1309 knockout mice. EGCG reduced the number of tumors in the stomach and the colon by 60 and 66%, respectively, but failed to do so in the small intestine. However, when the total tumor number was compared, no significant difference was observed between the EGCG and the control groups. In these

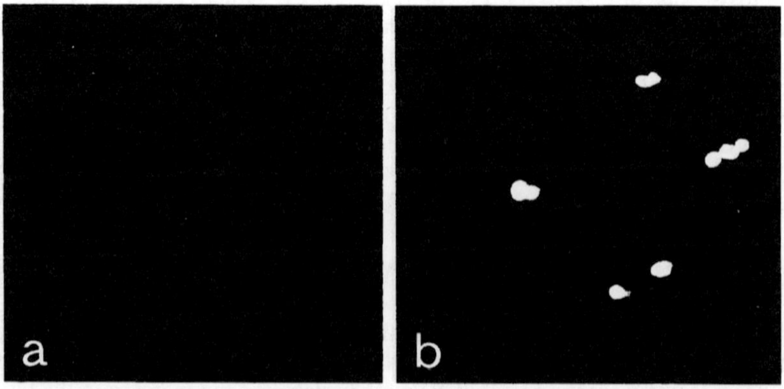

Figure 1. JB6 transformants cultured on cover slips were incubated with (b) or without (a) BTND at 80 μg /ml for 24 h. Apoptotic cells labeled fluorescently by the TUNEL method were detected using excitation at 492 nm and emission at 513 nm.

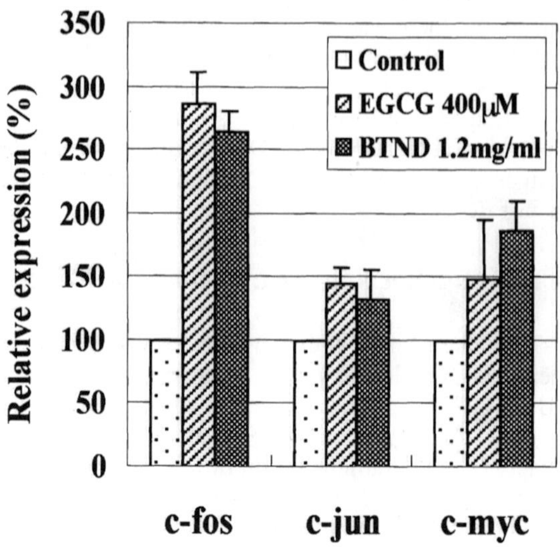

Figure 2. Effect of EGCG and BTND on expression of immediate-early response proto- oncogenes.

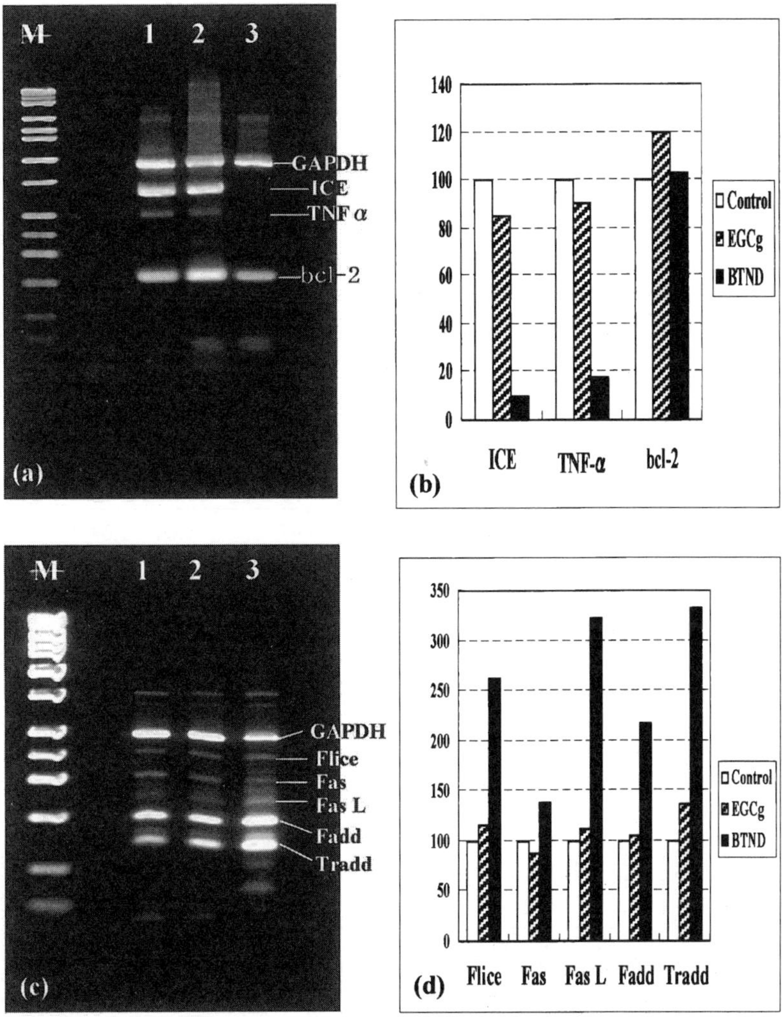

Figure 3. Effect of EGCG and BTND on mRNA expression. RT-PCR products from mRNA of control U937 cells (lane 1), cells incubated with EGCG at 200 μM (lane 2) or with 1.2 mg/ml of BTND (lane 3) were examined by agarose gel electrophoresis (a and c), and fluorescence intensity (ordinate) determined by FluoroImager (Molecular Dynamics Japan Inc., Yokyo, Japan) is expressed in percentage relative to that for glyceraldehyde-3-phosphate dehydrogenase, GAPDH (b and d). Primers used were sets for GAPDH, ICE, TNF-α, NF-κB, bcl-2, and I-κB (a) and for GAPDH, Flice, Fas, FasL, Fadd, and Tradd (c). M, DNA size marker.

Table I. Number of Tumors in Each Gastrointestinal Segment in APC 1309 Knockout Mice

Gastrointestinal segment	*Number of tumors per mouse*		
	Control	*EGCG group*	**GTND group**
Stomach	1.89±1.34	0.75±0.97	1.04±1.04
		(p <0.05)	(p <0.05)
Small intestine	27.78±11.92	23.58±12.09	20.08±9.77
		NS	(p <0.05)
Colon	2.00±1.73	0.67±0.65	1.08±1.10
		(p <0.005)	(p <0.05)
Total	31.67±12.95	25.00±11.80	22.21±10.03
		NS	(p<0.01)
No. of mice	27	12	24

Tumors ≧0.5 mm in size in the gastrointestinal tract were counted with a Video scope CF 200Z Magnifying Endoscope (Olympus Corp.). NS, not significant.

knockout mice, most of polyps were generated in the small intestine, and therefore, the change in the small intestine contributed mostly to the change in the total number.

GTND reduced the number of tumors larger than 0.5 mm in all tissues examined. When the polyp size was limited to the size larger than 3 mm, there was no difference between the control and the treated group either with EGCG or GTND (Table II). Because of the small number of polyps generated, further studies on evaluation of the effects is deemed necessary.

Lastly, the apoptosis in the tumor tissues was examined by the TUNEL method (Figure 4). In the untreated control group, tumor tissues larger than 0.5 mm, but smaller than 3.0 mm, had a smaller number of apoptotic cells than the tumor tissues larger than 3.0 mm. In contrast, the tumor tissues larger than 0.5 mm but smaller than 3.0 mm in the GTND-treated group tended to have the apoptosis index greater than that of tumors larger than 3.0 mm in this group, though not significant statistically. When tumor tissues larger than 0.5 mm but smaller than 3.0 mm in the control and GTND groups were compared, the apoptosis index in the GTND group was larger than that in the control with a statistical significance. These findings suggest that GTND induces apoptosis in the *in vivo* system, too, especially during the early stage of carcinogenesis.

In summary, the present study indicated that TNDs had anti-carcinogenic and apoptosis-inducing activities, and suggests that drinking of tea is beneficial for prevention of cancer of the digestive tract as has been suggested by epidemiological studies such as those by Oguni *et al.* (14) and Setiawan *et al.* (15).

Acknowledgements

This study was supported in part by Program for Promotion of Basic Research Activities for Innovative Biosciences from the Japan Science Society, by a Grant-in-Aid for Scientific research from the Ministry of Education, Science, Sports, and Culture of Japan (12660119), and by Goto Research Grant from University of Shizuoka.

We also thank greatly Dr. Tetsuo Noda for generous supply of APC1309 knockout mice.

References

1. Kuroda, Y.; Hara, Y. *Mutat. Res.* **1999**, *436*, 69-97.
2. Lin, J. K.; Liang, Y. C.; Lin-Shiau, S. Y. *Biochem. Pharmacol.* **1999**, *58*, 911-915.
3. Hibasami, H.; Achiwa, Y.; Fujikawa, T.; Komiya, T. *Anticancer Res.* **1996**, *16*, 1943-1946.
4. Saeki, K.; Sano, M.; Miyase, T.; Nakamura, Y.; Hara, Y.; Aoyagi, Y.; Isemura, M. *Biosci. Biotechnol. Biochem.* **1999**, *63*, 585-587.

Table II. Effects of EGCG and GTND on the Number of Gastrointestinal Tumors Larger than 3 mm

Treatment	*No. of mice*	*No. of tumors*
Control	27	3.30±2.27
EGCG	12	4.08±3.68
GTND	24	4.13±3.14

Mice were maintained on EGCG or GTND from 4 weeks until 14 weeks after birth. Data are presented as mean ±SD. The difference of tumor numbers between treated group and control group was not statistically significant.

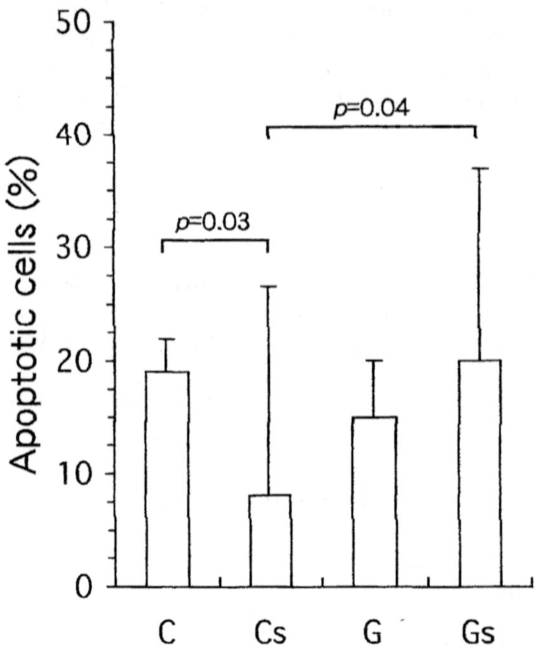

Figure 4. Apoptotic cell population in the tumors larger than 3.0 mm (C) and smaller than 3.0 mm but larger than 0.5 mm (Cs) of the untreated (control) APC1309 knockout mice or in the tumors larger than 3.0 mm (G) and smaller than 3.0 mm but larger than 0.5 mm (Gs) of the GTND-treated knockout mice.

5. Suganuma, M.; Okabe, S.; Sueoka, N.; Sueoka, E.; Matsuyama, S.; Imai, K.; Nakachi, K.; Fujiki, H. *Mutat. Res.* **1999**, *428*, 339-344.
6. Ahmad, N.; Cheng, P.; Mukhtar, H. *Biochem. Biophys. Res. Commun.* **2000**, *275*, 328-334.
7. Chen, Z. P.; Schell, J. B.; Ho, C. T.; Chen, K. Y. *Cancer Lett.* **1998**, *129*, 173-179.
8. Yang, G. Y.; Liao, J.; Kim, K.; Yurkow, E. J.; Yang, C. S. *Carcinogenesis* **1998**, *19*, 611-616.
9. Nakamura, Y.; Kawase, I.; Harada, S.; Matsuda, M.; Honma, T.; Tomita, I. In *Food Factors for cancer Prevention*; Ohigashi, H., Osawa, T., Terao, J., Watanabe, S., Yoshikawa, T., Ed.; Springer-Verlag: Tokyo, 1997; pp 138-141.
10. Nakamura, Y.; Matsuda, M.; Honma, T.; Tomita, I.; Shibata, N.; Warashina, T.; Noro, T.; Hara, Y. In *Plant Polyphenols 2: Chemistry, Biology, Ecology*; Gross, A., Ed.; Kluwer Academic / Plenum Publishers: New York, NY, 1999; pp 629-641.
11. Hayakawa, S.; Kimura, T.; Saeki, K.; Koyama, Y.; Aoyagi, Y.; Noro, T.; Nakamura, Y.; Isemura, M. *Biosci. Biotechnol. Biochem.* **2001**, *65*, 459-462.
12. Eliot, H. E.; Borner, M. M.; Sinha, B. K. *Anticancer Res.* **1995**, *15*, 729-733.
13. Abiko, Y.; Arai, J.; Mitamura, J.; Kaku, T. *Cancer Lett.* **1997**, *118*, 101-107.
14. Oguni, I.; Nasu, K.; Kanaya, S.; Ota, Y.; Yamamoto, S.; Nomura, T. *Japan J. Nutr.* **1989**, *47*, 93-102.
15. Setiawan, V.W.; Zhang, Z. F.; Yu, G. P.; Lu, Q. Y.; Li. Y. L.; Lu, M. L.; Wang, M. R.; Guo, C. H.; Yu. S. Z.; Kurtz, R. C.; Hsieh. C. C. *Int. J. Cancer.* **2001**, *92*, 600-604.

Other Food Factors

Chapter 34

Structural Modification to Improve Psyllium Functionality

Liangli Yu

Department of Food Science and Human Nutrition, Colorado State University, Fort Collins, CO 80523–1571

A novel procedure was developed to improve psyllium functionality by conducting a solid-state enzyme reaction. The procedure requires no special equipment/operation (such as freeze dry) and could be carried out without using any additional chemicals. To evaluate the solid-state enzymatic procedure, modified psyllium preparations were produced under selected reaction conditions, and analyzed for their water-absorbing capacity, gelling capacity, particle surface structure, and soluble and insoluble fiber contents. The results showed that structural modification improved psyllium functionality. Modified psyllium preparations had reduced water-absorbing capacity and less gelling ability. The reduced water-absorbing capacity may be explained by the decreased surface area of psyllium particles. In addition, the solid-state enzymatic treatments had much less effects on soluble fiber contents than the liquid phase enzymatic reactions.

Psyllium, the seed husk of the plant Plantago genus, is an excellent source of soluble and insoluble dietary fibers. Previous studies have shown that psyllium is a highly branched acidic arabinoxylan (*1*). The xylan backbone has both (1→4) and (1→3) linkages. Other monosaccharides presented in psyllium include D-rhamnose, D-galactose, D-galacturonic acid, 4-O-methyl-D-glucuronic acid, and 2-*O*-(2-D-galactopyranosyluronic acid)-L-rhamnose (*2*). A number of studies have been conducted to investigate the health benefits of psyllium and its applications in food and other consumer products such as hair-setting lotions (*2*). In addition to its cholesterol-lowering activity, psyllium also has laxative effects, can reduce the risk of colon cancer, treat gastric hypoacidity, and may be helpful in weight control (*3-7*). The application of psyllium in functional foods have received more attention since FDA approved that psyllium containing foods may have a health claim of reducing the risk of heart disease. However, its extremely strong water-uptaking and gelling capacities have limited the incorporation of psyllium in foods as well as its other applications.

There have been several physical/mechanical means developed to improve the functionality and sensory properties of psyllium, including controlling the range of particle size (*8*), mixing and extruding with other food ingredients (*9*), and coating and granulating psyllium with polyvinylpyrrolidone and polyethylene glycol (*10*). These previous investigations have indicated the potential possibility of improving the physicochemical/sensory properties of psyllium and to promote its applications in foods. However, none of them could sufficiently solve the strong gelling and extreme water-uptaking problems of psyllium. No structural modification has been conducted to improve the functional properties of psyllium until Yu and others (*1*) disclosed an enzymatic procedure to produce novel psyllium preparations with a reduced water-uptaking capacity and different gelling properties. Unfortunately, this procedure is not practically applicable since a freeze-dry step has to be involved to remove the water added for the enzyme reaction.

In this chapter, a solid-state enzymatic procedure for psyllium modification and the novel psyllium preparations with improved functionalities is discussed. This procedure requires no special operation, equipments and hazardous chemicals. This procedure also produces no chemical wastes.

Materials and Methods

Solid-state Enzymatic Reaction

A known amount of enzymes was added to 50 g raw psyllium (98% purity, 40 mesh, JB Laboratories). The enzyme preparations may contain cellulases, xylanases, hemicellulases, pentosanses, aribanases, and beta-glucanases but substantially free of amylase and protease activities (*1*). The reaction was conducted at 40-50°C and terminated by inactivating enzymes. The enzymes were inactivated according to the method described previously (*1*). The final product of the solid-state reaction was obtained after grinding the material through a 20 mesh sieve. Controls were performed using the above procedure without addition of enzymes.

Water Absorbing Capacity

Water absorbing capacity was determined gravimetrically using a modification of the method described by Elizalde *et al.* (*11*), with some modification. Briefly, all samples were equilibrated in a 10% relative humidity (RH) chamber for 48 hours. Then, samples were transferred into a 98% RH chamber and exposed to moisture for 5 min. The dry matter and the absolute amount of absorbed water were determined. All measurements were made in triplicate. The results were expressed as the mean ± SD in mg water absorbed by per gram of psyllium per minute.

Gelling Property

Gelling properties were analyzed using a TA-XT2 texture analyzer (Texture Technologies Corp, Scarsdale, NY), with a 25 mm diameter probe (*12*). 1.50 g of each psyllium preparation was added into 30 ml distilled deionized water and stirred for 30 seconds. After setting for 24 hours, gel samples were subjected to a double compression test. Measurements were performed with a pretest speed of 2.0 mm/sec, a test speed of 5.0 mm/sec, a post test speed of 5.0 mm/sec, and a distance of 6 mm. All measurements were made in triplicate. The results were expressed as the mean ± SD in gram force for Hardness and Adhesiveness.

Fiber Contents

Soluble and insoluble fiber contents in modified and raw psyllium were measured using a commercial kit purchased from Megazyme International Ireland Ltd (Wicklow, Ireland) according to the previously reported procedure (*13*).

Surface Structures

Scanning electron microscope (SEM) analysis was conducted to determine the surface structures of modified psyllium preparations using a Philips SEM 505 instrument (Holland).

Results and Discussion

A solid-state enzymatic procedure was developed for psyllium modification to improve the functionalities of psyllium and consequently to promote it applications in functional foods. Modified psyllium products from the solid-state reactions were powdered solid (Figure 1A) and required no additional steps for water removal. In contrast, a free-dry step has to be involved to remove water from the final gel materials (Figure 1B) obtained from the conventional liquid-phase enzymatic reactions (*1*). The weight based yield of the solid-state procedure is about 100%, which is much higher than that of the liquid-phase reactions (*1*).

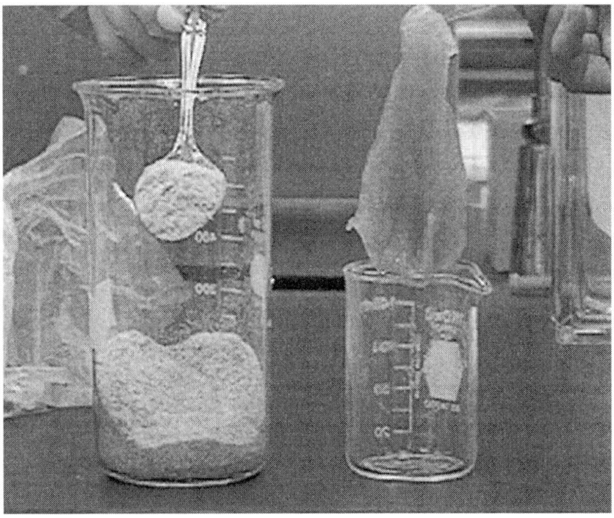

A B

Figure 1. Modified psyllium products from solid-state enzymatic reaction vs. conventional liquid-state enzymatic reaction. *A = modified psyllium at the end of solid-state reaction, and B = modified psyllium at the end of liquid state enzymatic reaction. Psyllium preparation A requires no additional water-removing step, while psyllium preparation B requires additional step to remove water.*

Psyllium prepared by the solid-state enzymatic procedure had reduced water-absorbing capacity (Figure 2). Increased levels of enzymes were not always associated with further reduction in water absorbing capacity. The lowest water-uptaking rate of modified psyllium by the solid-state procedure

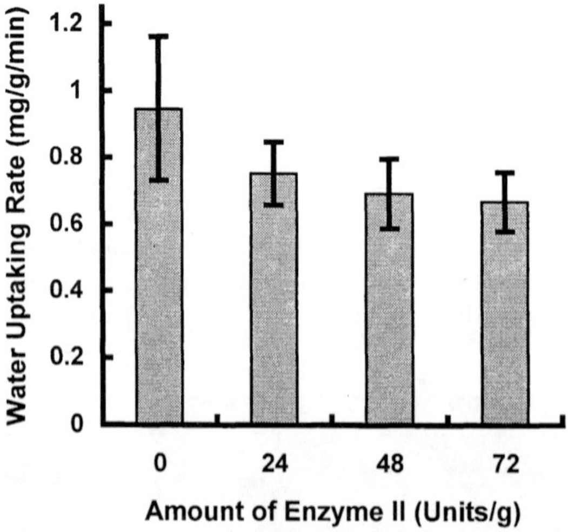

Figure 2. Effects of solid-state enzymatic treatment on water-absorbing capacity of psyllium.

was 41% of that of the control sample under the experimental conditions. Reduced water-absorbing capacity is preferred for food applications of the psyllium preparations (*1,8, 9*).

Solid-state enzymatic treatment reduced the gelling capacity of the modified psyllium preparations (Figure 3). Compared to raw psyllium, modified psyllium formed a weaker and less adhesive gel. Higher concentration of enzyme may further reduce the gelling capacity of modified psyllium (Figure 4). The psyllium preparations, with lower gelling ability, are much easier to incorporate into food formulae. These psyllium preparations also raise less concern about the undesirable sensory properties of the final food products containing significant levels of psyllium fibers.

To better understand the solid-state enzymatic reactions, the surface structures of the modified psyllium were analyzed and compared to that of raw psyllium using a scanning electron microscope (SEM). SEM results showed that modified psyllium had a smoother surface than raw psyllium (Figure 5). In another words, solid-state enzymatic treatment reduced the total surface area of the psyllium particles. This reduction may explain the reduced water-uptaking rate of the modified psyllium preparations, but not the improved gelling properties. More studies are needed to evaluate the effects of solid-state enzymatic modification on gel forming properties of psyllium.

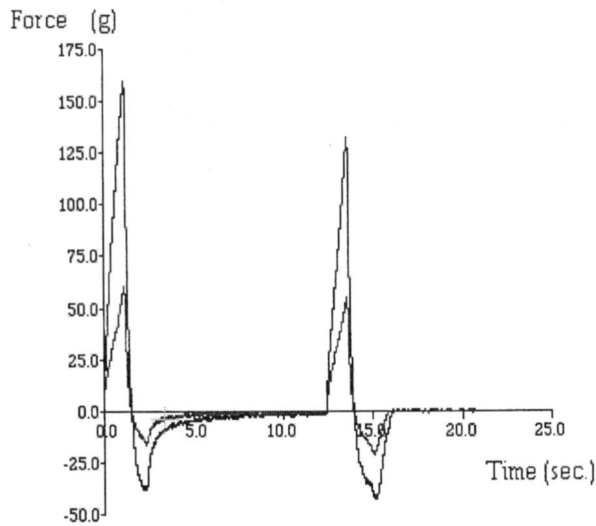

Figure 3. Effects of solid-state enzymatic treatment on gelling capacity of psyllium.

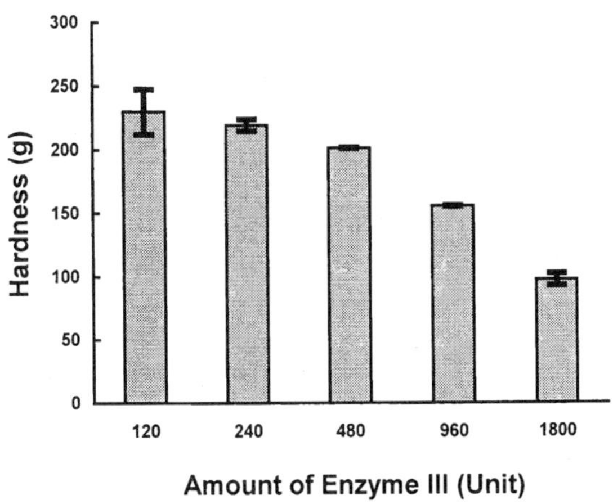

Figure 4. Effects of enzyme amount on gel hardness.

A B

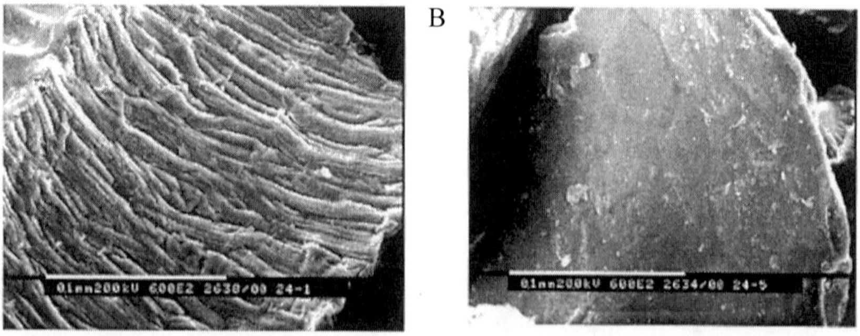

Figure 5. Surface structures of psyllium preparations determined by SEM. *A = surface structure of raw psyllium, and B = surface structure of modified psyllium.*

The soluble and insoluble fiber contents of the modified psyllium preparations were measured to estimate the effects of structural modification on the biological activities of psyllium including cholesterol-lowing activity, since the soluble fibers were believed to contribute to the cholesterol-lowing activity of raw psyllium (*1, 8, 9*). Compared to the liquid-phase enzyme reaction, solid-state enzymatic treatments showed less effect on soluble fiber contents of the modified psyllium preparations (Table 1), while both procedures had minor effects on insoluble fiber contents. Similar ratios of the selected enzyme resulted in about 15% reduction in soluble fiber content by the conventional liquid-phase enzymatic reaction (*1*), while only had less than 4% reduction in soluble fiber content under the solid-state reaction conditions. This is another advantage of the solid-state enzymatic procedure vs. the liquid-phase enzymatic reaction described previously by Yu et al. (*1*).

Table I. Soluble and insoluble fiber contents of modified psyllium

Enzyme II (U)	*Soluble fiber (g/100 g psyllium)*	*Insoluble fiber (g/100 g psyllium)*
120	72.9	12.4
240	77.3	12.6
480	75.9	13.2
960	73.1	11.9
1800	68.3	12.3
Raw psyllium	79.6	12.4

Acknowledgments

This study was supported by the Colorado Agricultural Experiment Station and the Colorado Wheat Research Foundation. The author would like to thank Dr. Mary Harris in the Department of Food Science and Human Nutrition at Colorado State University for her review of this manuscript.

References

1. Yu, L.; DeVay, G.; Lai, G.; Simmons, C.; Neilsen, S. 2001, US Pat. 6248373.
2. Chan, J.K.C.; Wypyszyk, V. *Cereal Foods World* **1988**, *33*, 919-922.
3. Park, H.; Deib, P.A.; Chung, O.K. *Cereal Chem.* **1997**, *74*, 207-211.
4. Hara, H.; Suzuki, K.; Kobayashi, S.; Kasai, T. *Nutr. Biochem.* **1996**, *7*, 549-554.
5. Ganji, V.; Kies, C. V. *J. Food Sci. Nutr.* **1996**, *84*, 595-597.
6. Arjmandi, B.H.; Craig, J.; Nathani, S.; Reeves, R.D. *J. Nutr.* **1992**, *122*, 1559-1565.
7. Anderson, J.; Deakins, D.A.; Floore, T.L.; Smith, B.M.; Whitis, S.E. *Crit. Rev. Food Sci. Nutr.* **1990**, *29*, 95-146.
8. Rudin, R. 1988, US Pat. No. Re. 32,811.
9. Wullschleger, R.D.; Creek B.; Chen, S.C.; Bowman, F.A.; Hawblitz, L.V. 1993, US Pat. 5,227,248.
10. Powell, D. R.; Patel, V. K. 1982, US Pat. No. 4,321,263.
11. Elizalde, B.E.; Pilosof, A.M.R.; Bartholomai, G.B. *J. Food Sci.* **1996**, *61*, 407-409.
12. Paraskevopoul, A.; Kiosseoglou, V. J. Food Sci. **1997**, *62*, 208-211.
13. Lee, S. C.; Rodriguez, F.; Storey, M.; Farmakalidis, E.; Prosky, L. *J. AOAC Int.* **1995**, *78*, 724-729.

Chapter 35

Effect of Antioxidants on Photosensitized Degradation of Methionine by Riboflavin

Shuichi Muranishi[1], Hideki Masuda[1], Susumu Kiyohara[1], Toshio Ueno[1], and Chi-Tang Ho[2]

[1]Material Research and Development Laboratories, Ogawa and Company, Ltd. 15–7, Chidori, Urayasushi, Chiba 279–0032, Japan
[2]Department of Food Science, Rutgers, The State University of New Jersey, 65 Dudley Road, New Brunswick, NJ 08901

Methionine and riboflavin are useful nutrients in foods, especially, dairy products. However, during light irradiation, methionine is well-known to produce sulfur off-odorants due to the participation of photosensitized riboflavin under neutral conditions. In this study, the important sulfur off-odorants were found to be methional, dimethyl disulfide, and dimethyl trisulfide, formed from methionine and riboflavin under acidic conditions during light irradiation. The inhibition effect of a variety of antioxidants on the formation of the off-odorants has also been studied.

Methionine and riboflavin, that is vitamin B_2, are important nutrients. However, these components are well-known to produce several sulfur compounds during irradiation with light (*1-4*). In general, the sulfur compounds have a characteristic odor and extremely low threshold for producing off-odors as well as being an important odor in foods (*5*). Therefore, it is important to prevent the off-odor formation as well as the decrease of nutritive value under the light irradiation. Some studies using dark containers to inhibit the transmittance of light were reported (*6-8*). On the other hand, as for additives to prevent the off-odor formation, such as antioxidants, there have been few studies (*9-11*). In addition, taking into account the fact that acidic dairy products are becoming very popular on the market and the lack of studies about the deterioration under acidic conditions, we have focused on the effect of additives preventing the off-odors formed from methionine and riboflavin during light irradiation under acidic conditions. The formation pathway of off-odors is also discussed in this report.

Experimental

Methionine and riboflavin were purchased from Nakaraitesc. Methyl methanethiosulfonate was purchased from Aldrich. 2-Propenal, dimethyl disufide, and methyl heptanoate were purchased from Tokyo-kasei. Dimethyl trisufide was purchased from Taste maker. Rutin, quercitrin, *p*-coumaric acid, ferulic acid, sinapinic acid, *p*-hydroxybenzoic acid, vanillic acid, syringic acid, gallic acid, protocatechuic acid, butylhydroxyanisol (BHA), and L(+)-ascorbic acid were purchased from Nakaraitesc. Rosmarinic acid was purchased from Funakoshi. Chlorogenic acid was purchased from Wako Pure Chemical. 6-Hydroxy-2,5,7,8-tetramethylchroman-2-carboxylic acid (Trolox) was purchased from Tokyo-kasei. (-)-Epicatechin, (-)-epigallocatechin and (-)-epigallocatechin gallate were purchased from Kurita.

A 3.35 mM methionine and 1.33 μM riboflavin acidic aqueous solution were prepared in the following way. One g of methionine, 10 mL of 0.266 mM riboflavin buffer solution, and 1 mL of 1% (w/v) methyl heptanoate (an internal standard) ethanolic solution were mixed and then the mixture was diluted with acidic buffer solution (pH=3.5) up to 2 L. The buffer solution was prepared by mixing a 0.1 M citric acid aqueous solution and 0.2 M sodium dihydrogen phosphate aqueous solution. For testing the antioxidant's effect, 0.5 mL of each 10 mM antioxidant solution in 50% (w/w) ethanol was added to the methionine-riboflavin acidic solution (total 50 mL) and sealed in a glass vessel. For testing the participation of singlet oxygen, sodium azide (0.154, 0.769 and 1.54 μM) were added to the 3.35 mM methionine and 1.33 μM riboflavin acidic aqueous solution. Each solution was irradiated with fluorescent light consisting of daylight color (40 W×15, 15,000 Lux) at 10°C for 3 hrs in an Eyela LST-300 light box apparatus. After the light irradiation, the degradation products were extracted with dichloromethane (30 mL×2). The extract was dried over sodium sulfate, evaporated (40°C/450mmHg), and concentrated to about 100 μL in a stream of nitrogen.

A GC-MS analysis was performed using a Hewlett-Packard 5890 Series II gas chromatograph equipped with a flame ionization detector (FID) and a DB-

WAX fused silica capillary column (60 m×0.25 mm i.d.; film thickness of 0.25 µm; J&W Scientific) was used. The operating conditions were as follows: injector temperature, 250°C; detector temperature, 250°C; nitrogen carrier gas flow rate of 1.2 mL/min; oven temperature program, 40°C (2 min), raised at 12°C/min to 210°C (20 min); 1 µL of sample was injected using a split ratio of 1:28. The amounts of the methionine degradation products were calculated by the ratios of the computed areas versus that of the internal standard (methyl heptanoate). The response factors between the all degradation products and methyl heptanoate were determined in advance.

The radical scavenging activity was assayed according to the following method. A 0.1 M citric acid-sodium dihydrogenphospate buffer (pH 3.5, 2 mL), 0.04 mM 1,1-diphenyl-2-picrylhydrazyl (DPPH) in ethanol (1 mL), and 2 mL of 5 µM antioxidant solution in 50% (w/w) ethanol were mixed. For the control, 2 mL of 50% (w/w) ethanol was added instead of the antioxidant solution. After allowing the mixture to stand at room temperature for 30 min, the absorbance at 517 nm was measured. The radical scavenging activity of each antioxidant (2 µM) was explained as the DPPH radical inhibition rate which is defined by the following formula: DPPH radical inhibition rate = (the absorbance at 517 nm of the addition sample of antioxidant)/(the absorbance at 517 nm of control sample). All tests were run in triplicate and averaged.

A GC-MS analysis was performed using a Hewlett-Packard 5890 Series II gas chromatograph equipped with an HP-5972 mass selective detector and a DB-WAX fused silica capillary column (60 m×0.25 mm i.d.; film thickness of 0.25 µM; J&W Scientific) was used. The operating conditions were as follows: injector temperature, 250°C; helium carrier gas flow rate of 1 mL/min; oven temperature program, 40°C (2 min), raised at 12°C/min to 210°C (20 min); 1 µL of sample was injected using a split ratio of 1:50; ionization voltage, 70 eV; ion source temperature, 140°C.

Results and Discussion

Some volatile sulfur compounds were obtained from methionine and riboflavin after light irradiation under acidic conditions (Table I). Methyl mercaptan seems to be one of the important off-odor components. At this time, because of using the solvent extraction with dichloromethane, the amount of highly volatile methyl mercaptan seemed to be low. Therefore, we focused the other off-odor components, that is, methional, dimethyl disulfide (DMDS), dimethyl trisulfide (DMTS) and methyl methanethiosulfonate (MMTS). In particular, DMTS is considered to be significant because of its extremely low threshold value. Figure 1 shows that the amount of DMDS and DMTS increased with decreasing pH value.

Table I. Sulfur Compounds Formed from Methionine and Riboflavin during Light Irradiation under Acidic Conditions.

Sulfur compound	*Yield* [a)]	*Odor description*	*Threshold value* [b)]
methional	30.4 (3.2)	cooked potate-like	0.2
DMDS	28.7 (2.7)	cooked cabbage-like, pickle-like	0.16-12
DMTS	7.3 (0.9)	cooked cabbage-like, pickle-like	0.005-0.01
MMTS	1.1 (0.1)	pickle-like	-
methyl mercaptane	trace	cabbage-like	0.02

[a)] µM (ppm). [b)] ppb; ref. in *12*.

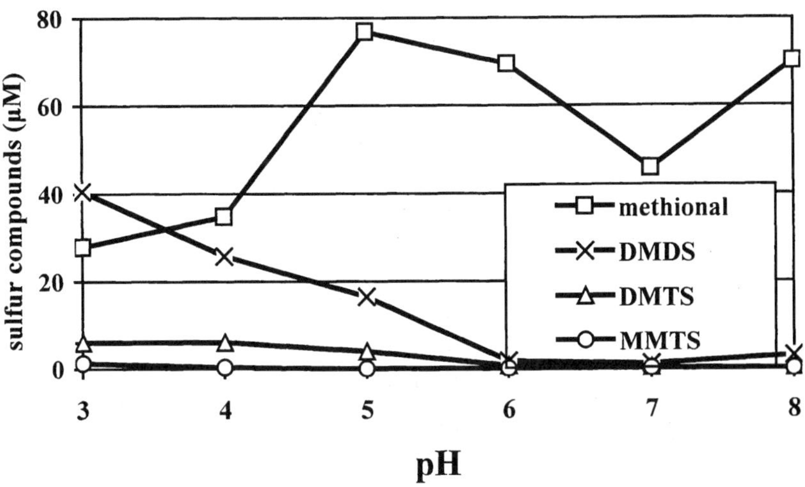

Figure 1. Relationship between the amount of sulfur compounds and the pH value.

Figure 2 shows that part of the antioxidants accelerated the formation of DMTS, however, most antioxidants inhibited the formation of all the sulfur compounds. Especially, the addition of catechin derivatives, that is (-)-epicatechin, (-)-epigallocatechin, (-)-epigallocatechin gallate, and rosmarinic acid were found to decrease the amounts of methional, DMDS, and DMTS at

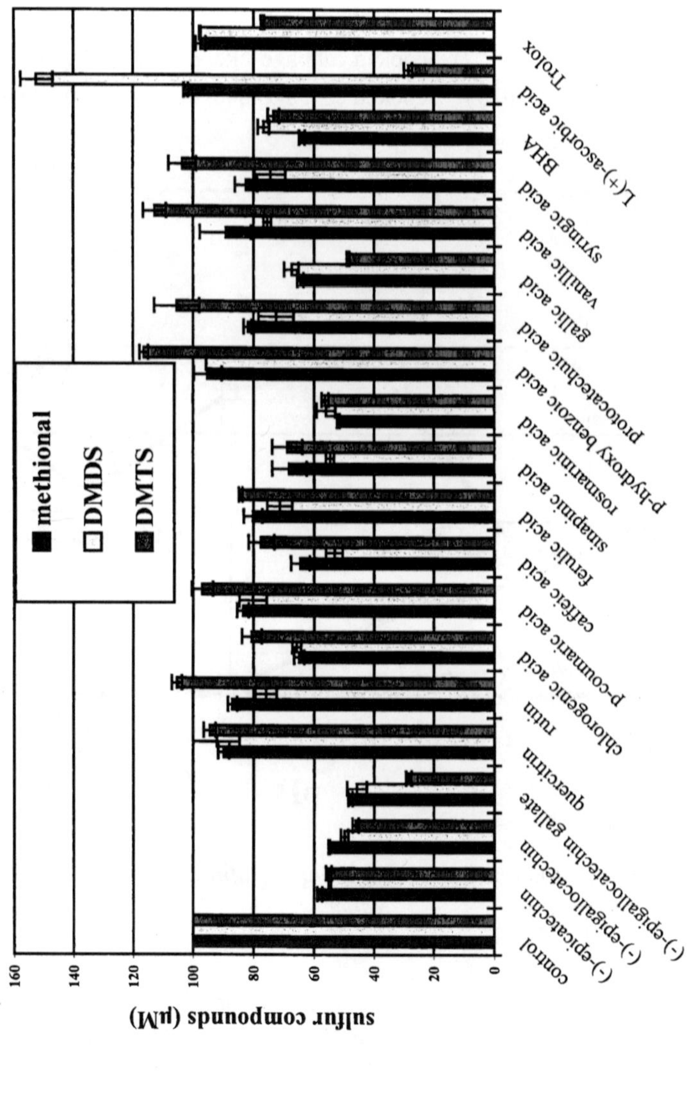

Figure 2. Effect of antioxidants on the amount of sulfur compounds.

less than 60% compared to those with no addition. As shown in Figure 3, the relationship between the DPPH radical scavenging activities of a variety of antioxidants and the amount of methional, DMDS and DMTS had a good negative correlation, respectively, when L(+)-ascorbic acid was ruled out as an outlying value. In addition, in order to study the action of the antioxidant in detail, we noted the behavior of all the sulfur compounds. Methional was reported to be formed via the Strecker degradation-like reaction of methionine by riboflavin (*13*). On the other hand, for the formation pathway of DMDS, it has been formed from methional and riboflavin during light irradiation (*14*). With the possibility of methional as the key precursor, the effect of methional addition into the reaction system of methionine and riboflavin on the amount of methional, DMDS, and DMTS was studied (Figure 4). Because there was no change in the amount of DMDS and DMTS by the addition of methional, methional appeared not to be a precursor of DMDS and DMTS. Furthermore, as for DMDS, singlet oxygen was reported to participate in its formation (*15,16*). In order to confirm the probable participation of singlet oxygen, sodium azide was added to the system of methionine and riboflavin under light irradiation. Sodium azide is well known to be a singlet oxygen quencher, however, it does not react with superoxide and the free radical species. The result in Figure 5, which shows the decreased tendency of DMDS and DMTS being greater than that of methional, supported the participation of singlet oxygen on the formation of DMDS and DMTS. Therefore, in order to evaluate the variety of antioxidant action, its quenching effect on singlet oxygen is considered to be also important as well as that on the free radical species.

Conclusion

Methional has been reported to be the most important off-odorant in the system of riboflavin and methionine under neutral conditions with light irradiation, however, under acidic conditions, dimethyl disulfide and dimethyl trisulfide in addition to methional were also the characteristic off-odorants. Most of the antioxidants used were found to be effective inhibitors of the formation of the sulfur off-odorants. Especilally, the catechin derivatives and rosmarinic acid were available. The scavenging ability of the antioxidant against the free radical seems to be related to the formation amount of methional, dimethyl disulfide, and dimethyl trisulfide. In addition to the radical species, singlet oxygen was also suggested to participate in the formation of dimethyl disulfide and dimethyl trisulfide from methionine and photosensitized riboflavin under acidic conditions.

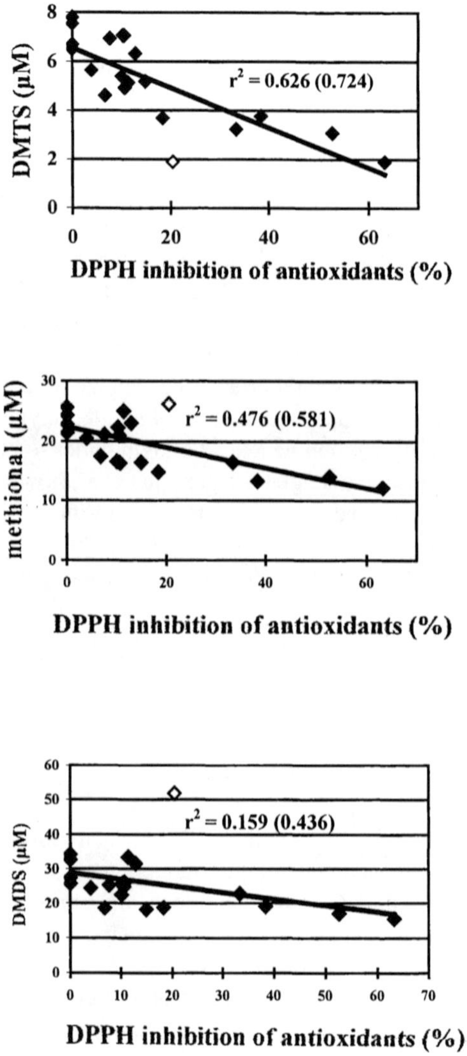

Figure 3. Relationship between the amount of dimethyl trisulfide (top) methional (center) and dimethyl disulfide (bottom), and the DPPH radical scavenging activities. Open symbols and filled ones represent the values for L(+)-ascorbic acid and those for other antioxidants, respectively. The r^2 values of parenthesis are those of all the antioxidants except for L(+)-ascorbic acid.

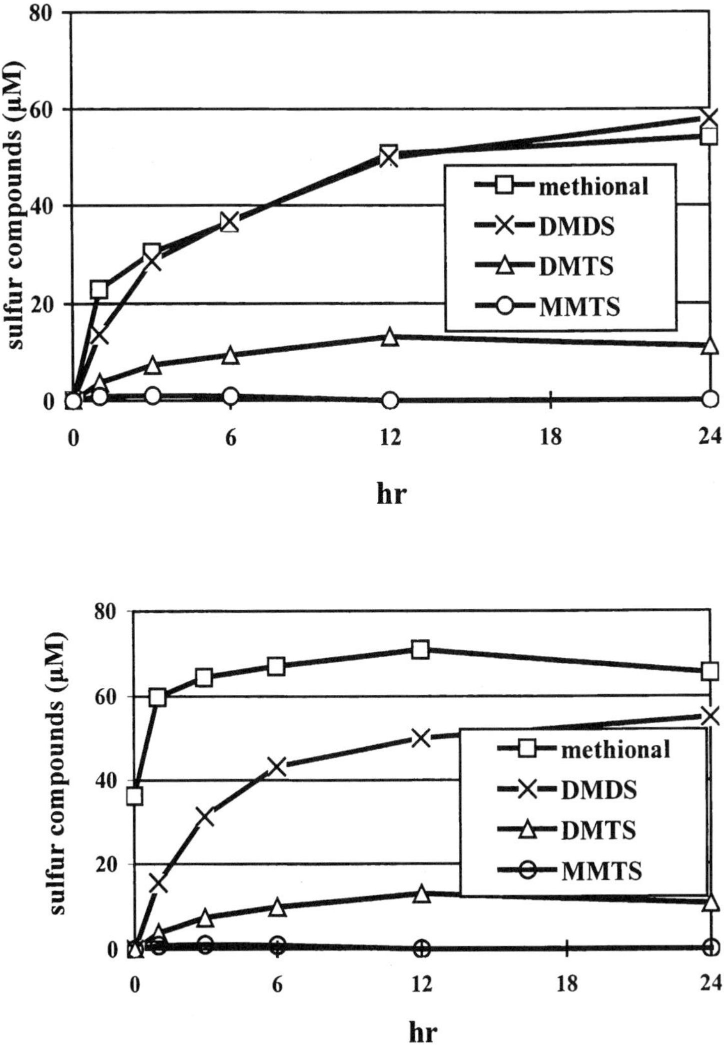

Figure 4. Effect of the addition of methional on the amount of sulfur compounds. Top: the non-addition of methional. Bottom: the addition of methional.

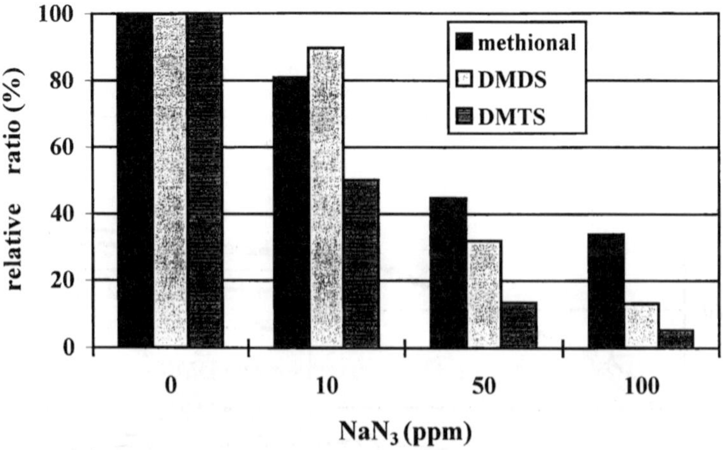

Figure 5. Effect of sodium azide on the amount of sulfur compounds.

References

1. Forss, D. A. *J. Dairy Res.* **1979**, *46*, 691-706.
2. Badings, H. T. In *Volatile compounds in foods and beverages*; Maarse, H., Ed.; Marcel Dekker, Inc.: New York, USA, 1991; pp. 91-106.
3. Azzara, C. D.; Campbell, L. B. In *Off-flavors in Foods and Beverages*; Charalabous, G., Ed.; Elsevier Science Publishers: Amsterdam, The Netherlands, 1992; pp.329-375.
4. Ott, A.; Fay, L. B.; Chaintreau, A. *J. Agric. Food Chem.* **1997**, *45*, 850-858.
5. Mussian, C. J.; Keelan, M. E., Eds. *Sulfur Compounds in Foods*. ACS Symp. Ser. 564; American Chemical Society: Washington, DC, 1994.
6. Dimick, P. S. *J. Milk Food Technol.* **1973**, *36*, 383-387.
7. Hoskin, J. C.; Dimick, P. S. *J. Food Prot.* **1979**, *42*, 105-109.
8. Fanelli, A. J.; Burlew, J.V.; Gabriel, M. K. *J. Food Prot.* **1985**, *48*, 112-117.
9. Bekbolet, M. *J. Food Prot.* **1990**, *53*, 430-440.
10. Kawamura, K.; Tanaka, K. Japan Patent 91, 272,643, **1991**.
11. Yamada, M.; Utena, M.; Hayashi, M.; Ezawa, K. Japan Patent 92, 21,450, **1992**.

12. Leffingwell, J. C.; Leffingwell, D. *Perfumer & Flavorist* **1991**, *16*, 1-19.
13. Dimick, P. S. *Can. Inst. Food Sci. Technol. J.* **1982**, *15*, 247-256.
14. Maujean, A. *Sciences Des Aliments* **1983**, *3*, 589-601.
15. Jung, M. Y.; Yoon, S. H.; Lee, H. O.; Min, D. B. *J. Food Sci.* **1998**, *63*, 408-412.
16. Bradley, D. G.; Min, D. B. *Crit. Rev. Food Sci. Nutr.* **1992**, *31*, 211-236.

Chapter 36

Comparative Study of Glycans in Lactoferrin-a and Lactoferrin-b

Zheng Wei and Toshihide Nishimura

Faculty of Applied Biological Science, Hiroshima University, Higashi, Hiroshima 739–8528, Japan

In lactoferrin-a, the glycans linked to Asn-233 and Asn-545 were of the high-mannose type, whereas those present at Asn-368 and Asn-476 were complex-type ones. These glycans possessed heterogeneous structures. HPLC analyses showed that the structures of glycans linked to Asn-368, Asn-476 and Asn-545 in lactoferrin-a were very similar to those in lactoferrin-b, and that the structure of glycan linked to Asn-233 was different between lactoferrins-a and –b. In addition, the glycan bound to Asn-281 present only in lactoferrin-a was complex-type one, which possessed the heterogeneous structures including Man3GlcNAc2, Man3GlcNAc4 and Man3GlcNAc4Fuc.

Lactoferrin (Lf) is an 80kDa iron-binding glycoprotein found in various biological secretions, mainly in milk (*1*) and in polymorphonuclear leukocytes (*2,3*). Biological properties ascribed to Lf include the regulation of absorption of metals, modulation of immunity and inflammation, and antimicrobial activity against bacteria and yeast (*4-,6*). Recently, other functions of Lf have been elucidated such as anti-virus, antioxidative, and anti-carcinogenic activities (*7-9*).

Bovine lactoferrin (bLf) consists of a 689-amino acid polypeptide chain to which complex and high-mannose type glycans are linked (*10*). These glycans are structurally heterogeneous and presented in four *N*-linked glycosylation sites, in which Asn-233 and -545 are linked with a high-mannose type glycan only, and Asn-368 and -476 with both complex or high-mannose type (*11*). However, a previous study clearly showed that a glycan is also present at Asn-281 potential glycosylation site in bovine lactoferrin-a (bLf-a) which possesses a higher molecular mass than regular lactoferrin-b (bLf-b) (*12*). This glycan resulted in the difference in molecular mass of bLf-a and bLf-b.

Recently, bLf-a was found to possess higher bactericidal activity against E. coli than bLf-b (*16*), however, the mechanism for this action is poorly understood. Therefore, it is important to clarify the structures of glycans in the five glycosylation sites of bLf-a.

In this chapter, the structures of glycans linked to five N-linked glycosylation sites in bLf-a were characterized, and compared with those from bLf-b.

Materials and Methods

Materials

BLfs-a and -b were purified from bovine colostrum by carboxymethyl cation exchange chromatography. Glycopeptides from bLfs-a and -b were separated by HPLC on a reverse-phase column (*12*).

Preparation of Glycans from Glycopeptides

The glycans were released from glycopeptides by gas phase hydrazinolysis (100°C, 2 hr) with Hydraclub C-206 (Honen Co., Tokyo, Japan), followed by *N*-acetylation. The pyridylamino (PA) derivatives of these glycans with 2-aminopyridine were prepared with a PALSTATION model 4000 (Takara Co. Kyoto, Japan) (*17*). The PA-glycans were purified by HPLC on a normal phase column.

Exoglycosidase Digestion of PA-glycans

The purified PA-glycans were digested with a GlycoSEQTM *N*-Complex Fit-Check Kit (Takara Co. Kyoto, Japan) in 20 μl of 0.5 M citrate-phosphate buffer (pH 5.0), at 37°C for 16 h. The GlycoSEQTM *N*-Complex Fit-Check Kit contained a glycosidase mixture of β-*N*-acetylhexosaminidase (from jack bean), β-galactosidase (from *Aspergillus*), neuraminidase (from *Arthrobacter*), α-1,3/4-fucosidase (from *Streptomyces*) and α-fucosidase (from beef kidney).

Endoglycosidase H Digestion of PA-glycans

The purified PA-glycans were digested with 5 mU endoglycosidase H (Endo H) in a citrate-phosphate buffer (pH 5.0), at 37°C for 16 h.

Analysis of PA-glycans on HPLC

The analysis of PA-glycans was carried out by JASCO GULLIVER HPLC system (Jasco, Co., Tokyo, Japan) with normal phase columns. HPLC was performed with a PALPAK Type-S column (Φ4.6mm*250mm: Takara Syuzo Co., Otsu, Japan) by a linear gradient, from 40 to 100 % B, which was run over a period of 50 min. Solvent A was 500 mM acetic acid- trimethylamine (pH 7.3) / acetonitrile / H_2O (10:75:15, v/v/v), and solvent B was 500 mM acetic acid-trimethylamine (pH 7.3) / acetonitrile / H_2O (40:50:10, v/v/v). Elution was performed at a flow rate of 1.0ml/min at 40°C, and the PA-glycans fluorescence was detected using excitation and emission wavelengths of 320 and 400 nm, respectively.

Results

Characterization of Glycans in BLf-a

The glycans linked to Asn-233, 368, 476 and 545 in bLf-a were analyzed by HPLC on a PALPAK Type-S column before and after endoglycosidase digestion for glycan.

Glycans at Asn-233 and Asn-545

As shown in Figure 1-A, the glycans bound to Asn-233 of bLf-a were separated into two major and several minor peaks by HPLC, suggesting that the glycan linked to Asn-233 possessed a heterogeneous structure. After a mixture of glycans was digested with Endo H, all glycan peaks shifted (Figure 1-B), suggesting that the glycan linked to Asn-233 was a high-mannose type glycan.

On the other hand, the glycan linked to Asn-545 was separated into one major peak and several minor peaks. These glycan peaks moved by treatment with Endo H. These results suggested that the glycan linked to Asn-545 was a high-mannose type glucan, and possessed a heterogeneous structure.

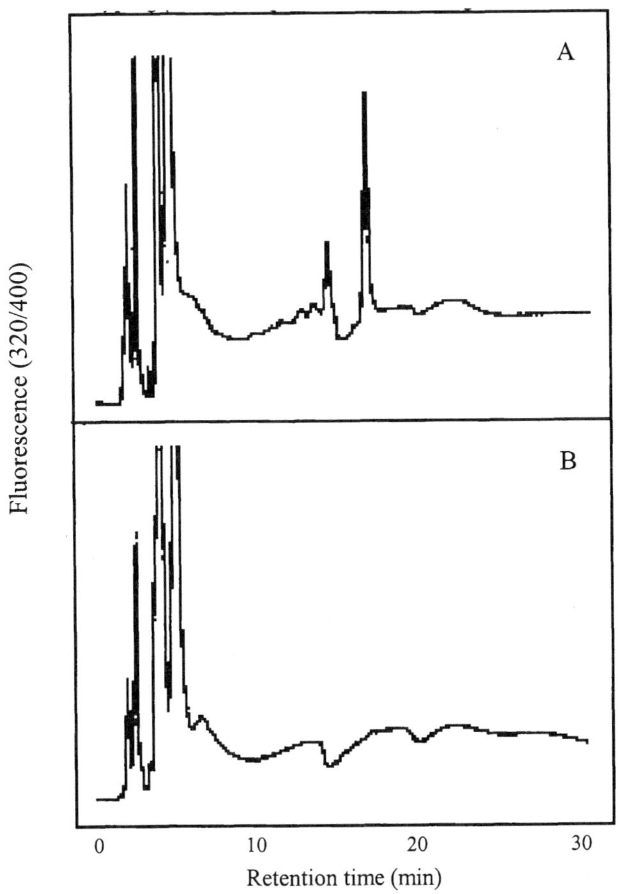

Figure 1. Analysis of glycans at Asn-233 of bLf-a by HPLC on a PALPAK Type-S column. A, PA-glycan at Asn-233; B, PA-glycan at Asn-233 after digestion with Endo H. The experimental details are given under materials and methods.

Glycans at Asn-368 and Asn-476

Several glycan peaks were detected in HPLC pattern for the glycan linked to Asn-368, suggesting that the structure of the glycan linked to Asn-368 was heterogeneous (Figure 2A). When these glycans were digested with a mixture of glycosidases, only one major peak whose elution position coincided with that of standard S1 was detected, indicating that the glycan linked to Asn-368 was a complex type glycan.

On the other hand, the glycan linked to Asn-476 was also separated into several peaks. As a result of treatment with a mixture of glycosidases, these glycan peaks moved to the peak possessing the same retention time as standard S1, indicating that the glycan linked to Asn-476 possessed a heterogeneous complex type structure.

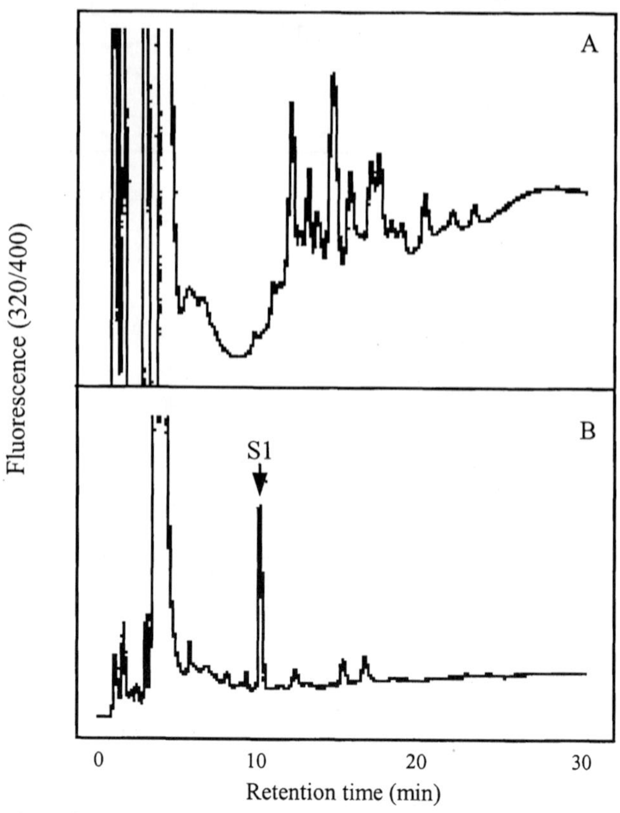

Figure 2. Analysis of glycans at Asn-368 of bLf-a by HPLC on a PALPAK Type-S column. A, P glycan at Asn-368; B, PA-glycan at Asn-368 after digestion with the mixture of exoglycosida Arrow indicate the elution position of standard PA-glycan (S1, $Man_3GlcNAc_2$-PA). T experimental details are given under materials and methods.

Glycan at Asn-281

The glycan linked to Asn-281 in bLf-a was analyzed by two-dimensional HPLC. The first dimension was reversed phase, and the second one was normal phase HPLC. Five standard PA-glycans S1 S2, S3, S4 and S5 were used. The structures of these standard glycans were $Man_3GlcNAc_2$-PA, $GlcNAc_2Man_3GlcNAc_2$-PA, $Gal_2GlcNAc_2Man_3GlcNAc_2$-PA, $GlcNAc_2Man_3GlcNAc_2Fuc$-PA, $Gal_2GlcNAc_2Man_3GlcNAc_2Fuc$-PA, respectively.

Five major peaks of glycans at Asn281 in bLf-a were detected, and the elution positions of three major peaks in both HPLC coincided with those of standard PA-glycans S1, S2 and S4, respectively, suggesting that these glycans possessed the same structure of standards. The proposed structures of glycans linked to Asn-281 in bLf-a were $Man_3GlcNAc_2$-PA, $GlcNAc_2Man_3GlcNAc_2$-PA, $GlcNAc_2Man_3GlcNAc_2Fuc$-PA.

Comparative Study of Glycans in BLf-a and BLf-b

Glycans linked to Asn-233, -368, -476 and -545 in bLf-b from colostrum were also analyzed, and compared to those in bLf-a. The elution pattern of glycans linked to Asn-368, -476 and -545 in bLf-a were very similar to those of bLf-b, suggesting that the structures of these glycans in bLfs-a and -b were very similar.

However, the elution pattern of glycans linked to Asn-233 in bLfs-a and -b were different, indicating that the structures of glycan linked to Asn-233 between in bLfs-a and -b were different.

Discussion

It was reported that in bLf, Asn-233 and -545 were linked with high-mannose type glycan only, and Asn-368 and -476 with complex or high-mannose type glycan (*11*). However, the relative proportions of these glycans in bLf varied with the period of lactation (*11*). In this study, glycans linked to bLf-a from bovine colostrum were characterized, suggesting that glycans linked to Asn-233 and -545 were high-mannose type, and glycans to Asn-368 and -467 were complex type. This result indicated that glycan biosynthesis might be controlled by hormones in the mammary gland, or that the folding of the protein inhibits the activity of the glycosyltransferases.

The glycans linked to Asn-233, -281, -368, -476 and -545 in bLf-a were found to possess heterogeneous structures. The structure analysis of glycan at Asn-281 in bLf-a showed that 5 kinds of major glycans were linked to Asn-281 with three of them possessing $Man_3GlcNAc_2$, $GlcNAc_2Man_3GlcNAc_2$, $GlcNAc_2Man_3GlcNAc_2Fuc$ structures. It is well known that glycans linked to bLf have highly heterogeneous (*18*), as those in transferrin family do. A previous study also showed that the glycan linked to Asn-281 in bLf-a was also heterogeneous. The heterogeneity of glycans in bLf-a might have occurred in the following process: 1) the rapid transportation of bLf through the Golgi apparatus resulted in the uncomplete trimming and synthesis of its glycans, or / and 2) exoglycosidases digestion of glycans occurred in bovine milk after secretion from the mammary gland.

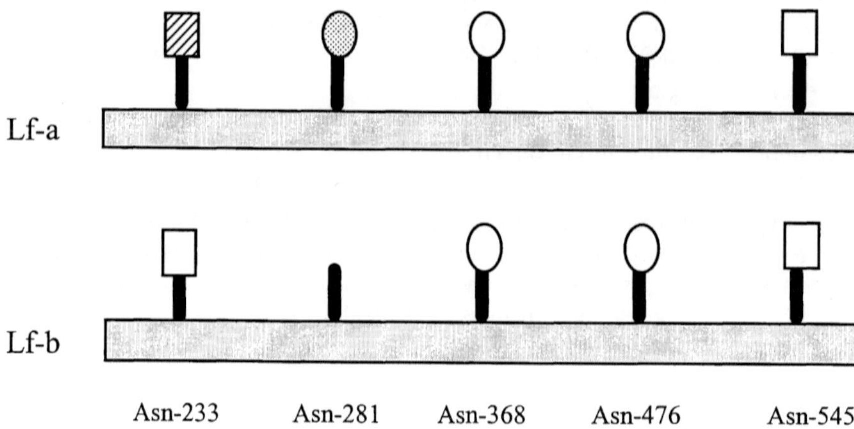

Figure 3. Distribution of N-glycans in bLf-a and bLf-b. ▨ , polypeptide chain of bLf; ▮, potential glycosylation site of bLf; ◯, complex type glycan; □ , high-mannose type glycan.

The glycans linked to Asn-368, -476 and -545 in bLf-a were very similar to those in bLf-b. However, the glycan bound to Asn-233 was different for bLf-a and bLf-b. The reason for the difference presented in the glycan linked with Asn-233 between two bLf has not yet been clarified. It has been proposed that glycosylation at one sequon might affect glycosylation at another site in the glycoprotein which possesses multi-glycosylation sites (*19*). In other words, the structure of polypeptide near the glycosylation site may influence the activity of the glycosylatransferases. Because the position of Asn-281 in bLf-a was very close to that of Asn-233 in primary structure, the glycosylation of Asn-281 might affect the processing of glycan at the nearest Asn-233.

Recently, the glycans in Lf were shown to play an important role in a multitude of biological functions of Lf. For example, the glycopeptides possessing high-mannose type glycan derived from bLf were found to strongly inhibit the hemagglutination activity of type 1 fimbriated *E. coli* and agglutinate these bacteria (*20*). A previous study showed that bLf-a had higher bactericidal activity against *E. coli* than bLf-b (*16*), indicating that the difference of glycans at Asn-233 in two bLf, or the presence of glycan in Asn-281 of bLf-a might cause the difference in antibacterial activity between both bLf. However, the specific role that glycan plays requires clarification.

REFERENCES

1. Fox, P. F. 1982. *Development in Dairy Chemistry-1*, Interspecies comparison of milk protein. Applied Science Publishers, New York, pp. 87-114.
2. Baggiolini, M.; de Duve, D.; Masson, P.L.; Heremans, J.F. *J. Exp. Med.* **1970**, *13*, 559.
3. Masson, P.L.; Heremans, J.F.; Dive, C. *Clin. Chim. Acta* **1966**, *14*, 735.
4. Lehrer, R.I.; Ganz, T.; Selsted, M.E.; Babior, B.M.; Curnutte. J.T. *Ann. Intern. Med.* **1988**, *109*, 127-142.
5. Masson, P.L.; Heremans, J.F.; Prignot, J.J.; Wauters, G. *Thorax* **1966**, *21*, 538-544.
6. Reiter, B. *Int. J. Tissue React.* **1983**, *5*, 87-96.
7. Brock, J. 1999. Page 13 *in* abstracts of the 4th international conference on lactoferrin. Univ. Hokkaido, Sapporo, Japan, pp.13.
8. Ikeda, M.; Sugiyama, K.; Tanaka, T.; Sekihara, H.; Kato, N. *Biochem. Bioph. Res. Co.* **1998**, *245*, 549-553.
9. Tsuda, H.; Sekine, K.; Ushida, Y.; Kuhara, T. 1999. Abstracts of the 4th international conference on lactoferrin. Univ. Hokkaido, Sapporo, Japan, pp. 52.
10. Pierce, A.; Colavizza, D.; Benaissa, M. *Eur. J. Biochem.* **1991**, *196*, 177-184.
11. Hutchens, T.W.; Rumball, S.V.; Lonnerdal, B. *Adv. in Exp. Med. & Biol.* **1994**, *357*, 21-32.
12. Wei, Z.; Nishimura, T.; Yoshida, S. *J. Dairy Sci.* **2000**, *83*, 683-689.
13. Tsuji, S.; Hirata, Y.; Matsuoka, K. *J. Dairy Sci.* **1989**, *72*, 1130-1136.
14. Yoshida, S.; Ye, X-Y. *J. Dairy Sci.* **1991**, *74*, 1439-1444.
15. Rejman, J.J.; Hegarty, H.M.; Hurley, W.L. *Comp. Biochem. Physiol.* **1989**, *93B*, 929-934.
16. Yoshida, S.; Wei, Z.; Shinmura, Y.; Fukunaga, N. *J. Dairy Sci.* **2000**, *83*, 2211-2215.

17. Kondo, A.; Suzuki, J.; Kuraya, N. *Agric. Biol. Chem.* **1990**, *54*, 2169-2170.
18. Coddeville, B.; Strecker, G.; Wieruszeski, J. M.; Vliegenthart, F.G.; Spik, G. Heterogeneity of bovine lactoferrin glycans. *Carbohydrate Res.* **1992,** *236*, 145-164.
19. Berkel, P.H.C.V.; Van Veen, H.A.; Geerts, M.E.J.; De Boer, H.A.; Nuijens, J.H. *Biochem. J.* **1996**, *319*, 117-122.
20. Teraguti, S.; Shin, K.; Fukuwatari, Y.; Shimamura, S. *Infection and Immunity,* **1996**, *64*, 1075-1077.

Chapter 37

Influence of Endopeptidases and Aminopeptidases on the Production of Taste Peptides and Free Amino Acids in Muscle Foods

Toshihide Nishimura

Department of Food Science, Faculty of Applied Biological Science, Hiroshima University, Higashi-Hiroshima-shi, Hiroshima 739–8528, Japan

Meat flavor as well as texture is improved during postmortem aging. The improvement of taste in meat flavor is due to the increase in free amino acids and peptides in meats during postmortem aging. The former increase contributes to enhancement of brothy taste including umami, while the latter increase is responsible for giving mildness. The increase in peptides is caused by the action of cathepsins B and L, and calpains on muscle proteins. On the other hand, the increase in free amino acids is caused by aminopeptidases C, H and P during postmortem aging. The levels of these protease activities in meats influence the production of taste peptides and free amino acids during postmortem aging.

Meat is one of the most nutritious and palatable foods. There are many factors involved in the palatability of meat. Meat color, marbling, texture and flavor play an important role in meat palatability. Although skeletal muscle immediately after death is soft, it soon becomes very tough and unpalatable by rigor mortis. Then, its toughness gradually decreases, and meat texture is improved during postmortem aging. Meat flavor as well as texture is improved during postmortem storage of meat at low temperatures. By these improvements during postmortem aging, muscle is converted to meat as food. In general, beef, pork and chicken are stored at 4°C for about 2 weeks, 1 week and 1 day, respectively, after slaughter.

Meat taste is one of the most important factors responsible for its palatability as described previously. It is mainly caused by chemoreception of water-soluble (non-volatile) compounds. The improvement of meat taste during postmortem aging is caused by changes in chemical components, which are catalyzed by several biochemical reactions in the muscle in the absence of oxygen after death.

In this chapter, the roles of peptides and free amino acids in the improvement of meat taste during postmortem aging is described. The mechanisms involved in the increases in these compounds are also introduced. Finally, the influences of proteases on their production during postmortem aging is provided.

Improvement of Meat Taste

Beef immediately after slaughter has been reported to elicit a sour taste and possess little beefy flavor even if it is cooked. However, postmortem storage of beef at a low temperature for 8 days gives it beefy and palatable flavor (*1*). (*2-5*) also observed that storage of beef after slaughter at a low temperature improves its flavor. On the other hand, Parrish *et al.* (*6*) observed that the storage of beef from 4 through 7 days after death had no influence on its flavor. Minks and Stringer (*7*) showed that the aging of beef at 2 C for 7 or 15 days did not improve its flavor. Field *et al.* (*8*) also showed that the aging of beef at 2 C for 2, 7 or 21 days after death had no influence on its flavor. Although there have been many studies on changes of beef flavor during postmortem aging, consistent results have not been obtained. As to pork, Bennett *et al.* (*9*) showed that the storage of pork loin from 2 to 6 days after slaughter at 2 C had no influence on its flavor. Harrison *et al.* (*10*) also observed that the aging of pork at 2 C for 1, 4, 8 and 12 days did not improve its flavor. Chicken flavor was reported to be more pleasant at 8-h postmortem than immediately after death (*11*). Thus, different results regarding the improvement of meat flavor have been observed among animal species. These differences may be caused by sensory evaluations conducted on flavor including both taste and aroma, indicating that taste and aroma should be evaluated separately.

There are few reports on the improvement of taste in flavor during the postmortem storage of meat. Changes in the brothy taste intensity of beef, pork and chicken during postmortem aging was examined (*12*). There was no significant difference in the brothy taste intensity of beef before or after aging. This result is inconsistent with that in reports by Caul (*1*) and Paul *et al.* (*2*). Therefore, it might be concluded that the aging of beef does not enhance brothy taste intensity, but suppresses sourness sensed immediately after slaughter. On the other hand, the brothy taste intensity of pork and chicken was significantly stronger after aging than prior to it. From this result, it is elucidated that the brothy taste of pork and chicken is enhanced and the meaty taste is improved during postmortem aging. The components that cause this improvement of meat taste during postmortem aging require attention.

Components Responsible for Improvement of Meat Taste During Postmortem Aging

There are many taste components in meat, which are non-protein nitrogenous compounds such as free amino acids and peptides, nucleotides, lactic acid, sugars and minerals. Among them, free amino acids and peptides in meat are shown to increase by proteolysis during postmortem aging, and improve meat taste.

Monosodium glutamate (MSG) or monosodium aspartate in free amino acids are well known to contribute to the umami taste in meat by a synergistic effect with inosine monophosphate (IMP) (*13*). Take and Otsuka (*14*) reported that the contents of free amino acids including Glu contribute to the umami intensity of chicken meat. Sensory analyses of the artificial meat soups prepared from free amino acids and IMP also showed that free amino acids including Glu are responsible for the intensity of umami and brothy taste in meat (*15*). Free amino acids, except for Glu and Asp, do not elicit umami. However, they have been shown to have a synergistic effect in the presence of IMP and MSG on umami, even if their contents are below their threshold values (*16,17*). These results suggest that the increase in free amino acids in meat during postmortem aging contributes to the improvement of meat taste.

Recently, the contribution of peptides to meat taste has been gradually clarified. The increase in peptides in beef is shown to be very significant during the cooking in vacuum at 60 C for 6 h (*18*). As shown in Figure 1, peptides, which

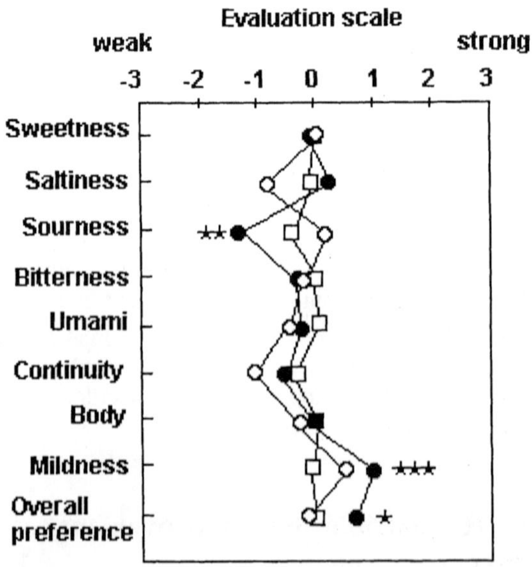

Figure 1. Effect of the addition of peptide fraction on taste of beef soup.
The basic extract was prepared from changed beef cooked in vacuum at 60 °C for 10 min. Peptide fractions were prepared from aged beef cooked in vacuum at 60 °C for 6h, separated by ultrafiltration, and added to the basic extract. Effect of the addition of each peptide fraction (○, MW500-1000; ●, MW1000-10000; □, MW more than 10000) on the taste of basic extract was examined by sensory evaluation. *, $p<0.05$; **, $P<0.01$; ***, $P<0.001$. (Reproduced with permission from Nishimura (1998))

possess molecular mass of 1,000-10,000 Da in this beef, suppress sourness and enhance the mildness of the unaged beef soup (*19*). Peptides in pork cooked in vacuum at 60 C for 6 h were also shown to suppress sourness and enhance umami. Peptides isolated from this pork possessed the following primary structure; APPPPAEVHEVV, APPPPAEVHEVVE, APPPPAEVHEVHEEVH. These sequences were shown to be similar to that of rabbit muscle troponin T. A synthesized peptide of APPPPAEVHEV, which is common sequence among three peptides, suppressed sourness, while APPPP had no suppression. Ueda (*20*) demonstrated the extraction of components enhancing brothy taste intensity from beef extract and derived from tropomyosin and collagen. Recently, peptides such as EE, EV, ADE, AED, DEE, SPE in chicken muscle hydrolysate by protease have been shown to enhance umami of inosinic solution (*21*). These results also indicate that the increase in peptides during the postmortem storage of meat is responsible for the improvement of meat taste. Thus, it is interesting to clarify in detail the relationships between the structure of peptides and their effects on meat taste.

Mechanism of the Increase in Peptides in Meat During Postmortem Aging

In the muscle, there are lysosomal cathepsins B, D, H and L, which are most active in acidic pH, sarcoplasmic m- and m-calpains, which are activated by Ca^{2+} and exhibit most activities in neutral pH, and a proteasome dependent on ATP for activation.

The storage of porcine muscle homogenate at various pHs and 4 C for 5 days showed that the increase in peptides was large in acidic pH below 5 even in the absence of Ca^{2+}; it was also large in neutral pH around 7 in the presence of Ca^{2+} (Figure 2). The former increase seems to be caused by the action of cathepsins B, D and L. On the other hand, the latter increase seems to be caused by the action of calpains.

It is reported that cathepsins B, D and L degrade myofibrillar proteins, while cathepsin H scarcely causes hydrolysis of these proteins (*22,23*). SDS-PAGE analyses show that a polypeptide with a molecular mass of 30 kDa is produced during the postmortem aging of meat (*24-28*). This was shown to be derived from a myofibrillar protein, troponin T. The peptide (APPPPAEVPEVHEEV) derived from troponin T is also reported to increase during the storage of beef (*29*).

Zeece *et al.* (*30*) and Lisa *et al.* (*31*) showed that calpain is involved in the degradation of myofibrillar proteins during the postmortem storage of meat. Calpain is also shown to degrade phosphorylase b, creatine kinase, and GAPDH in sarcoplasmic proteins (*32*). The action of calpain on GAPDH leads to the production of peptides, which contain the sequence (VPTPNVSVVDLT) of a peptide produced during postmortem aging.

From these results, it might be concluded that both m- and m-calpains and cathepsins B and L are responsible for the increase in peptides concentrations at the ultimate pH (5.5-5.8) during postmortem aging of meat.

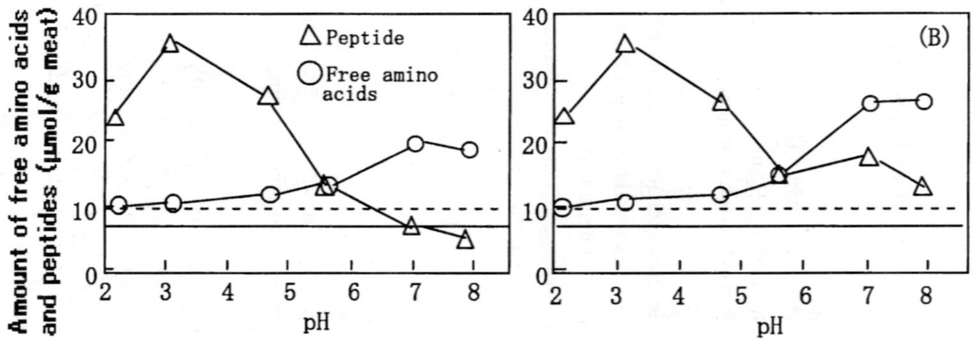

Figure 2. Increase in peptides and free amino acids during storage of porcine muscle homogenates prepared with buffers of various pHs at 4 °C for 5 days. (A) homogenates without Ca^{2+}. (B) homogenates with 1 mM Ca^{2+}. The solid and broken lines indicate the contents of peptides and free amino acids before storage respectively.

Mechanism of the Increase in Free Amino Acids in Meat During Postmortem Aging

The storage of porcine muscle homogenate at various pHs and 4 C for 5 days also shows that the increase in free amino acids is very small in an acidic pH region, while it is large under neutral pH (Figure 2). Since carboxypeptidase activities have been reported to be very slight in the muscle (*33*), the increase in free amino acids appears to be caused by the action of aminopeptidases which possess the optimal pH in the neutral region.

In chicken muscle, at least six aminopeptidases are detected upon ion-exchange column chromatography (*34*). Among them, aminopeptidases C and H have been suggested to be major contributors to the increase in free amino acids during postmortem aging. Because these activities are major and their substrate specificities show highest similarity with the pattern of free amino acids released during the postmortem storage of chicken.

The mechanism of the increase in free amino acids in meat during postmortem aging is clarified by purified aminopeptidases C and H (34-43). In the beginning, peptides are prepared from chicken myofibrillar (MF) and sarcoplasmic (SP) proteins by treatment of cathepsins (cath) and calpain (cal). As shown in Figure 3, the amounts of peptides (MF-cath- and SP-cath-peptides) from myofibrillar and sarcoplasmic proteins by the treatment of cathepsins are 2.68 and 2.68 mmol amino acids eq./g meat, respectively, while those (MF-cal- and SP-cal-peptides) from myofibrillar and sarcoplasmic proteins by the treatment of calpain are 1.45 and 1.05 μmol amino acids eq./g meat, respectively. After each peptide group (MF-cath-, MF-cal-, SP-cath- and SP-cal-peptides) was incubated with aminopeptidase C and H, the increase in free amino acids was determined. The amounts of free amino acids released from the MF-cath-, MF-cal-, SP-cath- and SP-cal-peptides by the treatment of aminopeptidases C and H are 1.54, 0.56, 1.30 and 0.68 μmol amino acids/ g meat (Figure 4). It is confirmed that both aminopeptidases are major contributors to the increase in free amino acids during the storage of meat. However, no release of Pro is detected by the action of both aminopeptidases. Aminopeptidase P (*44*), which releases an N-terminal amino acid from the peptide (X1-Pro-X2-X3-, Xi: amino acid) possessing Pro at the second position from its N-terminus, is suggested to contribute to the increase in Pro during the storage of meats, because aminopeptidases C and H do not exhibit such an action as described previously. The mechanism of the increase in Pro during the postmortem aging of meats was examined using aminopeptidases C, H and P isolated from the chicken skeletal muscle (*40*). A peptide, Tyr-Pro-Leu-Gly, was

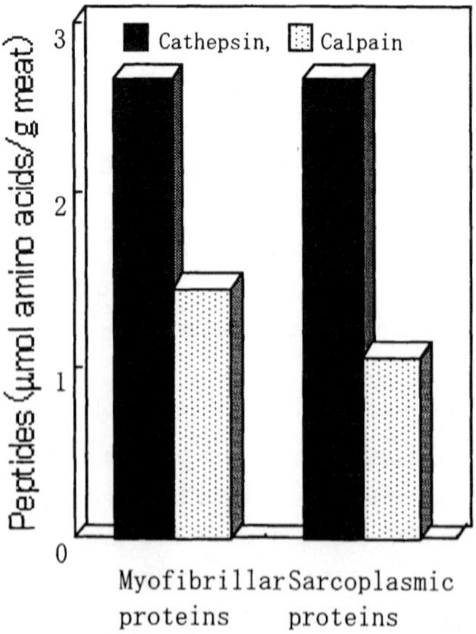

Figure 3. Amounts of peptides produced from myofiblillar and sarcoplasmic proteins by thr treatment with cathepsins and calpain. (Reproduced with permission from Nishimura (1998))

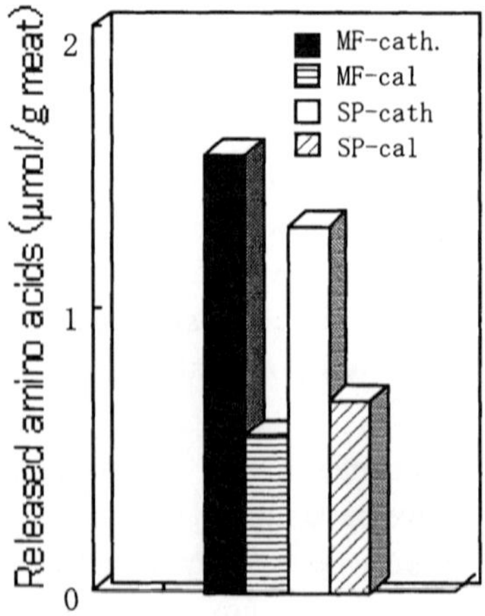

Figure 4. Amount of free amino acids released from peptides by aminopeptidases C and H MF-cath- and MF-cal-peptides indicate the peptides produced from myofibrillar proteins by cathepsins and calpain, respectively. SP-cath- and SP-cal-peptides indicate the peptides produced from sarcoplasmic proteins by these proteases.

incubated with these enzymes on the basis of the data regarding the content of each enzyme in the muscle. The incubation of a peptide, Tyr-Pro-Leu-Gly, with aminopeptidases C, H and P showed that Tyr was released at first by the action of only aminopeptidase P; Pro, Leu and Gly were then released by the action of aminopeptidases C and H (Figure 5).

It might be concluded that the increase in free amino acids in meats during postmortem aging was mainly caused by the action of aminopeptidases C, H and P on the peptides, which are produced from meat proteins by the action of cathepsins and calpains (Figure 6).

Influence of Endopeptidases and Aminopeptidases on the Production of Peptides and Free Amino Acids

The levels of endopeptidases and aminopeptidases contributing to the production of peptides and free amino acids are thought to influence meat taste improvement during postmortem aging.

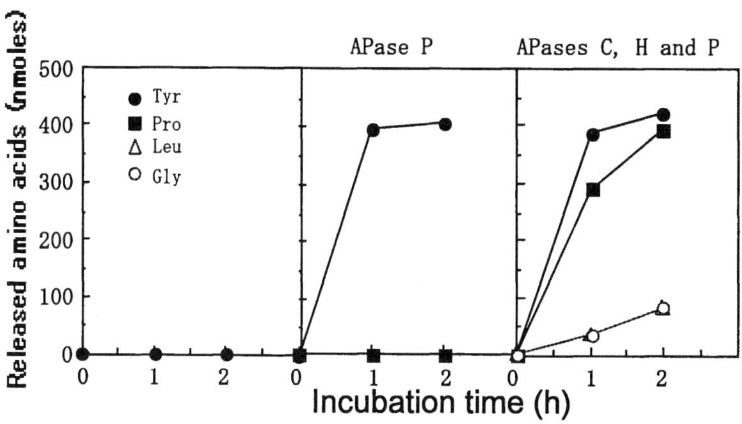

Figure 5. Action of aminopeptidases (Apases) C, H and P on Tyr-Pro-Leu-Gly. One millimolar substrate was incubated with 45.9, 21.4 and 104.1 mU of aminopeptidases C, H and P, respectively, in 0.4 ml of 50 mM Tris-HCl (pH 7.2)/1 mM $MnCl_2$/1 mM DTT at 37°C. (Reproduced with permission from Nishimura (1998))

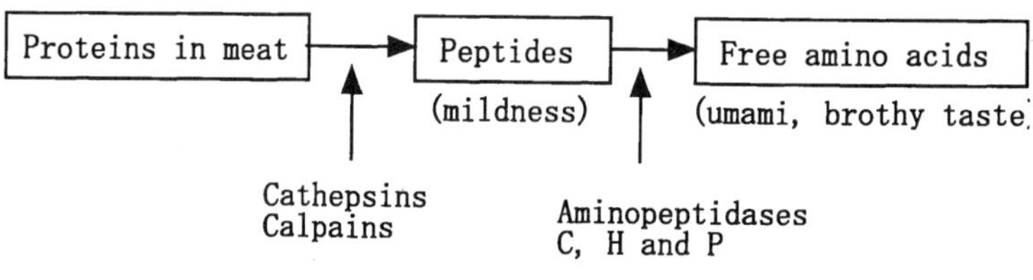

Figure 6. Mechanism involved in the increase in peptides and free amino acids during the postmortem aging of meats. (Reproduced with permission from Nishimura (1998))

The level in the activities of cathepsins B and L was estimated to be highest in porcine muscle among bovine, porcine and chicken and chicken muscle showed the lowest activities of cathepsins B and L (*45*). The measurement of calpain activity in beef, pork and chicken showed that chicken had the lowest activity among these three species.

Aminopeptidase activities in bovine, porcine and chicken muscle were measured using various amino acid-b-naphthylamides as substrates. Both porcine and chicken possessed the same aminopeptidase activities, while bovine muscle possessed only 2/3 the level of other muscle's activities (Table 1). This difference in aminopeptidase activities seems to cause that increment of free amino acids in beef was very small during postmortem aging and that brothy taste of beef was not enhanced during postmortem aging. Therefore, it seems that activities of proteases, including endopeptidases and aminopeptidases, influence the production of peptides and free amino acids during postmortem aging and may produce each specific meat taste.

Table 1. Aminopeptidase activities in bovine, porcine and chicken muscle

Amino acid - β-naphthylamimde	Activity (μmol amino acid/h/g meat)		
	Bovine	Porcine	Chicken
Ser	10.2	17.4	22.8
Glu	3.6	8.8	12.8
Pro	13.0	17.4	22.8
Gly	0.4	0.4	0.6
Ala	100.8	127.8	140.6
Val	2.4	2.8	3.4
Met	51.4	76.6	71.2
Leu	42.4	56.2	54.2
Lys	76.2	107.2	115.6
Total activity	300.4	414.6	444.2

Amino acid β-naphthyiamides were used to measure aminopeptidase activities of each muscle.

References

1. Caul, F. 1957. In "Survey Progr. Military Subsistence Problems. Ser.I. No. 9", Quarter Master Food and Container Inst., pp.152.
2. Paul, P.; Lawe, B.; McClurg, B.R. *Food Res.*, **1944**, *9*, 221-233.
3. Rodel, W. *Die Nahrung*, **1969**, *13*, 489-493.

4. Smith, G.C.; Culp, G.R.; Carpenter, Z.L. *J. Food Sci.*, **1978**, *43*, 823-826.
5. Okitani, A.; Matsuishi, M.; Negishi, H.; Yoshikawa, S. *Jpn. J. Zootech. Sci.*, **1990**, *61*, 990-997.
6. Parrish, Jr., F.C.; Rust, R.E.; Popenhagen, G.R.; Miner, B.E. *J. Animal Sci.*, **1969**, *29*, 398-403.
7. Minks, D.; Stringer, W.C. *J. Food Sci.*, **1972**, *37*, 736-738.
8. Field, R.A.; Riley, M.L.; Chang, Y.O. *J. Food Sci.*, **1971**, *36*, 611-612.
9. Bennett, M.E.; Bramblett, V.D.; Aberle, E.D.; Harrington, R.B. *J. Food Sci.*, **1973**, *38*, 536-538.
10. Harrison, D.L.; Bowers, J.A.; Anderson, L.L.; Tuma, H.J.; Kropf, D.H. *J. Food Sci.*, **1970**, *35*, 292-294.
11. Terasaki, M.; Kajikawa, M.; Fujita, E.; Ishii, K. *Agric. Biol. Chem.*, **1965**, *29*, 208-215.
12. Nishimura, T.; Rhyu, M.R.; Okitani, A.; Kato, H. *Agric. Biol. Chem.*, **1988**, *52*, 2323-2330.
13. Yamaguchi, S.; Yoshikawa, T.; Ikeda, S.; Ninomiya, T. *J. Food Sci.*, **1971**, *36*, 846-849.
14. Take, T.; Otsuka, H. *Niigatadaigaku Kyoikugakubu Kiyou*, **1967**, *9*, 97-101.
15. Kato, H.; Nishimura, T. 1987. In "Umami: a basic taste", ed. by Y. Kawamura and M.R. Kare, Marcel Dekker, Inc., New York and Basel, pp.289-306.
16. Tanaka, T.; Saito, N.; Okuhara, A.; Yokotsuka, T. *Nippon Nogeikagaku Kaishi*, **1969**, *43*, 171-176.
17. Yokotsuka, T.; Saito, N.; Okuhara, A.; Tanaka, T. *Nippon Nogeikagaku Kaishi*, **1969**, *43*, 165-170.
18. Ishii, K.; Tsuchida, M.; Nishimura, T.; Okitani, A.; Nakagawa, A.; Hatae, K.; Shimada, A. *J. Home Econ. Jpn.*, **1995**, *46*, 229-234.
19. Ishii, K.; Nishimura, T.; Okitani, A.; Tamura, Y.; Hatae, K.; Shimada, A. *J. Home Econ. Jpn.*, **1995b**, *46*, 307-312.
20. Ueda, Y. *Jpn. J. Taste and Smell Res.*, **1997**, *4*, 197-200.
21. Maehisa, K.; Matsuzaki, M.; Yamamoto, Y.; Udaka, S. *Biosci. Biotechnol. Biochem.*, **1999,** *63*, 555-559.
22. Okitani, A.; Matsukura, U.; Kato, H.; Fujimaki, M. *J. Biochem.*, **1980**, *87,* 1133-1143.
23. Ouali, A.; Garrel, N.; Obled, A.; Deval, C.; Valin, C. *Meat Sci.,* **1978**, *19*, 83-100.
24. Samejima, K.; Wolfe, F.H. *J. Food Sci.*, **1976**, *41*, 250-254.
25. Penny, I.F.; Ferguson-Pryce, R. *Meat Sci.*, **1979**, *3*, 121-141.
26. Negishi, H.; Yoshikawa, S. *Animal Sci. Technol.(Jpn),* **1994**, *65*, 882-889.
27. Negishi, H.; Yamamoto, E.; Kuwata, T. *Meat Sci.*, **1996**, *42*, 289-303.

28. Okumura, T.; Inuzuka, Y.; Nishimura, T.; Arai, S. *Anim. Sci. Technol. (Jpn.),* **1996**, *67*, 360-367.
29. Nakai, Y.; Nishimura, T.; Shimizu, M.; Arai, S. *Biosçi. Biotech. Biochem.*, **1995**, *59*, 2255-2258.
30. Zeece, M.G.; Robson, R.M.; Lusby, M.L.; Parrish, Jr., F.C. *J. Food Sci.*, **1986**, *51*, 797-803.
31. Lisa, D.F.; Tullio, R.D.; Salamino, F.; Barbato, R.; Melloni, E.; Siliprandi, N.; Schiaffino, S.; Pentremoli, S. *Biochem. J.*, **1995**, *308*, 57-61.
32. Okumura, T.; Nishiumi, T.; Nishimura, T.; Yoshida, S. 1997 Presented at the 92nd Annual Meeting of Japanese Society of Zootechnical Science., Tokyo, March 28-29, p.105.
33. Okitani, A.; Otsuka, Y.; Katakai, R.; Kondo, Y.; Kato, H. *J. Food Sci.*, **1981a,** *46*, 47-51.
34. Nishimura, T.; Okitani, A.; Rhyu, M.R.; Kato, H. *Agric. Biol. Chem.*, **1990**, *54,* 2769-2775.
35. Adachi, H.; Tsujimoto, M.; Fukasawa, M.; Sato, Y.; Arai, H.; Inoue, K.; Nishimura, T. *Eur. J. Biochem.*, **1997**, *245*, 283-288.
36. Nishimura, T.; Kato, Y.; Okitani, A.; Kato, H. *Agric. Biol. Chem.*, **1991a,** *55*, 1771-1778.
37. Nishimura, T.; Rhyu, M.R.; Kato, H. *Agric. Biol. Chem.*, **1991b,** *55*, 1779-1786.
38. Nishimura, T.; Kato, Y.; Rhyu, M.R.; Okitani, A.; Kato, H. *Comp. Biochem. Physiol.*, **1992,** *102B*, 129-135.
39. Nishimura, T.; Rhyu, M.R.; Kato, H.; Arai, S. *J. Agric. Food Chem.*, **1994,** *46*, 2709-2712.
40. Nishimura, T.; Rhyu, M.R.; Tajima, T.; Kato, H. 1996. In the proceedings of "The 42nd International Congress of Meat Science and Technology". Lillehammer (Norway), pp.412-413.
41. Okitani, A.; Nishimura, T.; Kato, H. *Eur. J. Biochem.*, **1981b**, *115*, 269-274.
42. Otsuka, Y.; Okitani, A.; Katakai, R.; Fujimaki, M. *Agric. Biol. Chem.*, **1976**, *40*, 2335-2342.
43. Rhyu, M.R.; Nishimura, T.; Kato, Y.; Okitani, A.; Kato, H. *Eur. J. Biochem.*, **1992**, *208*, 53-59.
44. Harbeck, H.T.; Mentlein, R. *Eur. J. Biochem.*, **1991**, *198*, 451-458.
45. Etherington, D.J.; Taylor, M.A.J.; Dransfield, E. *Meat Sci.*, **1987**, *20*, 1-18.

Author Index

Subject Index

B

E

G

H

I

N

O

P

Q

R

S

T

V

W

X